S0-BMA-239

MECHANISMS OF TINNITUS

MECHANISMS OF TINNITUS

Jack A. Vernon

Oregon Hearing Research Center

Aage R. Møller

University of Pittsburgh

Editors

ALLYN AND BACON

Boston • London • Toronto • Sydney • Tokyo • Singapore

Series Editor: Kris Farnsworth
Editorial Assistant: Christine M. Shaw
Editorial-Production Service: Walsh Associates
Cover Administrator: Suzanne Harbison
Composition Buyer: Linda Cox
Manufacturing Buyer: Louise Richardson

Copyright © 1995 by Allyn & Bacon
A Simon & Schuster Company
Needham Heights, MA 02194

All rights reserved. No part of the material protected by this copyright notice may be reproduced or utilized in any form or by any means, electronic or mechanical, including photocopy-
ing, recording, or by any information storage and retrieval system, without the written
permission of the copyright owner.

Library of Congress Cataloging-in-Publication Data

Mechanisms of tinnitus / Jack A. Vernon, Aage R. Møller, editors.
     p.   cm.
   Includes bibliographical references and index.
   ISBN 0-205-14083-1
   1. Tinnitus—Etiology.   I. Vernon, Jack A.   II. Møller, Aage R.
   [DNLM:1. Tinnitus—physiopathology.   WV 272 M4863 1994]
RF293.8.M43   1994
617.8—dc20
DNLM/DLC
for Library of Congress   94-27956
                                         CIP

Printed in the United States of America
10   9   8   7   6   5   4   3   2   1   00   99   98   97   96   95

It is with a feeling of gratitude and humbleness that we dedicate this book to Jean Marc Gaspard Itard, M.D. (1775–1838), the first to use masking for the relief of tinnitus.

Itard, J.M.G. "Traite des Maladies de l'Oreille et de l'Audition." Mequignon-Marvis, Paris, 1821.

Doctor Itard, better known for the "Wild Boy of Aveyron," recognized the seriousness the problem of tinnitus can impose. In discussing the matter, he emphasized that the tinnitus patient should be examined by a medical doctor to determine the possibility of a correctable medical cause for the tinnitus. He went on to add that in fully 95 percent of the cases no such cause would be found and therefore the tinnitus should be treated in a nonmedical manner. The technique he recommended is what we today term masking. Lacking the luxury of electronics, Doctor Itard instructed patients to produce sounds which would cover up their tinnitus. He often instructed patients to build a fire and listen to the sound it made. If the patient had a roaring-type tinnitus, that is, a low-pitched tinnitus, the fire was to be made with dry wood so that a roaring sound resulted. It the tinnitus was high-pitched, the fire was to be built with green or moist wood so that hissing sounds would result. He even encouraged one patient to live in a water mill so that the constant sound of the mill wheel could mask her tinnitus.

We are endebted to Dai Stevens for bringing Doctor Itard to our attention.

Stevens, S.D.G.: "Historical Aspects of Tinnitus." In J.W.P. Hazell (Ed.), *Tinnitus*, Churchill Livingston, Edinburgh, 1987.

Jack Vernon, Ph.D
Aage Møller, Ph.D.

CONTENTS

Tinnitus affects a large number of people, and the possibilities to cure or alleviate tinnitus are rather limited. One of the reasons why there is no cure for tinnitus is our lack of knowledge about the mechanisms of tinnitus. We know very little about why and how the auditory system, under certain circumstances, can produce a sensation that is similar to that of a sound while no external sound is present. We do not know how tinnitus is generated and we do not know whether tinnitus is generated in the ear or in the auditory nervous system.

Recent research on tinnitus has posed a number of questions: Why does tinnitus have widely different qualities? Why, in a study of 97 patients with tinnitus, is the quality of the tinnitus in 81.4 percent best matched by a single pure tone, in 9.0 percent to a noise, while the remaining 9.6 percent have a more complex form of tinnitus (Tinnitus Data Registry)? Does the tonal tinnitus suggest a restricted lesion on some tonotopic loci while a noise-type tinnitus is caused by a more extensive disruption along the tonotopic organization? Or do the various qualities of tinnitus imply completely different underlying mechanisms? Why do some patients with tinnitus also experience hypersensitivity to sound? Why can external factors such as alterations in atmospheric pressure produce a change in tinnitus in almost 10 percent of a series of 873 patients queried: 0.8 percent experienced relief of tinnitus while 9 percent experienced a worsening of their tinnitus? Most patients with relentless tinnitus experience the tinnitus constantly, but there are those for whom the intensity varies sharply and unpredictably. Still more confusing are those patients in whom the intensity of the tinnitus either increases or decreases only during sleep. Do these characteristics bear any relationship to the mechanisms that underlie tinnitus?

The perceived location of tinnitus can be at the ears, at various locations in the head, or even outside the body. In a study of tinnitus location involving 1033 patients from the Oregon Tinnitus Data Registry, 856 (83 percent) located their tinnitus at the ears, 146 (14 percent) located it in the head, and 31 (3 percent) indicated multiple locations. Do these different perceived locations of tinnitus suggest different underlying mechanisms?

Why can external masking sounds have a different effect on tinnitus than on a similar sound that reaches the ear? Tinnitus may be temporarily eliminated or suppressed for a brief period of time following masking (residual inhibition), which occurs in 83 percent of the patients tested for it.

Ordinary masking does not usually produce any after effect, whereas masking of tinnitus routinely produces the residual inhibition as mentioned. The time course of residual inhibition is different from the phenomenon of tone decay or adaptation, but we do not know what it is. What kind of tinnitus mechanism could account for these various effects?

There are chemical agents that can induce both permanent and temporary tinnitus. For example, quinine, in sufficient quantity, can induce permanent tinnitus. Aspirin can induce temporary tinnitus. In both cases the tinnitus persists long after the offending chemicals have cleared the body. What is the mechanism by which tinnitus is maintained when the offending chemical is no longer present? This persistence effect clearly disturbs us when we try to explain the underlying mechanisms of tinnitus.

Since the time of E.P. Fowler, it has been well established that the loudness of tinnitus, when measured in sensation level, is slight at best. In a sample of 1296 tinnitus patients from the above mentioned Tinnitus Data Registry, 1001 (77 percent) had a loudness match of 7 dB SL or less. The median value was 4.0 dB SL and the modal value was 3.0 dB SL. If we have measured the loudness of tinnitus correctly, we are forced to ask how such low values can be so intrusive in the life of the patient.

In several recent publications tinnitus has been likened to the phenomenon of pain. Because tinnitus can be associated with every known pathology of the entire auditory system, it has often been referred to as the "pain" signal of the hearing mechanism— that is, "auditory pain." These examples are sufficient to suggest that the attributes of tinnitus are complex.

There is an ancient and interesting account of three blind men describing an elephant. The man standing at the front described the elephant as the trunk of a tree; the man standing at the side likened the elephant to the side of a barn; and the man standing at the tail thought the elephant resembled a rope. All of their descriptions were correct and, of course, all of them were incorrect.

What follows in this book may somewhat resemble those efforts of the three blind men, that is, each author will probably devise a mechanism of tinnitus according to his or her experiences with this very troublesome problem. What the authors construct by way of a mechanism of tinnitus will, in a sense, represent a form of selective blindness. It could not be expected, however, that any one contributor would be able to satisfy all the various quandaries and the almost infinite variations and puzzles that tinnitus places before us. Moreover, with our present inadequate information it is highly unlikely that any one proposed mechanism can account for more than a select few of the many different forms and aspects of tinnitus.

We have asked each contributor to this book to *speculate* as to what he or she thinks is the underlying mechanism of tinnitus. Each contributor was encouraged to be as free in his or her speculations as wished. Each was given to understand that in this effort he or she had a unique opportunity: Each was given license and freedom without any responsibility, so if the suggested mechanisms are a bit "off the wall" blame us, the editors, and not the authors.

The speculations presented here will not provide the final answer as to the identity of THE MECHANISM of tinnitus, but we hope that they contribute to our understanding of the enigma of tinnitus and that others will be encouraged to continue this line of endeavor, which may ultimately lead to cures for tinnitus.

The various chapters' appearance is entirely haphazard, and we have not imposed any sequence to the presentations. No given presentation is propaedeutic to any other presentation.

ABOUT THE EDITORS

JACK ALLEN VERNON was born in Kingsport, Tennessee on April 6, 1922. He served as a bomber pilot (B-24s) and flight instructor during WWII. Vernon attended the University of Virginia, and obtained a PhD in Sensory Psychology in 1952. He taught at Princeton University from 1952 until 1966 in the Department of Psychology. Vernon currently serves as Professor of Otolaryngology and Director of the Hearing Research Center, Oregon Health Sciences University where he has been from 1966 to the present. His present research effort is mainly devoted to tinnitus and implantable hearing aids. Vernon's delayed retirement is planned for the winter of 1995.

AAGE MØLLER obtained his medical education from the Karolinska Institute in Stockholm, Sweden, Cand. Med. and Med. Dr. (Doctor of Medical Sciences). He was Assistant Professor in Physiology at the Karolinska Institute and Associate Professor at the Department of Otolaryngology at the University of Gothenburg. Dr. Møller has served the University of Pittsburgh School of Medicine in several positions since 1978: Research Professor of Otolaryngology and later of Neurological Surgery, and from 1988 to present, he has been Professor of Neurological Surgery. From 1984 until the present, Dr. Møller has served as Adjunct Professor in the Department of Communications University of Pittsburgh School of Arts and Sciences. His research has mainly been in the area of auditory physiology, but he has done work in other areas of neurophysiology. He has published over 300 papers (of which 150 were in referred journals), written three books, edited (or co-edited) two books. Dr. Møller is a member of many professional and scientific societies and he served as President of the American Society for Neurophysiological Monitoring between July 1991 and July 1992.

CONTRIBUTING AUTHORS

ROBERT C. BILGER received a PhD in Experimental Psychology from Purdue University in 1954. He is currently Professor of Speech and Hearing Science and of Psychology at the University of Illinois at Urbana-Champaign. In addition to his research concerning spontaneous otoacoustic emissions and their heritability, he studies the effects of aging on speech perception. His work is supported by a grant from the National Institute of Deafness and Other Communication Disorders (DC00174).

RAIMUND BRIX, PhD, was born in Vienna, Austria in 1948. His 1972 doctoral dissertation was on the "Objectivation of concept discrimination and concept formation in electroencephalogram." Since 1973, Dr. Brix has served as Assistant Professor of ENT at the University Clinic in Vienna, and since 1992 in the University Clinic ENT, General Hospital Vienna. In 1983 he served as university lecturer in Otoneuropsychology. His research and professional work have been in the areas of audiology and neuropsychology; he has developed subjective and objective audiological tests, and conducted research in imagery and EEG ("imagination potentials"), frequency discrimination, tinnitus, cochlear implants, and evoked response audiometry.

ROBERT E. BRUMMETT received his PhD in 1964 from the University of Oregon Medical School with a major in pharmacology and minors in biochemistry and physiology. He became interested in auditory physiology through the efforts of Dr. Jack A. Vernon. From this alliance, he became interested in the effects of drugs on the auditory system. Since 1968 the majority of his research efforts, as reflected in his publications, have been on the topic of ototoxicity, mainly that of the aminoglycosides and the loop inhibiting diuretics. Much of his work has been in collaboration with Dr. Kaye E. Fox.

ROSS R.A. COLES qualified in medicine in 1952. After seventeen years in the Royal Navy, much of it researching on noise-induced hearing loss, Dr. Coles spent ten years as head of the audiology group at Southampton University's Institute of Sound and Vibration Research. His final twelve years in the workplace was at the MRC Institute of Hearing Research at Nottingham doing research, conducting clinics, and teaching on tinnitus. Following "retirement" in 1992, he continues his tinnitus and occupational deafness work privately.

JOS J. EGGERMONT received an MSc in experimental physics (1967), and a PhD in (bio)physics in 1972 from the University of Leyden, The Netherlands. He has served as Research Associate in the ENT department of Leyden University Hospital, head of the Department of Biophysics at the University of Nijmegen, and has served as Professor in the Department of Psychology at the University of Calgary, Canada, from 1986 until the present. Dr. Eggermont received the C.J. Kok Prize from the University of Leyden for Excellence in Medical Research in 1973, and the Guyot Prize from Groningen University in 1984 for outstanding achievements in otology research. He was elected a corresponding member of the Royal Netherlands Academy of Arts and Sciences in 1989, and a member of the Collegium ORLAS in 1986. He is a member of the Editorial Boards of Hearing Research and the International Journal of Pediatric Otolaryngology.

ARNE ERNST, MD, PhD, was born in 1958, and is an ENT specialist who served as an Associate Professor at the University of Tübingen with Professor Zenner from 1989 to 1993. From 1993 to present, he is at the Medical University of Hannover, Germany with Professor Lenarz. His research fields are the cochlea (micromechanics, ion transport, molecular mechanisms of drug ototoxicity), tinnitus, implantable hearing and aids, and cochlear implants in children.

HARALD FELDMANN, MD, PhD, was born in Germany in 1926. He received his MD in 1956, with medical training in ENT in Heidelberg. He obtained his PhD in 1963, and became an Associate Professor. From 1976 to 1991, Feldmann was Professor and Director of the Otolaryngological Department of the University of Münster, Westphalia, Germany. In 1991, he was named Professor emeritus. Dr. Feldmann's fields of research include audiology, tinnitus, otosurgery, the history of medicine, and medicolegal aspects in ENT.

JOHN GRAHAM, an ex-classicist, was a general surgeon and is now practicing general ENT with an interest in the physiology of hearing and tinnitus. He is the founding President of the British Association for Paediatric Otorhinolaryngology and consultant at the University College London Hospitals (previously U.C.H. and The Middlesex). John Graham's interest in tinnitus grew from close professional association with Jonathan Hazell, Royal National Institute For the Deaf, and was fostered by a period of static river dwelling in the pioneer territory of one of England's previous colonies.

JONATHAN W.P. HAZELL is a Senior Lecturer and Consultant Otologist at the University College of London Hospital and Head of the Medical Research Unit at the Royal National Institute for Deaf People in London. He has researched tinnitus mechanisms for the last twenty years. His work in London is linked with that of the tinnitus center in Baltimore, where Dr. Hazell is Visiting Professor. He has run a weekly tinnitus clinic since 1976, is the author of a book on tinnitus, and has published over fifty papers on the subject.

PAWELL J. JASTREBOFF received a PhD in Neurophysiology from the Polish Academy of Sciences. He is currently a Professor of Surgery and Physiology at the University of Maryland at Baltimore, School of Medicine, and Director of the University of Maryland Tinnitus and Hyperacusis Center. Dr. Jastreboff has been involved in the study of tinnitus since 1983. His research, sponsored by grants from the NIH/NIDCD, focuses on the mechanisms of tinnitus and finding new methods of tinnitus alleviation.

NELSON YUAN-SHENG KIANG was born in WuXi, China, and came to the United States in 1934. After receiving a PhD from the University of Chicago in 1955, he went to the

Massachusetts Institute of Technology. In 1956, Dr. Kiang was asked to start the Easton-Peabody Laboratory and became interested in the clinical implication of auditory physiology. He also is currently teaching at the Massachusetts Institute of Technology and Harvard.

MAASAKI KITAHARA, MD, completed medical school at Kyoto University, and in 1978 joined Shiga University of Medical Science as Professor and Chairman, Department of Otolaryngology. From 1986–1991, he served as Director of the Vestibular Disorders Research Committee, organized by the Ministry of Health and Welfare, Japan. In 1990, he was named to the International Tinnitus Advisory Board, and 1988, Dr. Kitahara served as President of the 50th Annual Meeting of Practica Otologica, where the International Symposium on Tinnitus was held. Co-authors Hiroya Kitano, Mikio Suzuki, and Kazutomo Kitajima are studying Neurotology under Professor Kitahara at the Department of Otolaryngology, Shiga University of Medical Science.

Dr. THOMAS LENARZ studied medicine at the Universities of Tübingen, Erlangen, Heidelberg, and London. He is currently Chairman and Professor in the Department of Otolaryngology at the Medical University of Hannover, Germany. Some of his fields of interest include cochlear implants in children and adults, implantable hearing aid research, auditory evoked potentials, otoacoustic emissions, acoustic neuromas, intraoperative monitoring, and tinnitus with special reference to the spontaneous activity within the auditory system and neuropharmacology of the auditory system. The Department of Otolaryngology at the Medical University of Hannover is the main center for all kinds of implants in otology in Germany.

ERIC LEPAGE has a PhD in auditory physiology from the University of Western Australia (1981), and has held research posts at Washington University Medical School in St. Louis, Boston University, and the University of Tübingen. He is currently a senior research scientist at the National Acoustic Laboratories in Sydney, Australia.

Dr. ROBERT LEVINE is presently Assistant Professor of Neurology at Harvard Medical School, Assistant Neurologist at the Massachusetts General Hospital, and Assistant in Otolaryngology (Neurology) at the Massachusetts Eye and Ear Infirmary, where he has been conducting a tinnitus clinic since 1986. Besides tinnitus, his research interests include brainstem mechanisms in human hearing and preservation of hearing during treatment of acoustic neuromas.

WILLIAM HAL MARTIN earned a BS degree in Biological Sciences, with honors in research, from the University of California at Irvine in 1975. His PhD was granted in Speech and Hearing Sciences, with emphasis in Auditory Neurophysiology, from the Universities of California at Santa Barbara and San Francisco in 1983. He performed a Postdoctoral fellowship in Behavioral Biology and Neuroscience at the Technion in Haifa, Israel from 1983–1985. He is presently an Associate Professor of Otorhinolaryngology, Bronchoesophagology, and Physiology, and Director of Audiology and the Garfield Auditory Research Laboratory, at the Temple University Medical

School. He is an Adjunct Professor in the Temple University Speech-Language-Hearing program and in the Speech and Hearing Sciences program of the City University of New York Graduate School. Dr. Martin's current interests include neurophysiologic processes related to hearing and hearing disorders. He is currently directing projects involving signal processing, multidimensional evoked potentials, and mechanisms of tinnitus.

MARY B. MEIKLE received her PhD from the University of Oregon Medical School in physiological psychology. She is a member of the faculty of the Departments of Otolaryngology and of Medical Psychology, School of Medicine, Oregon Health Sciences University. Her research interests include electrophysiology of the mammalian auditory system and epidemiological studies of tinnitus. Dr. Meikle established the Tinnitus Data Registry, which houses medical, audiological, and tinnitus-related information and constitutes the most comprehensive source of tinnitus information available to date.

MERRILYNN J. PENNER received an undergraduate degree in mathematics from Harvard University in 1966, and her doctoral degree in experimental psychology from the University of California at San Diego in 1970. She is currently a professor at the University of Maryland at College Park. Her research has been funded by the National Science Foundation, the National Institutes of Health, the American Association of University Women, and the Burrows-Wellcome Foundation. Dr. Penner is a fellow of the Acoustical Society of America, the American Association for the Advancement of Science, and the American Psychological Society. Her research interests include mathematical models of temporal processing of auditory stimuli, acoustic emissions, and tinnitus. She is presently funded by the National Institutes of Health to study tinnitus in patients with sensorineural hearing loss.

CHRISTOPH E. SCHREINER, PhD, MD, completed his training in Physics and Medicine at the University of Goettingen, Germany, then relocated to the University of California, San Francisco. There he began an exploration of the ensemble activity of the auditory nerve to low-frequency stimulation and spontaneous activity under normal and pathological conditions. In parallel, he investigated the effects of peripheral electrical stimulation on the ensemble response in animals, and the perception of tinnitus in patients with cochlear implants. In addition, he is studying the representation of complex acoustic signals in the auditory cortex of cats and monkeys, with special consideration for the signals from cochlear implants.

YVONNE SININGER received a BA in Speech and Hearing (1972), and an MA in Audiology (1973) from Indiana University, then her PhD in Hearing Science (1984) from University of California, San Francisco. From 1973 to 1979, she served as Assistant Professor of Otolaryngology, University of Cincinnati Medical Center, from 1984–1991, Research Associate, Electrophysiology Laboratory, House Ear Institute. From 1991 to present, Dr. Sininger is Director, Children's Auditory Research and Evaluation Center, House Ear Institute.

RUSSELL L. SNYDER, PhD, was trained as an anatomist and has published research on the auditory and somatosensory system. For the last fifteen years his research has concentrated on the anatomy and physiology of the auditory system. His current research focuses on the anatomical connections between the cochlea and cochlear nuclei as well as the physiological consequences of chronic electrical stimulation of the cochlea via cochlear prostheses.

JUERGEN TONNDORF, MD, was born in Goettingen, Germany the son of otolaryngology professor Waldemar Tonndorf. During World War II he served as a medical officer aboard submarines in the German Navy. After World War II he came to the United States and devoted himself to fulltime research initially with the School of Aviation Medicine at Randolph Field, then at the University of Iowa, and finally at Columbia University. Experience aboard submarines led him to study the effects of pressure changes on hearing. He also made numerous contributions in the areas of middle ear and inner ear mechanics. He was one of three founding fathers who established the Association for Research in Otolaryngology, an outgrowth of the Forum for Research in Otolaryngology that he had also helped to establish. Late in his career, Dr. Tonndorf became interested in the clinical problem of tinnitus; he was working on this subject when chronic renal failure caused his demise in 1989 at the age of 75.

HANS-PETER ZENNER received his MD and his PhD from the University of Mainz, Germany. He is currently Professor and Chairman in the Department of Otolaryngology at the University of Tübingen. His research interests and experiences include neurobiological hearing research, immunology, cell and tissue culture, hybridoma techniques, monoclonal antibodies in diagnosis and treatment of head and neck carcinomas, head and neck surgery, and ear surgery.

CHAPTER 1

PSYCHOPHYSIOLOGICAL DIMENSIONS OF TINNITUS

RAIMUND BRIX

University of Vienna Medical School

Greek legend has it that Eos, the rose-fingered goddess of the dawn, had fallen in love with Tithonos, king of Troy. So dearly did she love him that she asked Zeus to give him immortality. But in her zeal she forgot to beg for eternal youth for her lover. So, as time went by, the king grew older and older and smaller and smaller; his body shriveled and shrank, until all that was left of him was a disembodied voice: the sharp chirp of the cicada.

The term "tinnitus" refers to auditory sensations that are not consciously attributed to any external source, that is, to extracorporeal sounds or to "body sounds". These "internal auditory sensations" should be distinguished from auditory sensations caused by the perception of external stimuli. While the latter are physiologic, tinnitus as a rule occurs when the auditory system is functionally abnormal or diseased. Whether it may also occur in persons with a normal, intact auditory system all but defies clarification because of the masking effects of environmental noise or body sounds generated by breathing, movements, or the like in a camera silens.

METHODOLOGICAL CONSTRAINTS

Numerous structures within the auditory system and in neighboring anatomical regions may contribute to the generation of tinnitus. Causative mechanisms can be classified topographically by larger anatomical units, by substructures within these units, and by their functions. While physiologic and pathophysiologic processes are mainly studied in animals, psychological aspects are exclusively investigated in man. Particularly in the research of tinnitus this is a major problem, because observations made in animal experiments cannot readily be applied to humans and vice versa. In addition, the complexity of the auditory system and its limited investigability constitute almost insurmountable barriers to a scientific approach to tinnitus. When interpreting research data and models, it should be remembered that, although the use of sophisticated examination techniques has substantially advanced our understanding of the physiology and the pathophysiology of hearing, a causal relation between measurable functions and the true substrate of tinnitus has so far not been proven scientifically.

To compound matters, tinnitus may just be a sign of a dysfunction or hearing disorder or a symptom associated with them. The mechanisms involved in the development of hearing disorders generally affect more than one structure. In all likelihood, they give rise to functional sequels which may well contribute to the occurrence of tinnitus. Acoustic impulse trauma, for instance, affects not only the mechanical and electrical properties of the stereocilia and other structures of the outer hair cells, but also produces morphological changes of the afferent and efferent nerve endings (Spoendlin 1987). Whether the tinnitus reported by patients sustaining an acoustic impulse trauma is due to mechanical irritation or to secondary biochemical derangements cannot be decided without an adequate understanding of the pathophysiology involved. But even if adequate insights will be gained from future studies, it is quite unlikely that tinnitus as a psychological phenomenon will ever be assignable to specific structures or functions.

The multiplicity of possible sites of origin (middle ear, blood vessels, cochlea, retrocochlear regions, such as the VIIIth nerve, and central areas—brainstem to cortex) and the practical experiences made in the diagnosis of tinnitus and in attempts at treating it suggest that a distinction between "monocausal" and "multicausal" types of tinnitus is permissible, and at the same time, more realistic. After all, the search for a single mode of treatment for what is, in actual fact, a multimodal condition is bound to be futile (A.R. Møller 1987).

In light of the above, precise definitions or at least precise descriptions are needed in this difficult area of research to differentiate the phenomena to be investigated. A painstaking assessment of the parameters characteristic of tinnitus both in qualitative and in quantitative terms will, no doubt, yield more conclusive information on retrospective analysis. Years of experience with a psychophysiologically oriented approach to the study of tinnitus have shown this strategy to be useful, particularly for establishing the value of supposedly new modes of treatment. Both for research purposes and for practical work we have used a classification based on psychological factors for collecting data about tinnitus.

QUALITATIVE DIFFERENTIATION BETWEEN TINNITUS AND OTHER AUDITORY SENSATIONS

1. True tinnitus is a spontaneous and consciously experienced sensation which is auditory in nature, and should be distinguished from
2. "auditory perceptions" as mentioned at the outset, from
3. remembered events (memories), as well as from
4. so-called imagined events ("auditory imaginations" [Brix 1987]).

When asked to describe how they subjectively experienced episodes of tinnitus, patients often find it difficult to allocate them to these four categories. In the presence of "intermittent" tinnitus, spontaneous episodes may alternate, in the patient's mind, with episodes just past, but remembered during the free intervals. This pattern should be distinguished from "auditory imaginations" which, while containing remembered elements, represent a new sensation derived from imagination and association. This implies that someone who has never been exposed to spontaneous tinnitus is well capable of imagining it as an auditory sensation. When collecting and evaluating data about tinnitus, this distinction is rarely made. As a result, the value of a given mode of treatment is often misjudged.

If tinnitus can be differentiated from other auditory sensations in qualitative terms, it makes sense to consider such quantitative characteristics as the intensity of tinnitus and the severity of subjective impairment (suffering) caused by it.

SEVERITY OF TINNITUS

Vernon (1984) proposed to distinguish between "severe tinnitus" and "tinnitus secondary to some other primary complaint". In our group tinnitus is graded by its objective psycho-acoustically assessed intensity in "low-intensity tinnitus" (up to 0.2 sones) and "high-intensity tinnitus" (more than 0.2 sones) and by the patient's subjective coping potential in "compensable" and "non-compensable" tinnitus (Ehrenberger and Brix 1983). Shulman (1987) also proposed a comprehensive system of nomenclature and a classification by clinical types.

Most patients suffer from low-intensity tinnitus, and for most of them the tinnitus is compensable. However, its intensity and compensability are not consistently correlated. Often enough psychological factors, such as anxiety because of an inadequate understanding of the condition, reactive or endogenous depression, neurosis, organic psychosyndrome, and the like, determine whether or not the tinnitus is compensable. Depending on the patient's personality, tinnitus of low intensity by objective evidence or of intermittent occurrence may result in psychological "decompensation". In this event psychological interventions should be prescribed with critical discretion: Patients with contractions of the cervical muscles may respond well to autogenous training or physiotherapy. In other types of tinnitus the excessive concentration on, and preoccupation with, the symptom may be counterproductive. As a rule, a combination of medical and psychological interventions will help patients to cope with their condition.

ADAPTATION AND HABITUATION

Aside from the above qualitative and quantitative factors, the psychophysiology of adaptation and habituation should be considered. Adaptation is a normal peripheral process which occurs in the sensory organ itself, while habituation is a centrally controlled process which also plays a role in learning. Because of adaptation and habituation, a reduction in the intensity of tinnitus reported during treatment may no longer be experienced as such at a later time—patients may feel that their tinnitus has become louder again, even though psychoacoustic tests fail to substantiate this sub-

jective impression. What has actually happened in such cases is that the patients have become used to the new tinnitus level and have reset their subjective "rating scale" by it. Since they no longer remember the previously higher intensity level, their tolerance threshold is also reset.

Since the phenomenon of tinnitus all but defies precise description, patients should be followed up by repeated testing.

PSYCHOACOUSTIC TESTS
AND PLACEBO TESTS

In order to improve the accuracy of descriptive approaches to tinnitus and to provide for statistical analyses, audiologic tests and suitable psychoacoustic procedures were recommended. But their mere use does not guarantee the desired accuracy and validity of the data recorded. Only a well balanced test battery with built-in checks and counterchecks and an adequate number of repeat runs will enhance the reliability of the subjective data or at least make them evaluable (Brix and Ehrenberger 1987).

When placebo tests are used, it should be remembered that, psychologically, the active and the sham medication are attributed the same intrinsic value. In tinnitus types that remain stable over longer periods of time, the outcome of treatment is more easily evaluable than in types taking a variable course with intermittent episodes or highly variable intensities. In the latter case a set of adequate baseline data should, therefore, be obtained.

However, these rules are not consistently followed by all investigators. As a result, treatment modalities advocated for years may eventually turn out to be ineffective once they have been evaluated internationally.

In spite of these methodological constraints, it is both necessary and permissible to define concepts and models explaining the underlying physiology and the mechanisms involved in the development of certain types of tinnitus, using data from animal experiments as a corollary.

CONCEPTS OF TINNITUS

Topographic Concept of Tinnitus

Except for "objectively detectable" tinnitus, which is usually pulsatile in nature, the site from which tinnitus originates is generally not identifiable. Observations made by our group (Ehrenberger and Brix 1983; Brix and Ehrenberger 1984) after administering L-glutamic acid diethyl ester (L-GDEE) and L-glutamic acid (L-Glu) by IV infusion may well point to the site of origin of "cochlear" tinnitus: In patients with impaired hearing—with idiopathic sudden hearing loss or presbyacusis—adequate doses of L-GDEE and/or L-Glu (Ehrenberger and Brix 1987) reduced or suppressed the tinnitus for weeks and months. The changing quality of the sensations the patients reported while still receiving infusions was found to correlate with cochlear function assessed by the latency of the cochlear compound action potential (CAP = wave I (WI) of the brainstem evoked potentials) of the auditory nerve: A reduction in the intensity of the sensations correlated with a reduced latency of WI. Inappropriate doses increased the intensity and prolonged the latency (Brix and Ehrenberger 1984). On the basis of these observations a working hypothesis was drawn up: Assuming that Glu acted as a neurotransmitter at the afferent nerve endings of the cochlea, the tinnitus associated with the above conditions was felt to be "synaptic" in nature. This hypothesis is supported by micro-iontophoretic studies in guinea pigs (Ehrenberger and Felix 1991) and by therapeutic trials in humans (Denk, Brix, Felix, and Ehrenberger 1991).

Analogous topographic evidence was also found for some types of "retrocochlear" tinnitus in patients with acoustic nerve neurinomas or with vascular loops, where the sensations ceased postoperatively after microvascular decompression (M. Møller 1987; Jannetta 1987).

In this context, theories on the origin of tinnitus in the auditory nerve fibers following auditory nerve damage and resultant alterations of the myelin sheath gain increasing importance (A.R. Møller 1987). In the presence of neuronal damage, abnormal correlations of neural activity may not be confined to the course of the ascending auditory nerve, but may already occur in the periphery at the level of the spiral ganglion (Spoendlin 1987). Abnormal synchronization and distorted phase locking of nerve conduction would be the consequences.

Other Concepts of Tinnitus Generation

In most hearing disorders it has so far been impossible to relate the effects of treatment to a specific mechanism of tinnitus development. The tinnitus present in Ménière's disease may, for instance, be elicited both by damage to the outer hair cells and by abnormalities associated with the rupture of the membranous labyrinth (e.g., the mixing of endolymph and perilymph) (Spoendlin 1987). Similar interactions between mechanical forces and biochemical processes are likely to be operative in partial decoupling of hair cells from the tectorial membrane (Tonndorf 1981).

The effects produced by the glycerol test may, thus, not only be explainable in terms of osmolarity effects. They may just as well be mediated by a modification of the contractility of the outer hair cells (Zenner 1987).

The discovery of otoacoustic emissions (Kemp 1978) raised new hopes of finding an objective basis for certain types of tinnitus (e.g., mechanical damage). But several studies, among them that by Zwicker (1987), have so far failed to show a correlation between the parameters of emissions and those of tinnitus.

TREATMENT-RELATED CONCEPTS

Given the current state of inner ear research, models based on the functional interactions between afferents and efferents are at best speculative (Hazell 1987). While tinnitus maskers, hearing aids, and functional masking by electrostimulation may produce subjective benefits in some patients, they cannot help to elucidate the causative mechanisms involved. Their efficacy is explainable psychologically in terms of intermodal and intramodal masking. Muscle relaxants also fall into the group of general measures with numerous indirect interactions. Psychoactive drugs with a central sedating action also affect other brain functions. A specific drug which would exclusively act on the central component of tinnitus without producing side effects has so far not been found.

The example of patients who have been deaf for years shows that memories of tinnitus may be centrally stored, presumably in some subcortical or cortical areas. These patients report having vivid memories of voices, sounds, or noises that usually occur in dreams and are said to be quite similar to those experienced before deafness. This supports the concept that central excitatory circuits may develop during long-term stimulation or persistent tinnitus. At the same time, it implies that even if future studies will shed light on the causative mechanisms of tinnitus and suggest specific therapeutic approaches, there will be at least one type of tinnitus, the central type, which will presumably never be treatable, unless the specific memory in the brain is completely erased.

The concepts elaborated in this contribution cannot claim to offer an exhaustive explanation of the phenomenon of tinnitus. By addressing some arbitrarily selected aspects, the ideas in this chapter are intended to bring us closer to our goal—to relieve the suffering of those afflicted by tinnitus.

REFERENCES

Brix, R. 1987. "Die Objektivierung akustischer und optischer Vorstellungen im Elektroenzephalogramm." *Archives of Oto-Rhino-Laryngology*, *218*, 209–219.

Brix, R. and Ehrenberger, K. 1984. "Hirnstammpotentialmessungen im Rahmen von Glutaminsäure- und Glutaminsäurediäthylester-Infusion bei Tinnituspatienten." *Archives of Oto-Rhino-Laryngology*, *Supplement II*, 74–75.

Brix, R. and Ehrenberger, K. 1987. "Subjective and Objective Methods for Tinnitus Therapy Control." In H. Feldmann (Ed.), *Proceedings III International Tinnitus Seminar, Munster 1987* (pp. 170–173). Karlsruhe: Harsch Verlag.

Denk, D.M., Brix, R., Felix, D., and Ehrenberger, K. 1992. "Tinnitus Therapy with Transmitters." In J.-M. Aran and R. Daumann (Eds.), *Proceedings of the Fourth International Tinnitus Seminar, Bordeaux 1991*. Amsterdam: Kugler (in press).

Ehrenberger, K. and Brix, R. 1983. "Glutamic Acid and Glutamic Acid Diethylester in Tinnitus Treatment." *Acta Otolaryngolica (Stockholm)*, *95*, 599–605.

Ehrenberger, K. and Brix, R. 1987. "Tinnitus Treatment: Intravenous Administration of Glutamate and its Antagonist Glutamic Acid Diethylester." In H. Feldmann (Ed.), *Proceedings III International Tinnitus Seminar, Munster 1987*. (pp. 331–333). Karlsruhe: Harsch Verlag.

Ehrenberger, K. and Felix, D. 1991. "Glutamate Receptors in Afferent Cochlear Neurotransmission in Guinea Pigs." *Hearing Research*, *52*, 73–80.

Hazell, J.W.P. 1987. "A Cochlear Model for Tinnitus." In H. Feldmann (Ed.), *Proceedings III International Tinnitus Seminar, Munster 1987* (pp. 121–128). Karlsruhe: Harsch Verlag.

Jannetta, P.J. 1987. "Microvascular Decompression of the Cochlear Nerve as Treatment of Tinnitus." In H. Feldmann (Ed.), *Proceedings III International Tinnitus Seminar, Munster 1987* (pp. 340–347). Karlsruhe: Harsch Verlag.

Kemp, D.T. 1978. "Stimulated Acoustic Emissions from within the Human Auditory System." *Journal of the Acoustical Society of America*, *64*, 1386–1391.

Møller, A.R. 1987. "Can Injury to the Auditory Nerve Cause Tinnitus?" In H. Feldmann (Ed.), *Proceedings III International Tinnitus Seminar, Munster 1987* (pp. 58–63). Karlsruhe: Harsch Verlag.

Møller, M. 1987. "Vascular Compression of the VIIIth Nerve as Cause of Tinnitus." In H. Feldmann (Ed.), *Proceedings III International Tinnitus Seminar, Munster 1987* (pp. 340–347). Karlsruhe: Harsch Verlag.

Shulman, A. 1987. "Subjective Idiopathic Tinnitus—Clinical Types—A System of Nomenclature and Classification." In H. Feldmann (Ed.), *Proceedings III International Tinnitus Seminar, Munster 1987* (pp. 136–141). Karlsruhe: Harsch Verlag.

Spoendlin, H. 1987. "Inner Ear Pathology and Tinnitus." In H. Feldmann (Ed.), *Proceedings III*

International Tinnitus Seminar, Munster 1987 (pp. 42–49). Karlsruhe: Harsch Verlag.

Tonndorf, J. 1981. "Stereociliary Dysfunction, a Case of Sensory Hearing Loss, Recruitment, Poor Speech Discrimination and Tinnitus." *Acta Otolaryngolica (Stockholm)*, 9, 469–479.

Vernon, J. 1984. "Identification of Tinnitus: A Plea for Standardization." *British Journal of Laryngology and Otology (Supplement) 9*, 45–54.

Zenner, H.P. 1987. "Modern Aspects of Hair Cell Bio-chemistry, Motility and Tinnitus?" In H. Feldmann (Ed.), *Proceedings III International Tinnitus Seminar, Munster 1987* (pp. 52–57). Karlsruhe: Harsch Verlag.

Zwicker, E. 1987. "Objective Otoacoustic Emissions and Their Uncorrelation to Tinnitus." In H. Feldmann (Ed.), *Proceedings III International Tinnitus Seminar, Munster 1987* (pp. 75–82). Karlsruhe: Harsch Verlag.

CHAPTER 2

A MECHANISM FOR TINNITUS?

ROBERT F. BRUMMETT
Oregon Health Sciences University

Tinnitus is an abnormal perception of sound. The characteristics of tinnitus sounds are not those of meaningful sounds, such as words or music—they usually take the form of white or pink noise, pure tones, or some combination of these sounds. The anatomic origin of tinnitus is sometimes discussed as an attempt at diagnostic and/or treatment strategies. Because objective sensorial hearing loss generally accompanies tinnitus, the anatomic site of the generation of the tinnitus is usually reported to be the same as the anatomic site of the accompanying hearing loss. This is an unproven assumption with no basis in fact. Therefore, in this chapter, I will not attempt to separate central from peripheral tinnitus, but will allow for the contribution of both. My proposed mechanism of tinnitus is that peripheral damage in the auditory system results in a depressed GABA-mediated inhibiting effect on neural activity entering the inferior colliculus. The extraneous activity that escapes to the auditory cortex is perceived as tinnitus.

The basis of my proposed mechanism for tinnitus is from assumptions derived from studies of drugs used to treat tinnitus. Most of the studies discussed will only be those that have been randomized, double-blind, and placebo-controlled. However, because of the paucity of such reports, I will include others as well. The first study to be considered involves the drug alprazolam (Brummett, Johnson, and Schleuning 1992). In this study, thirteen of seventeen patients who completed the study and were receiving alprazolam had a reduction in their perceived tinnitus loudness as judged both by a visual analog scale and by a tinnitus loudness match using an external tinnitus-like sound. Only one of the nineteen patients receiving the placebo who completed the study reported a decline in tinnitus. It was concluded from this investigation that alprazolam could reduce the intensity of tinnitus, although it did not disappear completely in any patient.

Alprazolam is a benzodiazepine drug related chemically to Valium® and Atavan®, or pharmacologically to Miltown®. These drugs are all selective central nervous system depressants. They all appear to have their mechanism of action ascribed to an ability to enhance the action of Gamma Amino Butyric Acid (GABA) in the central nervous system (CNS) (Hindmarch, Beaumont, Brandon, and Leonard 1990). The effect is mediated by the binding of the benzodiazepine to receptors that are activated by GABA. When GABA activates these receptors, the end result is inhibition of nerve activity. The effect of the benzodiazepine activating the benzodiazepine receptors on the GABA receptors is to enhance the inhibiting effect of GABA.

GABA has been found in the inferior colliculus of the central auditory pathway (Faingold, Gehlbach, and Caspary 1991). Furthermore, the enzyme responsible for GABA synthesis, glutamic acid decarboxylase (GAD), and the genetic information necessary for the synthesis of GAD has also been found in the inferior colliculus (Figure 2-1) (Adams and Wenthold 1979; Najlerahim, Harrison, Barton, Hefferman, and

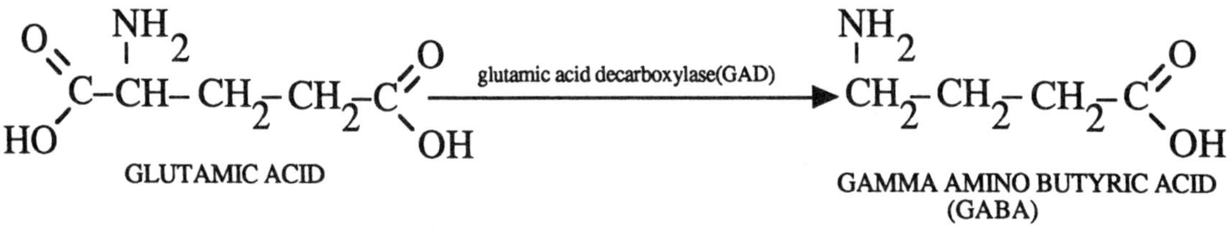

$$O \backslash \underset{HO}{\overset{O}{\diagup}} C{-}CH{-}CH_2{-}CH_2{-}C \overset{O}{\underset{OH}{\diagdown}} \quad \xrightarrow{\text{glutamic acid decarboxylase(GAD)}} \quad \underset{CH_2{-}CH_2{-}CH_2{-}C}{\overset{NH_2}{|}} \overset{O}{\underset{OH}{\diagdown}}$$

GLUTAMIC ACID

GAMMA AMINO BUTYRIC ACID
(GABA)

FIGURE 2-1. GABA synthetic pathway

Pearson 1990). GABA transaminase an enzyme responsible for the degradation of GABA, has been found in the inferior colliculus (Fisher and Davis 1976), as have GABA and benzodiazepine receptor binding (Bristow and Martin 1988; Seighart 1986). Therefore, GABA and the metabolic machinery for its synthesis and degradation have been found in the central auditory pathways. Furthermore, binding sites for GABA and benzodiazepines have been found in the same structures.

The physiological function of the inhibitory GABAergic activity in the inferior colliculus is not thoroughly understood. In one sense, this lack of data makes it easier to speculate about what might happen. It has been shown that GABA activity in the inferior colliculus is involved in sharpening the tuning curves of at least some neurons (Yang and Pollak 1992; Pollak and Park 1992; Park and Pollak 1992). These data are indirect because what was demonstrated is that when GABA activity is blocked by bicucculine, the tuning curves that were originally sharply tuned became much broader, although the tips of the tuning curves were not altered. Bicucculine is an antagonist to GABA (Gilmans, Rall, Nies, and Taylor 1990). It could be implied that GABAergic activity is involved in inhibiting extraneous activity from progressing to the auditory cortex. How the GABAergic activity is activated to do this in the normal operation of the auditory system is not known.

Most individuals who have tinnitus also have a demonstrable hearing loss (Vernon 1984). In those few who do not appear to have a hearing

loss, it is quite conceivable that there may be some defect at frequencies other than those tested. It has been reported that glutamic acid decarboxylase activity in the inferior colliculus is decreased after cochlear lesions (Adams and Wenthold 1979). If this is the case, the result would be a reduced capability of the inferior colliculus to synthesize GABA. Finally, the reduced GABAergic activity would interfere with the ability of the inferior colliculus to inhibit unwanted neural activity. It is my hypothesis that this unwanted activity that escapes inhibition in the inferior colliculus is perceived as tinnitus when it reaches the auditory cortex. For such a hypothesis to hold water, it should be able to explain some of the known characteristics of tinnitus, such as residual inhibition due to masking.

Masking, or the ability of one sound to inhibit the perception of another, is an often observed phenomenon found in tinnitus patients where environmental or artificially generated sounds are able to reduce or abolish the perception of tinnitus. The mechanism of masking is not known.

According to my hypothesis, sound-induced or spontaneously occurring nerve activity normally results in an increased GABAergic shaping of the nerve activity when it reaches the inferior colliculus. If a patient who is experiencing tinnitus is exposed to a masking tone of sufficient intensity, this masking sound could result in an increase in GABAergic activity in the inferior colliculus. Masking sounds that produce residual inhibition must be close to the frequency of the tinnitus to mask the tinnitus effectively in most individuals. This would probably mean that the nerve activity in the inferior colliculus resulting from the masking sound would be processed near the area where the tinnitus neural activity is escaping GABAergic inhibition. That is, the inhibitory response in the inferior colliculus to shape nerve activity induced by the masking sound could also affect the tinnitus. Residual inhibition due to masking could be produced by prolonged activity of the masking-sound-induced released GABA.

Aminoxyacetic acid (AOAA), an inhibitor of GABA transaminase, has been shown by Guth and colleagues (Guth, Risey, Briner, Blair, Reed, Bryant, Norris, Housley, and Miller, 1990) in a controlled study to decrease tinnitus. Because GABA transaminase is responsible for GABA degradation, the effect would be to prolong the inhibitory activity of released GABA.

Nortriptyline, a tricyclic antidepressant has been extensively investigated in a very carefully controlled clinical trial in depressed patients (Sullivan, Dobie, Sakai, and Katon, 1989). Investigators found that the nortriptyline helped the patients cope with their tinnitus, but did not reduce its intensity as measured by a visual analog scale and a tinnitus loudness match. Nortriptyline is not known to affect the GABA system.

Furosemide, a loop-inhibiting diuretic, has also been found by Guth and colleagues (Guth, Risey, Amedee, and Norris 1992) to decrease tinnitus in some patients. The rationale for the trial of furosemide was that aminoxyacetic acid has already been shown to decrease the endocochlear potential as does furosemide. However, it is not known if furosemide in any way affects GABA activity. It does not appear to do so as furosemide has not been reported to be associated with CNS depression.

It is easy to speculate about mechanisms of biological phenomena, such as tinnitus, relative to the known mechanisms of drug action. While this exercise is often attempted, as has been done here, it is fraught with many pitfalls. If a drug is known to have an established mechanism of action producing one effect—such as benzodiazepines enhancing the activity of GABA in producing CNS depression—it is easy to speculate that enhancing the action of GABA is responsible for all of its effects. This may be true. However, there is no guarantee. Most drugs are known to have a multiplicity of effects often mediated by different mechanisms. Thus, it could be possible that the benzodiazepines, AOAA, and furosemide all have some other effect that is not shared with nortriptyline in depressing tinnitus. Since drugs are often used to explore the mechanism of the action of biological effects, this pitfall must be kept in mind.

If all tinnitus was produced by the same mechanism, it might be assumed that every individual with tinnitus would respond to the same treatment. In the studies conducted so far, this has not been the case, suggesting that there is more than one basic tinnitus mechanism. This guess is supported by the observation that tinnitus appears to have many different causes. It may also be the case that in the drug treatment studies mentioned here, the dose of drug may not have been sufficiently large to affect everyone, or, as in the case of masking or electrical stimulation procedures, we do not know how to apply the treatment so that it is effective for everyone.

REFERENCES

Adams, J.C. and Wenthold, R.J. 1979. "Distribution of Putative Amino Acid Transmitters, Choline Acetyltransferase and Glutamate Decarboxylase in the Inferior Colliculus." *Neuroscience, 4,* 1947–1951.

Bristow, D.R. and Martin, I.L. 1988. "Light Microscopic Autoradiographic Localization in the Rat Brain of the Binding Sites for the $GABA_A$ Receptor Antagonist [3H]SR 95531: Comparison with the [3H] $GABA_A$ Receptor Distribution." *European Journal Pharmacology, 148,* 283–288.

Brummett, R.E., Johnson, R., and Schleuning, A. 1992. "Alprazolam (Xanax) for Tinnitus Relief." (Abstract 398) *Association for Research in Otolaryngology,* Feb. 2–6, p. 134.

Faingold, C.L., Gehlbach, G., and Caspary, D.M. 1991.

Functional Pharmacology of Inferior Colliculus Neurons." In R.A. Altschuler, R.P. Bobbin, B.M. Clopton, and D.W. Hoffman (Ed.), *Neurobiology of Hearing: The Central Auditory System*, pp. 223–251. New York: Raven Press.

Fisher, S.K. and Davis, W.E. 1976. "GABA and Its Related Enzymes in the Lower Auditory System of the Guinea Pig." *Journal of Neurochemistry*, 27, 1145–1155.

Gilmans, G.A., Rall, T.W., Nies, A.S., and Taylor, P. (Eds.) 1990. *The Pharmacological Basis of Therapeutics* (8th edition), p. 258. New York: Pergamon Press.

Guth, P.S., Risey, R., Amendee, R., and Norris, C.H. 1992. "A Pharmacological Approach to the Treatment of Tinnitus." In J.-M. Aran and R. Dauman (Eds.), *Proceedings of the Fourth International Tinnitus Seminar, Bordeaux, France, 1991*, pp. 1–3. Amsterdam/New York, R. Kugler Publications.

Guth, P.S., Risey, J., Briner, W., Blair, P., Reed, H.T., Bryant, G., Norris, C., Housley, G., and Miller, R. 1990. "Evaluation of Amino-oxyacetic Acid as a Palliative in Tinnitus." *Annals of Otology, Rhinology, and Laryngology*, 99, 74.

Hindmarch, I., Beaumont, G., Brandon, S., and Leonard, B.E. (Eds.). 1990. *Benzodiazepines: Current Concepts*, p. 45. New York: John Wiley & Sons.

Najlerahim, A., Harrison, P.J., Barton, A.L., Hefferman, J., and Pearson, R.A. 1990. "Distribution of Messenger RNA's Encoding the Enzymes Glutaminase, Aspartate Aminotransferase and Glutamic Acid Decarboxylase in Rat Brain." *Molecular Brain Research*, 7, 317–333.

Park, T.J. and Pollak, G.D. 1992. "The Role of GABA in Shaping Binaural Properties and Receptive Fields of E-1 Neurons in the Inferior Colliculus." (Abstract 237) *Association for Research in Otolaryngology*, p. 79.

Pollak, G.D. and Park, T.J. 1992. "The Role of GABA in Shaping Monaural Properties of Neurons in the Interior Colliculus." (Abstract 236) *Association for Research in Otolaryngology*, p. 79.

Seighart, W. 1986. "Comparison of Benzodiazepine Receptor in Cerebellum and Inferior Colliculus." *Journal of Neurochemistry*, 47, 920–923.

Sullivan, M.D., Dobie, R.A., Sakai, C.S., and Katon, W.J. 1989. "Treatment of Depressed Tinnitus Patients with Nortriptyline." *Annals of Otology, Rhinology, and Laryngology*, 98, 867–872.

Vernon, J.A. 1984. *Tinnitus in Hearing Disorders* (2nd edition), p. 291. Boston/Toronto: Little Brown and Co.

Yang, L.C. and Pollak, G.D. 1992. "The Role of GABA in Sharpening Tuning Curves of Neurons in the Mustache Bat's Inferior Colliculus." (Abstract 190) *Association for Research in Otolaryngology*, p. 63.

CHAPTER 3

CLASSIFICATION OF CAUSES, MECHANISMS OF PATIENT DISTURBANCE, AND ASSOCIATED COUNSELING

BY ROSS R.A. COLES, EMERITUS
Medical Research Council, Institute of Hearing Research,
Nottingham, United Kingdom

Tinnitus has in fact many possible mechanisms, simply because it is a symptom rather than a diagnostic entity. I think it most helpful, therefore, to classify type and causation of tinnitus according to site of the underlying disorder leading to the tinnitus (Coles 1987). Such a classification of the more common forms of tinnitus and speculation on some of the mechanisms is described in the first section of this chapter, together with some relevant epidemiological data on the factors influencing the prevalence of tinnitus.

The second section will look at how and in what ways tinnitus may trouble the patient. Having a model of this is of great value in deciding the most appropriate line(s) of management for each particular patient. It also highlights the need to explain to the patient how his or her tinnitus has been generated, and I will give some examples of how I do this for patients with various types and degrees of hearing disorders.

CLASSIFICATION BY SITE OF DISORDER LEADING TO TINNITUS

Cochlear Disorders, Causing Sensorineural Tinnitus

Tinnitus is most commonly associated with disorder or damage or degeneration in the internal ear, most common in the form of age-related hearing loss (ARHL) or noise-induced hearing loss (NIHL). One cause of cochlear disorder seems to be associated with tinnitus just about as frequently as any other, with the notable exception of classical Ménière's disease where tinnitus is present by definition. It may be slightly more frequent also when the causative disorder is sudden, as from acute acoustic, mechanical, or barometric trauma. However, what really seems to govern prevalence of tinnitus, in population terms, is how much cochlear disorder is present.

The evidence for this has been published elsewhere (Coles, Davis, and Smith 1990). The data are from the UK National Study of Hearing, a multiphase, multicenter cross-sectional study of hearing and hearing disorders, the most relevant parts of which were carried out in 1980 to 1985. In an initial analysis of the influence of demographic factors and personal history, the most important determinant of tinnitus prevalence was the report of a hearing problem. Other significant factors were age and noise exposure; gender and socioeconomic group were not significant.

On the other hand, when reported hearing difficulty was replaced by actual measurements of hearing threshold level (HTL), especially by those at high frequencies, age and noise exposure (either occupational or from gunfire) as separate determinants of moderately or severely annoying tinnitus became nonsignificant. HTL remained as the only significant determinant. Figure 3–1 shows the odds ratios for prevalence of such tinnitus for different degrees of HTL at 4 kHz in the better ear. Compared with its prevalence where there is less than 10 dB HTL, there is a threefold increase in odds for 20-29 dB HTL, eightfold increase for 40-49 dB HTL, and twenty-sevenfold increase for 80+ dB HTL.

This does not mean that absolutely all moderately or severely annoying tinnitus is associated with hearing impairment at 4 kHz in the better ear. For instance, it was present in 1.3 percent of those with hearing thresholds less than 10 dB HL. And it

is also probable that in some cases the tinnitus was associated with hearing impairment at other frequencies or in the worse ear. Indeed unilateral tinnitus is more common in the worse-hearing ear in noise-exposed persons (Chung, Gannon, and Mason 1984) and in clinical practice. But in the general population, hearing in the worse ear was not found to be as powerful a determinant of moderately or severely annoying tinnitus as hearing in the better ear.

In individuals it seems likely that there is some critical degree of disorder for the development of tinnitus that is particular to each individual and ear, and that in cochlear disorders this is largely independent of cause. If this is so, a variety of

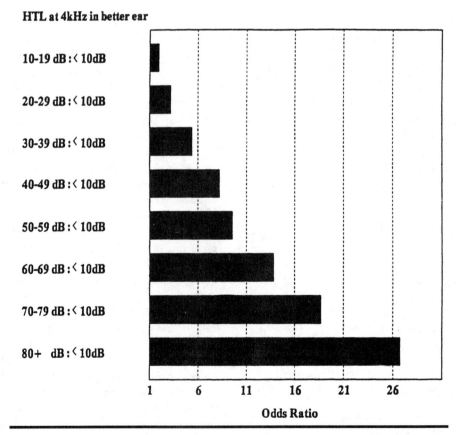

FIGURE 3-1. Determinates of moderately or severely annoying tinnitus (NSH, Phases 1, 2 and 3 combined, n = 2522)

causes of cochlear disorder may occur simultaneously or sequentially until their combined degree is large enough to lead to tinnitus.

This lends strong support to the clinical dictum that whatever factors caused the hearing loss most probably caused the tinnitus, too. This may seem obvious, but it is quite often forgotten in the assessment of cases of NIHL, who are claiming compensation for noise-induced tinnitus as well. Thus, if NIHL is present, it needs strong contrary evidence for tinnitus to be diagnosed as due to something else.

There is a further implication of practical importance here. If the onset of tinnitus is determined primarily by the amount of cochlear disorder, then just as several causes of such disorder can combine to produce greater hearing loss, so they can also combine to produce tinnitus. For instance, when ARHL occurs after the onset of earlier noise damage, the eventual hearing difficulty and/or tinnitus can be attributed at least in part to the earlier noise damage.

The concepts outlined above lead to a model of the effects of cochlear disorders in general, irrespective of whether the disorder is due to damage, degeneration, or any other noxious influence. The model is shown in Figure 3-2, and indicates the three main types of dysfunction present in cochlear disorder. These can occur separately or in different degrees in individual cases. I have often found this model very helpful in clinical counseling, as well as in medico-legal argument and teaching.

The first dysfunction is a reduction of sensitivity, normally measured as an elevation of the puretone HTL. The otological and occupational medical literature is dominated by this effect, because it gives a fairly accurate quantification of the damage, provides useful diagnostic information, is relatively simple to test, and can be precisely calibrated and standardized. On the other hand, individuals with

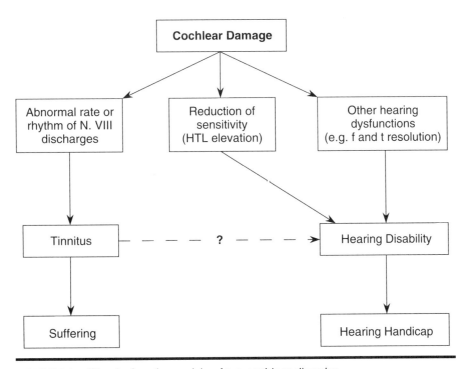

FIGURE 3-2. The dysfunctions arising from cochlear disorder

similar pure-tone audiograms sometimes have wide differences in hearing disability, either self-rated or measured by various forms of speech identification task. Reasons for this variability are probably different amounts of the second type of dysfunction, such as a reduction of frequency resolution ability and of temporal resolution ability, and probably other forms of disturbance as yet unidentified.

The third type of cochlear dysfunction relates to the mechanism of generation of tinnitus. It may be summarized broadly as an abnormal rate or rhythm of spontaneous discharges in the auditory nerve fibers; that is, abnormal relative to the normal state in quiet or in low levels of steady ambient noise. Since the brain interprets modulations of the spontaneous discharging as sounds, some ongoing abnormality in rate or rhythm is likely to be appreciated as a continuous sound, that is, tinnitus.

These three types of dysfunction, frequently accompanied by hyperacusis in cases of tinnitus, tend to occur in varying degrees of prominence relative to one other. Thus, tinnitus may be the first or the dominant effect, either or both of the dysfunctions causing hearing difficulty may be dominant, or all three may occur equally.

There are two additional complications in clinical work. One is that in many cases the hearing impairment demonstrable by pure-tone audiometry is of insufficient degree for hearing difficulty to be realized by the patient. The other is that although a hearing difficulty is recognized by the patient, it is often attributed to the tinnitus. The result is that the patient comes to fear the tinnitus, as if it were a disease of its own, rather than seeing it merely as a symptom of a hearing disorder, itself usually quite harmless.

The balance of evidence suggests that tinnitus does not cause hearing disability directly, for instance, by masking of speech sounds. But it can interfere with concentration in listening to what people are saying. And in turn this interference in concentration complicates an actual underlying reduction in speech identification ability associated with presence of one, other, or both of the other two forms of cochlear dysfunction.

Before leaving sensorineural tinnitus, I should not omit to mention the peripheral neural subdivision of sensorineural. Tinnitus of that origin occurs quite infrequently, for example, due to acoustic neuroma, although mechanical interference with VIIIth nerve function arising from vascular loops compressing the nerve or its blood supply (Møller 1987) and thus causing tinnitus may be rather more common than we realize.

Middle-Ear disorders

The term "conductive tinnitus" can be used to describe tinnitus associated with, or exacerbated by, conductive hearing loss. In most cases the tinnitus arises by the revealing or enhancing of an underlying tinnitus. Much of this is probably due to reduction of the normal masking effect of ambient noise, the reduction being due to the attenuating effect of the conductive hearing loss. Sometimes the enhanced or revealed sounds are physiological hum or due to extra-auditory abnormality causing, for example, vascular pulsing, muscular clicking, or respiratory blowing sounds. But much more commonly they are associated with an underlying sensorineural tinnitus. This may be due to a sensorineural disorder that is coincident with, but independent of, the middle-ear disorder causing the conductive hearing loss, for example, due to ARHL or NIHL; or it may be consequent on it, for example, in mixed stapedial and cochlear otosclerosis or in cochlear involvement in otitis media.

Kemp (1981) has postulated that pure conductive hearing losses may occasionally be associated with cochlear mechanical tinnitus. By this theory, the conductive disorder attenuates the transmission of intracochlear oscillations, otherwise measurable as spontaneous otoacoustic emissions, causing internal reflection and possibly magnification thereby.

Auditory Deprivation Tinnitus

In some cases it is difficult to explain the tinnitus accompanying a conductive hearing loss by the mechanisms just described. An example is when the tinnitus is not reduced following prosthetic or surgical restoration of hearing, when the patient should benefit from an increase in masking of tinnitus by ambient noise. Since it is difficult to imagine how a middle-ear disorder per se could produce tinnitus, it seems likely that there is some other mechanism of tinnitus generation in such cases. The most likely candidate for that is what I describe as an auditory deprivation effect (Coles 1987).

I conceive this as the central auditory nervous system reacting to lack of neural stimulation from the ear by increasing its "attentiveness" to the auditory neural signals that do reach it, with consequent awareness of sounds arising from previously subliminal abnormal neural activity in the system. Once established, the hearing of such tinnitus tends to continue, although it may gradually diminish with time following restoration of more normal auditory sensitivity—just as the hyperacusis after a successful stapedectomy gradually adapts. This auditory deprivation mechanism, or something akin to it, probably explains not only the particular cases of conductive tinnitus already referred to, but probably, at least in part, some cases of sensorineural tinnitus, too. It can also help to explain the hyperacusis that so often accompanies tinnitus, and how this hyperacusis and/or the tinnitus may gradually be desensitized by means of prolonged use of a tinnitus masker (Hazell and Sheldrake 1992).

Central Influences and Central Tinnitus

Apart from auditory hallucinations, which in fact come within most definitions of tinnitus but are obviously of very different nature and outside the present scope, disorders within the auditory central nervous system only rarely seem to cause tinnitus. Examples are the tinnitus that occasionally follows a stroke or occurs in cases of brain tumor. Presumably the majority of intracranial disorders do not involve the auditory tracts, and even if they do they probably have to have some particular characteristics in order to cause tinnitus.

On the other hand, the brain plays a major secondary role in almost all other forms of tinnitus (Jastreboff 1990), a role which will be described elsewhere in this book. It is sufficient for me to remind the reader here that tinnitus could not occur if we did not have a brain to sense the abnormal input from the peripheral auditory system. Hypothetically, a decerebrate person might still have auditory brainstem reflexes, but would not 'hear' anything. Moreover, as outlined later in this chapter, all the distressing effects of tinnitus are in the psychological domain; that is, they depend on cerebral attention.

SOAE-Associated Tinnitus

When SOAEs were first identified, our hope was that they corresponded to their owner's tinnitus and thus, at long last, we could measure tinnitus objectively. Disillusionment soon followed when it was observed that most people with SOAEs could not hear them, that they only occurred where at least part of the audiogram was close to normal, and that in patients having both SOAEs and tinnitus, their pitches only seldom coincided. The pendulum of opinion swung, too far in fact, to believing that SOAEs had nothing to do with tinnitus.

Now, thanks to the suppression/masking test developed by Penner and Burns (1987), it is easier to identify whether a measured SOAE is responsible for all or part of a patient's tinnitus. In addition, Penner (1990) has performed surveys herself as well as analyzing collectively those of other workers, and from these has estimated that SOAEs are responsible for at least part of the tinnitus in 4(1-9) percent of tinnitus patients. Our own subsequent studies (Baskill and Coles 1992) suggest the figure is about 2 percent. In most of SOAE tinnitus, the emissions appear to be somewhat variable in frequency and/or amplitude, and it is probably this that causes them to be audible (Penner 1992), counteracting the tendency to subjective adaptation to them. Indeed, SOAEs are measurable in about 50 percent and 30 percent of normal-hearing women and men respectively, but in the large majority they are not heard by their owners.

Interestingly, in the last two years, while routinely checking those of my tinnitus patients having fairly normal hearing for SOAEs, I have seen five young persons whose tinnitus came on immediately after exposure to high levels of sound in a discotheque and was subsequently identified (Penner and Burns 1987) as being due to SOAEs, somewhat variable ones. I believe that the overstimulation by loud music caused a slight degree of cochlear damage. This was not enough to take their hearing thresholds anywhere near the lower limit of hearing at which SOAEs can occur, 10 dB at their best-hearing frequency (Baskill and Coles 1992), but the damage probably caused one or more pre-existing SOAEs to become unstable and thus audible.

Apart from academic interest, SOAE-associated tinnitus has clinical importance, since such patients can be very positively and reassuringly counseled by explaining that SOAEs are essentially a sign of normal hearing. The SOAEs can easily be masked with a broadband noise masker, if needed. And if even that fails, they may be amenable to pharmacological control with aspirin (Penner and Coles 1992), and perhaps quinine. Further, it seems possible that such treatment may result in long-term reduction of the tinnitus (Baskill and Coles 1992), perhaps as a result of a minimal degree of ototoxic damage to the cochlea sufficient to alter the SOAEs but not cause any measurable hearing loss.

THE TROUBLESOME EFFECTS OF TINNITUS

To decide what line(s) of management is most appropriate for a particular tinnitus patient, it is essential to ascertain what it is about the tinnitus that is most troubling. In turn it is useful to look on such effects in light of a model (Coles, Davis, and Smith 1990), as shown here in Figure 3–3, the original concept of which was suggested by S.C. Jakes (personal communication, ca 1985).

Although the tinnitus itself is usually real and due to an organic disorder, its effects, as already pointed out, are in the psychological domain and hence are potentially reversible—note the upward arrow on the lefthand side of the figure. Such reversal can be assisted by psychological treatments, such as medical counseling by physicians and paramedical staff (3a in the figure), counseling by literature (3b), by lay counselors and tinnitus self-help organizations (3c), relaxation training therapy (3d), and cognitive therapy (3e). About 20 percent of tinnitus clinic patients in fact need no more than medical counseling (3a); that is, they are not troubled by the tinnitus itself but are worried about its cause and/or prognosis. We will return to the components of such medical counseling, since they involve explanations of the mechanisms of the patient's tinnitus.

But before that, the other types of management indicated by the numbers on Figure 3–3 will be outlined. First (1) comes prevention. Of course, this is not possible in an established case of tinnitus, but at least advice on control or prevention of further hazardous noise exposure may prevent further damage and possibly worse tinnitus. Next (2) is treatment of the cause—wax removal, hearing aid, or surgery to restore more normal degrees of masking of tinnitus by ambient noise, drug withdrawal, drug reinstatement, more gradual withdrawal in cases of tinnitus resulting from too-rapid benzodiazepine withdrawal, and treatment of pulsatile tinnitus due to hypertension, anemia or some localized vascular disorder.

Management 4 is tinnitus masking, either by a wearable masker or use of some environmental device, such as a radio. If all else fails, or the patient is in acute agitation or depression, drugs (5) can be used. These fall into two classes: (a) for short-term reduction of the effects of the drugs—tranquilizers, nocturnal sedatives, anti-depressants; (b) for attempting to reduce the tinnitus itself. Benzodiazepines, such as Xanax or clonazepam, seem to help in some cases, but great care has to be taken with such drugs due to risks of long-term dependency. On the other hand, frusemide (furosemide) has a more direct effect on the ear by reducing the endocochlear potentials and appears to be useful in some cases of tinnitus arising from an internal-

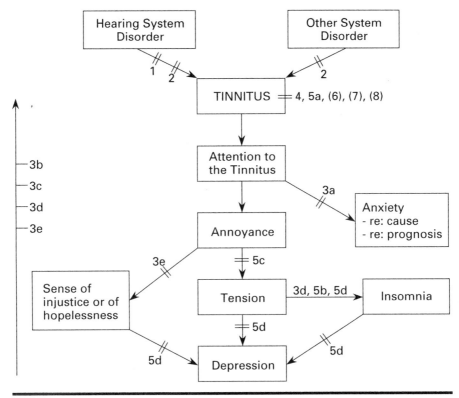

FIGURE 3-3. Causation, effects and management of tinnitus (see text for brief explanation of the numbers, which indicate methods of management)

ear disorder (Guth, Risey, Amedee, and Norris 1992).

Managements 6, 7 and 8 are less common, and are thus shown in parentheses in the figure. They are surgery, electrical stimulation, and suppression of SOAEs.

Medical Counseling

Whatever the effects of the tinnitus and whatever line(s) of management may be selected, there is in all cases a need for careful counseling by medical and/or paramedical staff. This must cover the following: (1) Diagnosis and explanation of its benign nature, as compared with fears of brain tumor, disease, or impending madness; (2) dem-

onstration of the audiogram, especially in cases of tinnitus associated with hearing losses of sufficiently small degree that they are not causing hearing difficulties recognized as such by the patient; (3) explanation of a realistic mechanism by which the disorder causing the hearing loss is causing the tinnitus. (4) A brief outline of the population prevalence (Coles et al. 1990) and a reassuring description of the generally favorable prognosis for the tinnitus (Coles et al. 1990).

So how should we explain to the patient how his or her tinnitus is being generated? If noncochlear in origin, then of course its source is explained. But for the cochlear cases, the large majority of tinnitus patients, I do not in fact have a standard explanation. This is because what one can say depends to a considerable extent on the degree and pattern of audiometric abnormality. It also depends on my estimate of the patient's ability to understand biological matters, his or her apparent degree of interest or concern, and, I have to admit, on how much time I have available for explaining.

By far the most common case is one of slight to severe cochlear hearing loss. I use a copy of a simple diagram of the ear to show the patient exactly where the disorder is, and I write down its name, otosclerosis, for example. The patient is later encouraged to keep the diagram. I then explain the transducing function of the hair cells, and that hearing a sound depends on the brain recognizing sound-induced changes in the rate or rhythm of the spontaneous trains of nerve impulses going up the nerve of hearing from the hair cells to the brain. I then explain that he or she probably had about 11,500 of these cells in each ear to start with, and now may have about xxx remaining, a number I judge crudely from the audiogram.

What I then say concerning the peripheral mechanism depends on whether the pitch match frequency is in or close to the area of maximum hearing loss, or whether it is in an area of relatively good hearing often below the frequencies most involved in the hearing loss. In the former case, I describe the tinnitus sensation as being due to a reduction in the normal firing rates in the nerve fibers coming from the zones of the cochlea showing the hearing loss. But where the tinnitus pitch is lower than the zone of hearing loss, I explain the efferent nervous control of cochlear sensitivity and how this is altered as an automatic adjustment to counteract the reduction in the nerve activity arising from the part of the cochlea affected. This in turn results in overactivity in adjacent parts, the latter then being appreciated as tinnitus.

With either explanation of the peripheral mechanism, I now add reference to the importance of the brain, explaining that it too increases in its sensitivity in response to a diminished input. This concept helps to explain the frequently coincident hyperacusis, and also provides a framework for explaining how use of a masker at a low level for many hours a day for a long period may gradually cause the brain to turn down its sensitivity, with consequent long-term reduction in tinnitus, hyperacusis, or both.

With total hearing loss, one cannot really utilize the efferent overactivity concept, since the ear is believed to be completely functionless. But the reduced input from the periphery can easily be explained as the cause of the sensation of tinnitus. What is worrying about this theory, and indeed the theories in relation to partial hearing loss, too, is the fact that sizable proportions of the hearing impaired do *not* have tinnitus.

And finally, how about a tinnitus that is present without there being any detectable hearing loss or pathology? Some of these cases are now being identified as due to SOAEs, leading to an easy and encouraging explanation as already described. Others, and indeed possibly most of the remainder, may be due to "internal tones", SOAE-like activity but without measurable emissions (Penner 1992). However, until this is proven and the presence of internal tones is more readily identifiable, I will continue to rely on my present explanation. By this, the very fact of there being tinnitus must mean that there is some disorder—even though it is so slight that it cannot be identified. I give a cause if one is evident or likely, such as those occurring since a loud noise exposure. I counsel that the normal audiogram shows how slight the causative disorder really is, but that the patient is unlucky in that this very minor disorder has revealed itself by causing tinnitus. I go on to explain that the general prospects favor reduction or even disappearance of the tinnitus, and it is very unlikely that it is the precursor of some progressive disorder of hearing.

Perhaps one day we will fully understand all aspects of tinnitus generation. But it will be too complicated to explain to most patients in detail. So something like the simple explanations given above will probably still be needed, though perhaps modified in places in light of further understanding of the underlying mechanisms.

REFERENCES

Baskill, J.B. and Coles, R.R.A. 1992. "Current Studies of Tinnitus Caused by Spontaneous Otoacoustic Emissions and Tinnitus." In J.-M. Aran and R. Dauman (Eds.), *Proceedings of the Fourth International Tinnitus Seminar, Bordeaux, France, August 27–30, 1991*. Amsterdam: Kugler.

Coles, R.R.A. 1987. "Tinnitus and Its Management." In S.D.G. Stephens (Vol. Ed.), *Scott-Brown's Otolaryngology*, Vol. 2, (pp. 368–414). Guildford: Butterworths.

Coles, R.R.A., Davis, A.C., and Smith, P.A. 1990. "Tinnitus—Its Epidemiology and Management." In J.H. Jensen (Ed.), *Presbyacusis—and Other Age Related Aspects* (pp. 377–402). Proceedings of the 14th Danavox Symposium, Danavox Jubilee Foundation, Copenhagen.

Chung, D.Y., Gannon, R.P., and Mason, K. 1984. "Factors Affecting the Prevalence of Tinnitus." *Audiology*, 23, 441–452.

Guth, S., Risey, J., Amedee, R., and Norris, C.H. 1992. "A Pharmacological Approach to the Treatment of Tinnitus." In J.-M. Aran and R. Dauman (Eds.), *Proceedings of the Fourth International Tinnitus Seminar, Bordeaux, France, August 27–30, 1991*. Amsterdam: Kugler.

Hazell, J.W.P. and Sheldrake, J.B. "Hyperacusis and Tinnitus: Mechanisms and Management." In J.-M. Aran and R. Dauman (Eds.), *Proceedings of the Fourth International Tinnitus Seminar, Bordeaux, France, August 27–30, 1991*. Amsterdam: Kugler.

Jastreboff, P.J. 1990. "Phantom Auditory Perception (Tinnitus): Mechanisms of Generation and Perception." *Neuroscience Research*, 8, 221–254.

Kemp, D.T. 1981. "Physiologically Active Cochlear Micromechanisms—One Source of Tinnitus." In D. Evered and G. Lawrenson (Eds.), *Tinnitus: Ciba Foundation Symposium 85* (pp. 54–81). London: Pitman.

Møller, M.B. 1987. "Vascular Compression of the Eighth Nerve as a Cause of Tinnitus." In H. Feldmann (Ed.), *Proceedings III International Tinnitus Seminar, Munster, 1987*. (pp. 340–347). Karlsruhe: Harsch Verlag.

Penner, M.J. 1990. "An Estimate of the Prevalence of Tinnitus Caused by Spontaneous Otoacoustic Emissions." *Archives of Otolaryngology—Head and Neck Surgery*, 116, 418–423.

Penner, M.J. 1992. "Linking Spontaneous Otoacoustic Emissions and Tinnitus." *British Journal of Audiology*, 26, 115–123.

Penner, M.J. and Burns, E.M. 1987. "The Dissociation of SOAEs and Tinnitus." *Journal of Speech and Hearing Research*, 30, 396–403.

Penner, M.J. and Coles, R.R.A. 1992. "Indications for Aspirin as a Palliative for Tinnitus Caused by SOAEs: A Case Study." *British Journal of Audiology*, 26, 91–96.

CHAPTER 4

CORRELATED NEURAL ACTIVITY AND TINNITUS

JOS J. EGGERMONT
The University of Calgary

YVONNE SININGER
House Ear Institute, Los Angeles, California

CORRELATION, THE BASIC MECHANISM OF THE BRAIN

The brain explores the sensory environment in a multitude of ways and uses the information obtained to guide its behavior. In doing so, correlation is its main mechanism to evaluate the environment, to guide motor actions and to learn (Eggermont 1990b). Correlation of neuronal activity can be done in many ways—it can be based on the coincidences in the times of firing of two or more nerve cells, or on the covariation of their instantaneous firing rates (as in the synchronization of burst firing in cortical neurons). Correlations can be found between the activity patterns of neuronal groups within the same cortical column (Gray and Singer 1988), between columns with similar orientation preferences from different cortical areas (Gray, König, Engel, and Singer 1989), or between neuronal groups with similar orientation preferences found in different hemispheres (Engel, König, Kreiter, and Singer 1991). Coincidence detection provides a way to assess correlated activity in afferent fibers and thereby allows inferences about the environment. Our thesis is that the cortex, and most other parts of the brain, are designed to detect correlated neural activity. We believe that correlation among the activity of different neural elements or neuronal groups is the only way to make sense out of inherently noisy neural activity patterns.

A major task of the central nervous system (CNS) is to determine whether a particular spike pattern in afferent neurons is caused by an external stimulus or whether it must be attributed to spontaneous activity. For instance, the activity caused by an external stimulus will produce a percept; spontaneous activity will not. In addition, stimulus intensity discrimination requires that the difference in afferent neural activity for two intensities can be distinguished from spontaneous fluctuations. Several strategies could be employed. The first requires the evaluation of the number of spikes that a neuron produces over a certain time period and estimation of a mean firing rate. This estimate is then compared with a stored "norm" of spontaneous rates for that particular neuron. A decision is based on the probability that the spike rate is above the norm. Because of the stochastic nature of the neural firings, this decision making must be a statistical process and may require lengthy evaluation periods to increase accuracy and sensitivity. This evaluation can be performed faster by an ensemble of neurons: Because the spontaneous rate of the ensemble will be less variable than the rate for individual neurons, the comparison can be made in shorter time with greater precision. The problem of how and where the "norm" is stored remains, however. This comparison mechanism is implicitly assumed in optimal processor theories (Viemeister 1983).

An alternative strategy is to compare the detailed firing patterns of at least two neurons with the same characteristic frequency (CF): When the neurons fire at about the same time an external stimulus is very likely. The decision will be more reliable as more neurons are simultaneously compared. Comparisons within a small ensemble of otherwise independently firing afferent neurons may thus result in a fast and reliable indication for the presence of an external stimulus. For instance, a typical inner hair cell in the basal turn of the cat is innervated by about twenty independently firing auditory nerve fibers (Johnson and Kiang 1976) with different spontaneous rates and threshold values. Activation of the hair cell will automatically result in synchronous release of the transmitter at some of its synapses and therefore in the synchronization of the firings of some of these neurons (Young and Sachs 1989). The amount of synchronization in the auditory nerve fibers increases with intensity and will be largely determined by the hair cell depolarization. One may assume, for moderate stimulus levels, that six to seven nerve fibers innervating a particular hair cell will be simultaneously active.

Spontaneous activity in the auditory system is normally inaudible because the auditory nerve fibers fire independently and may fail to produce sufficient synchronous firings to activate certain cochlear nucleus cells. Stimulus-induced changes may be audible because neighboring nerve fibers start firing more synchronously with the stimulus so that their firings become correlated. This correlation either increases the level of activity in higher centers or allows synchronous activity to proceed up to the cortex, causing correlated activity between distinct auditory cortical areas.

Our senses appraise the outside world in a parallel fashion that results in neural activity patterns organized in topographic maps (such as the various tonotopical maps in auditory cortex) of the brain (Figure 4-1). Neurons that have overlapping receptive fields, that is, auditory neurons innervating the same haircell, will show a covariance in instantaneous firing rate as well as a coincidence in the occurrence of spikes as a result of stimulation. The topographic mappings will ensure that coincidences in firing times will occur predominantly between neighboring units. Coincident firings generally form a subset of the firings of a group of neurons and may allow us to extract the relevant information from the neural "noise". For example, in the case of rather broadly tuned auditory neurons in the midbrain of the frog, the subset of coincident firings was found to represent particular stimuli (Eggermont and Epping 1987).

We will show that tinnitus can be understood on the basis of induced correlations in the firings of neighboring auditory nerve fibers by certain pathologies, a correlation that is normally absent under no-stimulus conditions (Johnson and Kiang 1976), and/or on the basis of correlations between groups of neurons in distinct, tonotopically organized, auditory cortical areas. How the tinnitus-causing disorder produces that correlation is not clear, but we speculate that abnormalities in the extra- or intracellular calcium concentrations could be a major factor.

WHY NORMAL SPONTANEOUS NEURAL ACTIVITY IS INAUDIBLE

Spontaneous neural activity has been considered at times as just neuronal noise (Siebert 1965), which limits the detection capabilities and sensitivity of our senses and obscures stimulus-related activity, but is inaudible in itself. The problem for the brain in analyzing the messages carried by the firing pattern in the nerve fibers was seen as similar to the problem of detecting a signal in a noisy communication channel. Another viewpoint held spontaneous activity to be the main process in the central nervous system upon which the sensory input acted as a modulator (Rodieck, Kiang, and Gerstein 1962). The main function of the stimulus was regarded as modulation of the interval statistics of the spontaneous activity by reorganizing

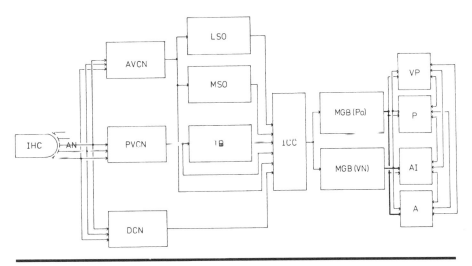

FIGURE 4-1. Parallel organization of the auditory nervous system. Parallel transmission of activity occurs from the most peripheral part of the nervous system to the interconnection of the various auditory cortical areas. The innervation of a single inner haircell with about 20 auditory nerve fibers, with different spontaneous rates and different thresholds, represents a way to convey different aspects of the sound in parallel fashion to the cochlear nucleus complex. Each single auditory nerve fiber sends collaterals to three subdivisions of the cochlear nucleus: the anteroventral cochlear nucleus (AVCN), the posteroventral cochlear nucleus (PVCN), and the dorsal cochlear nucleus (DCN). Each of these divisions contains various cell types that analyze different aspects of sound, for example, through spatial and temporal integration in bushy and stellate cells respectively, and through different membrane properties and innervation patterns of these cells (Oertel, Wu, and Hirsch 1988). Cells from the AVCN of both ears project the same information to two brainstem structures specialized in extracting directional information about sound, the superior olivary complex consisting of the lateral (LSO) and medial (MSO) nuclei. They supposedly analyze interaural-intensity, specifically interaural-time differences (Yin and Chan 1988). Output from all three sections of the cochlear nucleus also bypasses these binaural structures either partially (AVCN) or completely (DCN) to input directly to the inferior colliculus, where it is joined by the output of the MSO and LSO. This binaural information entering the inferior colliculus is used to construct neural maps of auditory space in the deep layers of the superior colliculus. The central nucleus of the inferior colliculus (ICC) is presumedly specialized in the first analysis and topographic representation of temporal properties of sound (Schreiner and Langner 1988). Input from the ICC is into both the ventral nucleus (VN) and the lateral part of the posterior group of nuclei (Po) of the thalamus. Each of these thalamic areas projects upon the tonotopically organized cortical fields A, AI, P, and VP; the dominant projection from VN is upon AI and that from Po is upon field A (Imig and Morel 1988). There are strong topographic interconnections among all four tonotopically organized cortical areas, illustrating the massive parallelism at nearly all levels of the auditory system.

the timing of the spike firings without necessarily increasing the overall firing rate. Such reorganization accompanies the sensation of sound. Evidence for such a modulatory action of the stimulus can be found in the auditory system: Nerve fibers with high spontaneous activity and characteristic frequency below 5 kHz display a much lower threshold (approximately 20 dB) to stimuli when a measure of synchronization to the stimulus is considered than when a certain (percentage) increase in firing rate is a criterion (Javel, McGee, Horst, and Farley 1988).

In general, spontaneous activity is most pronounced (in terms of mean rate) in the periphery of the auditory system and is commonly attributed to the spontaneous transmitter release from the haircells (Koerber, Pfeiffer, Warr, and Kiang 1966; Sewell 1990). An argument that favors this mechanism is that destruction of cochlear function destroys spontaneous activity in auditory nerve fibers. Only the integrity of the inner haircells appears to be required for normal spontaneous activity in auditory nerve fibers (Dallos and Harris 1978).

In the auditory nerve a clear distinction can be made among three groups of fibers on basis of their spontaneous firing rates. These firing rates correlate well with the size of the dendritic terminals of the nerve fibers as well as with their threshold for auditory stimulation. The larger the size of the dendritic terminal, the higher the spontaneous rate; higher spontaneous rate fibers have lower thresholds than low spontaneous rate fibers. Small, medium, and large terminals are found on all haircells; generally one haircell is contacted by about twenty auditory nerve fibers with various synaptic areas (Liberman and Oliver 1984). These findings support the idea that the amount of transmitter spontaneously arriving at the auditory nerve fiber and roughly proportional to the terminal size is a major determinant of the spontaneous rate. Spontaneous rates of up to 150 spikes per second are not unusual in the cat's auditory nerve (Kiang, Watanabe, Thomas, and Clark 1965) but are absent in the auditory cortex, where about 50 percent of the cells discharge with less than one

spike per second and the remainder at rates of 1 to 35 spikes per second (Goldstein, Hall, and Butterfield 1967; Eggermont in press).

It is assumed that, in the absence of mechanical stimulation, the hair cell is partially depolarized as a result of a leaking K^+-current flowing through the transduction channels at the top of the hair cells (Hudspeth 1989). This steady depolarization opens Ca^{2+} channels at the base of the haircell. The entry of Ca^{2+} ions results in spontaneous transmitter release. Blocking the Ca^{2+} channels reduces the spontaneous firing rate proportional to the concentration of the extra cellular blocking agent (e.g., Co^{2+} or Mn^{2+} ions[13]). In contrast, a reduction of the extracellular Ca^{2+} concentration to very low levels has been shown to result in an increase of the spontaneous activity with bursting behavior in *Xenopus* lateral line afferents (Russell 1971). Reducing the intracellular calcium concentration in cortical neurons, with, for example, chelating agents, results in bursting behavior as well (Friedman and Gutnick 1989).

In the auditory nerve of the guinea pig, nearly all fibers show spontaneous activity that can be described by exponential interval distributions with dead times ranging from 0.8 to 1.6 ms (Manley and Robertson 1976) and with the intervals independent of each other (Kiang et al. 1965). Thus, all necessary conditions are fulfilled to view spontaneous activity of auditory nerve fibers as a realization of a Poisson process with dead time.

In the auditory cortex, the spontaneous firing patterns are not that simple; unimodal, bimodal, and multimodal interval histograms can be found. The dominant modes are in the region of 1 to 10 ms and between 75 to 150 ms; the value of the latter depends on the specific cortical layer (Eggermont, unpublished observations). In cortical areas of other sensory modalities, firing properties for intervals exceeding 30 ms have been described by a Poisson shower (burst process) gated on and off by some other Poisson-like process. This results in bimodal, interval histogram distributions (Smith and Smith 1965; Pernier and Gerin 1975). Nearly all cells in the primary auditory cortex demonstrate an excess of short intervals (< 30 ms), compared to the exponential interval distributions. This bursting is a feature of many cortical neurons (Legendy and Salcman 1985), especially in layers IV and V (McCormick, Connors, Lighthall, and Prince 1985).

From this review we conclude that spontaneous activity is a prominent property of the auditory nervous system. The answer to the crucial question, Why don't we perceive this spontaneous activity as a sound? could be that we don't hear spontaneous activity because sound perception relies on correlations in the activity patterns of neighboring neurons. This inter-neuron or inter-neuronal group synchrony is absent under normal conditions. One effect of low level sound stimulation is to induce this correlation through synchronization of the firings to the stimulus.

THE EFFECT OF LOW-LEVEL
SOUND STIMULATION

In auditory nerve cells with CF < 5 kHz, low-level stimulation with continuous tones or noise evokes a change in the interval statistic of the firings and, at higher intensities, also in the mean firing rate. The change in interval statistic is caused by the tendency of the firings to become phase-locked to the period of the tone or to the band-pass filtered (by the tuning curve characteristic) noise (Eggermont, Johannesma, and Aertsen 1983). Thus, exponential interval distributions tend to be replaced by more symmetric ones. For high CF units, without phase-locking, an increase in firing rate is the most obvious single cell characteristic for the presence of a low-level continuous sound. In addition to the changes discussed, transient sounds such as clicks, noise or tone bursts, and speech segments, cause adaptation of the firing rate that to some extent depends on intensity (Smith 1988). The firing rate of auditory nerve fibers tends to follow the amplitude modulation of (complex) sounds in auditory nerve fibers up to modulation rates of about 1 to 3 kHz (Møller 1976; Javel 1981). This pattern also causes deviations of the Poisson character of the nerve fi-

ber discharges. On this basis, one could argue that both the mean firing rate (a zero-order statistic) and the interval histogram (a first-order statistic) carry information about the presence or absence of sound in single auditory nerve units. Higher-order statistics (e.g., serial dependence between intervals) that determine deviations from the renewal properties of auditory nerve fibers, may be important as well.

The emergence of correlated activity in neighboring auditory nerve fibers as a result of increased stimulus levels may lead to the activation of certain cochlear nucleus cells, such as the bushy cells, whose activation depends on such coincident input from different auditory nerve fibers (Oertel et al. 1988). Other cells in the cochlear nucleus, such as the stellate cells, which may receive the same input as the bushy cells, can be asynchronously activated and show temporal integration over larger intervals. A coincidence detection mechanism, therefore, can detect not only the presence of an external signal but also can enhance stimulus detection in noisy backgrounds. We have demonstrated such detection for neurons in the auditory midbrain (Epping and Eggermont 1987). The strength of the correlation may reflect the relative strength of the stimulus. Again, the cooperative effort of several nerve cells will enhance the speed and accuracy of this process and will extend the dynamic range of an output neuron if a certain range of threshold values is present for the input neurons.

A correlation mechanism combined with a spike count mechanism that transmits only sufficiently coincident spikes to higher order nuclei may reduce the spontaneous firing rate in higher auditory nuclei and extend the dynamic range of the neurons as well as the range of their threshold values. Thus the role of spike synchrony may diminish relative to the role of spike rate when advancing into the central nervous system. A sound sensation in this view is related to a "sufficiently strong" activation of the higher centers of the auditory nervous system. This "combination theory" still requires a mechanism that determines what is "sufficiently strong" activation.

Increasing the sound intensity to above threshold levels causes an increase in the firing rate in some cortical neurons and a decrease in others. Strong suppression effects are found and most cortical neurons respond only in an onset fashion to continuous stimulation. When transient stimuli of moderate length (e.g., with a duration of about 100 ms) are used, the average firing rate over the stimulus duration is rarely elevated above the spontaneous rate. This rate constancy is due to a pronounced reorganization of the firing times into an onset response followed by a relatively long post-activation suppression that is the cause of this. Phase-locking to the carrier frequency of a complex sound has not been demonstrated in cortical neurons. However, cortical pyramidal neurons can follow amplitude modulations up to modest frequencies (Schreiner and Urbas 1986; Phillips 1989; Eggermont 1991), usually below 32 Hz, which covers the range of amplitude modulations in speech (Javel et al. 1988).

Correlations between neuron pairs in primary auditory cortex can be found in at least 60 percent of the pairs recorded either on single electrodes or on dual electrodes separated by up to a few mm (Dickson and Gerstein 1974). Thus, the phenomenon of correlated neural activity in the primary auditory cortex will not be sufficient in itself to decide whether a stimulus is present or not. Changes in correlation strength may be involved. This returns to the problem of how much change is required to decide on the presence or absence of a stimulus.

To avoid comparison of correlated activity within the primary auditory cortex with a threshold, we propose a mechanism that evaluates the synchrony in activity of neuronal groups in different auditory cortical areas (A, AI, V, VP) in one hemisphere that receive parallel projections from the medial geniculate body (see Figure 4-1). We assume that spontaneous cortical activity is not synchronized among different cortical areas and that stimulus-driven activity is. A potential additional function of stimulus-induced synchrony

may be to "bind" the particular stimulus features analyzed in parallel by the various cortical areas (for related ideas in the visual system, see Gray and Singer 1988, Legendy and Salcman 1985). If pathologically induced correlations in the activity of auditory nerve fibers cannot be distinguished from stimulus-driven activity, then the subsequent intracortical synchronization will result in a sound sensation. Because tinnitus sensations are generally perceived independently from phantom sensations in other sensory modalities, it is hard to assume that the sole cause is in the cortex. A peripheral origin is therefore more logical, particularly in relation to the reported suppression of tinnitus by electrical currents of the correct polarity (Aran and Erre 1987).

FINDINGS IN ANIMAL MODELS OF TINNITUS

Acoustic Trauma

Tinnitus is commonly associated with inner ear pathology (Spoendlin 1987). A few studies have obtained spontaneous activity measures for single units in animals with induced cochlear hearing loss. Cats subjected to acoustic trauma showed changes in spontaneous activity, especially in regions where thresholds of the fibers were increased to above 60 dB SPL. In those regions, fibers with spontaneous rates of 10 to 30 spikes/second were more abundant than in the normal cochlea; however, fibers with a spontaneous rate larger than 30 spikes/second were observed less frequently (Liberman and Kiang 1978).This finding suggested that the high spontaneous rate population was differentially affected by the noise trauma and the firing rate of these fibers was reduced. Apart from a decrease in the mean spontaneous rate, changes in the temporal aspects of the spontaneous firings of a neuron have been found, especially for neurons innervating inner hair cells that are at the border of the noise-damaged region. The pitch of tinnitus in noise-induced hearing loss frequently correlates with the characteristic frequency of this region. The interval histograms for these nerve fibers can no longer be described as exponential, and the generation of a spike is no longer independent from the generation of the previous one. Cats with acoustic trauma may even have auditory nerve fibers that do not respond to sound yet remain spontaneously active. In these fibers, spontaneous activity of the Poisson type as well as of highly abnormal type was found. For example, double spikes or bursts of spikes that repeated every 50 ms or so were common after noise trauma (Liberman and Kiang 1978).

Endolymphatic Hydrops

In animal models of endolymphatic hydrops (as presumably occurs in Ménière's disease), Harrison and Prijs (1984) found that the spontaneous rate of auditory nerve fibers with threshold elevations did not differ from the normal firing rate. Fibers without spontaneous activity were occasionally found. Abnormal bursting activity was found in both spontaneous and stimulated conditions. Bursts were composed of intermittent groups of spikes with very short intervals, often less than 1 ms. In endolymphatic hydrops, the calcium concentration in the endolymph appeared to be increased (Sterkers, Bernard, Ferrary, Sziklai, Tran Ba Huy, and Amiel 1988); this could give rise to an increased calcium flux into the hair cell. In the saccular hair cell of the bullfrog, Hudspeth and Corey (1977) found a modest increase of the extracellular Ca^{2+} concentration to activate slow-acting voltage dependent channels, which occasionally led to fairly large (up to 40 mV), slow (5-10 ms rise time) spikes. These spikes were not altered by sodium blockers and were thought to be the result of the action of voltage dependent Ca-channels. If, for some reason, there are many more of these "Calcium spikes" in inner hair cells of pathological cochleas, they could be at the basis of a tinnitus-generating mechanism. Model studies have provided some support for this idea (Eggermont 1990a).

Salicylates

Short bursts of spikes in the spontaneous activity of auditory nerve fibers in cats treated with large doses of salicylates have been reported by Evans and colleagues (Evans, Wilson, and Borerwe 1981). The inter-spike-interval histograms for those fibers were usually bimodal and pairs of spikes were quite common. Drug treatment also resulted in a slight increase in the mean firing rate, especially for the subpopulation of units that showed high spontaneous rates before the salicylate application. For a mean preapplication rate of 59 spikes per second, an increase in rate of 10 to 20 spikes per second was observed after application of salicylate. Temporal abnormalities in the spike patterns as determined from the inter-spike-interval histograms were reportedly found in 63 percent of the nerve fibers.

Recently Stypulkowski (1990) reported the absence of significant changes in spontaneous firing rate of auditory nerve fibers in both the high spontaneous rate group (mean rate 53.2 spikes/s) and in the low spontaneous rate group (mean rate 6.2 spikes/s) after salicylate application in the cat. Several methodological differences exist between the Stypulkowski's (1990) and Evans and colleagues' (1981) studies which may help to explain their different results. Compared to Evans and colleagues, the range of the fiber's CFs in Stypulkowski's study was slightly lower. He also used a lower dose of salicylate.

Schreiner and Snyder (1987), recording from the auditory nerve in cats, noted that, after salicylate application, the spectrum of the spontaneous ensemble activity greatly increased in the range around 200 Hz. This increase suggests synchronous effects in the ensemble firing rate with an average period of 5 ms.

Comparison of spontaneous activity in the inferior colliculus of guinea pigs before and after salicylate administration showed a substantial increase in the modal firing rate, as determined from the mode of the interval histograms, from 29 to 83 spikes per second. Temporal changes in the spike trains for these midbrain neurons were noted but not specified (Jastreboff and Sasaki 1986).

Eggermont (in press) reported preliminary results in 91 control condition cortical neurons (in five cats, two of which received salicylate) and in 142 neurons recorded post salicylate (same dose as in the Evans et al. 1981). The main findings were: (1) The distributions of spontaneous firing rates from cells recorded across all cortical layers before application and from those postapplication, which were exclusively obtained from layer IV, were not significantly different. (2) For cells recorded pre- and postapplication in layer IV of the primary auditory cortex, the regression line of spontaneous firing rate on time relative to application had a significant positive slope which was caused mainly by the increase in firing rate post application (Fig-

ure 4-2). (3) The interval histograms typically showed a relative increase of counts for intervals in the range from 5 to 100 ms (Figure 4-3) and changed little for both shorter and longer intervals. (4) Only in 1 of 5 single units, recorded before and within a few hours after the application was the maximum postapplication spontaneous rate significantly enhanced above the presalicylate rate.

On basis of previously published data in cat auditory nerve (Evans et al. 1981) and guinea pig inferior colliculus (Jastreboff and Sasaki 1986) a substantial increase in firing rate for cortical neurons was expected. This did not materialize; firing rates in layer IV increased somewhat after salicylate application but not dramatically. It is not easy to conceive a model with a modest (Evans et al. 1981) or minimal change in spontaneous rate (Stypulkowski 1990) in (cat) auditory nerve fibers

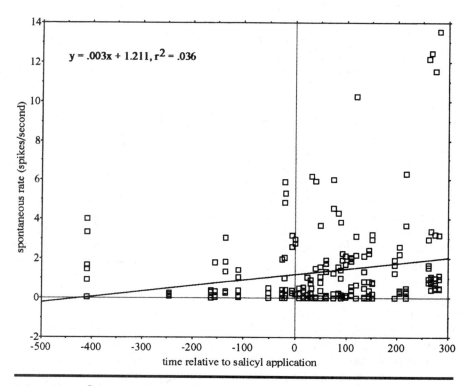

FIGURE 4-2. Spontaneous firing rate for neurons recorded in layer IV of two cats as a function of time before and after salicylate application.

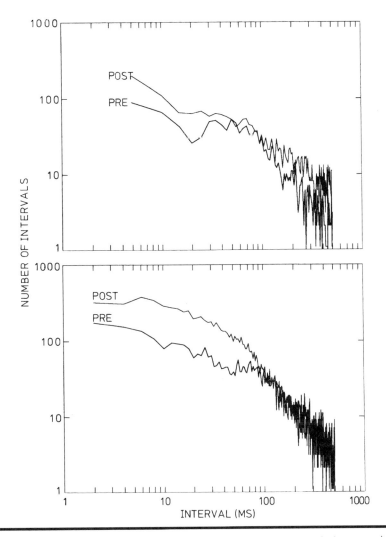

FIGURE 4-3. Interspike interval histograms for two neurons recorded pre- and postsalicylate application. Both ordinate and abscissa are on logarithmic scales. In both cases, the number of intervals with value below 100 ms increases.

and a dramatic increase in (guinea pig) inferior colliculus neuron modal spontaneous rate (Jastreboff and Sasaki 1986) resulting in, at most, a modest increase in firing rate for (cat) cortical neurons. A species difference in sensitivity to salicylate between cat and guinea pig would provide a possible explanation. It is noteworthy, however, that the effects of salicylate on spontaneous firing

rate for the auditory nerve and for the auditory cortex of the cat were compatible.

FINDINGS IN HUMANS SUPPORTIVE OF A CORRELATION MECHANISM

Recently we (Sininger, Eggermont, and King in press) reported recordings of spontaneous electrical activity from the eardrum in normal and tinnitus subjects. In a subgroup of the tinnitus subjects, we found a significant enhancement in the variance and extreme values of the second order autocorrelation function of the recorded activity, which was normalized at unit variance. This finding could be interpreted as an indication for spontaneous synchronous activity in the auditory nerve in some tinnitus subjects but not in normal ears.

A PHYSIOLOGICAL SUBSTRATE FOR TINNITUS

If one is looking for a unified correlate for tinnitus at the single neuron level, obviously a change in firing rate is not a likely candidate. Temporal changes in the firing pattern seem to be more uniformly present in animal models of tinnitus than changes in firing rate. The theory that changes in temporal patterns of neural activity may be a factor associated with tinnitus has been suggested previously (Eggermont 1984, 1990a).

However, the sense of hearing is not based on changing temporal activity patterns in independently active neurons. It is even debatable whether one could actually hear with one auditory nerve fiber: What would be the reference for the central nervous system (CNS) to decide that the firings were due to an outside, sensory event and not due to an occasional bout of high spontaneous activity? An investigator can characterize an auditory nerve fiber by its spontaneous rate and compare any stimulated activity to it, such as in defining the criterion for a tuning curve as a 20 percent increase above spontaneous firing rate. In addition, the experimenter uses the knowledge of the type and timing of the applied stimulus to choose an analysis method appropriate to elicit stimulus-response relationships. For instance, the investigator could determine the rate-intensity function or the dependence of amount of phase-locking as a function of intensity (Javel et al. 1988); the value of the estimated threshold level for these two methods could differ by about 20 dB.

However, the CNS can evaluate the activity of an auditory nerve fiber's activity only by means of the relationship of that activity with the instantaneous firing rates and/or timing of the spikes of other nerve fibers. Detection of temporal correlations between the discharge patterns of different auditory nerve fibers could therefore be a mechanism leading to sound sensations including tinnitus (Eggermont 1990a,b; Møller 1984). This mechanism would enable detection of sounds near threshold without reliance on stored values of the normal spontaneous rate. Temporal correlations could result from a more or less simultaneous occurrence of firings in a small group of nerve fibers, for example, originating from the same hair cell or from neighboring hair cells. Such synchrony could be enhanced through abnormal temporal firing patterns in the individual neurons. If synchronized firings of such nerve fibers innervating a few neighboring hair cells occurred, one would experience a tonal tinnitus with the pitch determined by the place of the hair cells in the cochlea. If the temporal synchronization of the activity of nerve fibers extends over larger parts of the cochlea and the firings do not exhibit a periodic pattern, a noise-like tinnitus will result.

Synchronized firings of neighboring auditory nerve fibers could also occur through ephaptic interaction between these fibers as a result of damage to the myelin sheath, caused, for instance, by acoustic neuroma or vascular compression (Eggermont 1990a; Evans et al. 1981; Møller 1984). In this condition, the electric field of an action potential in one nerve fiber may be large enough to induce sufficient depolarization in a neighboring nerve fiber to facilitate the generation of an action potential in that fiber.

Inter-neuron synchronization could also occur as a result of changes in the synaptic region of the hair cell or through changes in extracellular ion concentrations as in Ménière's disease, for example. Changes in extracellular ion concentrations could cause the membrane potentials of the neurons to be consistently close to the threshold of firing, thereby causing the generation of bursts of spikes that, in turn, increase the probability of synchronous firing.

One of us recently investigated the occurrence of neural pair correlation under stimulus and no-stimulus condition for cells across all layers in the primary auditory cortex of the cat (Eggermont, unpublished results). Two independently moving electrodes, spaced about 0.5 to 2 mm, were used. Correlations between cells recorded on the same electrode (for technical details, see Eggermont 1991) were obtained somewhat more frequently than between cells on different electrodes at the same depth below the dura surface. About 90 percent of 173 neuron pairs studied under stimulus conditions, with corrections for stimulus-related synchrony by use of the shift predictor (Perkel, Gerstein, and Moore 1967), showed neural correlation dominantly of the common excitation type. In 157 different pairs under spontaneous firing conditions, correlated neural activity was found in 76 percent of the pairs. By comparison, Dickson and Gerstein (1974) and Frostig and colleagues (Frostig, Gottlieb, Vaadia, and Abeles 1983) found that neural correlation in auditory cortex, both of the shared-input and unidirectional-excitation type, occurred in 60 percent and 86 percent of the pairs investigated (for a review of the presence of neural correlation in other cortical areas with similar findings, see Eggermont 1990b).

In two cats (Eggermont, unpublished results), the effect of salicylate on the frequency of occurrence of neural correlation in layer IV of the primary auditory cortex was studied. In the presalicylate stage, we obtained evidence for neural correlation under spontaneous firing conditions in 26 of 41 neuron pairs (60 percent), a number somewhat lower than the average across all layers in our control cats. Postsalicylate recordings were made from 121 pairs, only 56 (46 percent) of which showed evidence for neural correlation. This difference is not significant at the 95 percent confidence level ($\chi^2 = 2.80$, df=1). Thus, salicylate does not seem to affect the frequency of shared input between cortical cells. Enhanced or decreased incidence of correlations among neuronal pairs in the same or neighboring cortical columns of the primary auditory cortex are therefore not likely to be a cause of tinnitus.

Most primary auditory cortical neurons show correlations in their firings due to shared input with an abundance of other cortical neurons. The percentage of neurons showing correlations is not affected by salicylate application. Thus, the effect of peripheral synchronization of neighboring nerve fibers can be detected only as a result of increased strength of the neural correlation (which again requires a "norm"), or by correlations in the firings of neuronal groups in distinct auditory cortical areas. Accordingly, sound sensations may arise when two or more cortical areas (A, AI, V, VP) are synchronously active, most likely as a result of synchronous activation of a group of auditory nerve fibers (Figure 4-1).

We hypothesized (Eggermont 1990a) that a calcium homeostasis deficit resulting in an increase in the Ca^{2+} conductance through the hair cell membrane or an increase in extracellular Ca^{2+} could cause a transient increase in the internal Ca^{2+} concentration of the hair cells. The resulting calcium spikes cause a synchronous release of transmitter substance in all synapses of a single hair cell. These events may be one cause of an increase in spontaneous activity and in the synchronization of auditory nerve fiber activity in the absence of a sound and could be a peripheral cause for tinnitus.

As mentioned, a reduction of the extracellular Ca^{2+} concentration to very low levels has also been shown to result in an increase of the spontaneous activity with bursting behavior in *Xenopus* lateral line afferents (Russell 1971). As a cause for central tinnitus, a similar mechanism is likely at work: A reduction in intracellular Ca^{2+} (Friedman and Gutnick 1989) can result in an increase in bursting activity in cortical cells, which may result in significant neural correlation because bursting activity between groups of neurons can easily synchronize (Legendy and Salcman 1985). Thus, both an increase in the calcium-ion concentration surrounding the hair cells, as in experimental endolymphatic hydrops (Meyer zum Gottesberge 1988), for example, and a decrease in extracellular calcium could give rise to abnormal spiking behavior in peripheral and central neural elements.

An explanation of our findings in cortical neurons after salicylate application could be based on the postulate that Ca^{2+}-activated K^+-currents are blocked or diminished by the action of the salicylate. The moderating influence of this current on the firing rate of a cell is thereby abolished, which could lead to an increase in both overall spontaneous firing rate and the number of interspike-intervals between 5 and 100 ms. Since the afterhyperpolarization due to the Ca^{2+}-activated K^+-current is specific for the principal cells in the thalamus and for the pyramidal cells in the cortex, this suggests a central component to salicylate-induced tinnitus. To cause these changes in the Ca^{2+}-activated K^+-currents, one needs a decrease in the intracellular Ca^{2+} concentration. This could be caused by a reduced transmembrane conductance for Ca^{2+} or for K^+ through the action of salicylate.

Manny Don critically read the manuscript and provided valuable feedback.

REFERENCES

Aran, J.-M. and Erre, J.-P. 1987. "Effects of Electrical Currents Applied to the Cochlea." In H. Feldmann (Ed.), *Proceedings of the III International Tinnitus Seminar, Munster, 1987*, pp. 400–409. Karlsruhe: Harsch Verlag.

Dallos, P. and Harris, D. 1978. "Properties of Auditory Nerve Responses in Absence of Outer Hair Cells." *Journal of Neurophysiology, 41*, 365–383.

Dickson, J.W. and Gerstein, G.L. 1974. "Interaction between Neurons in Auditory Cortex of the Cat." *Journal of Neurophysiology, 37*, 1239–1261.

Eggermont, J.J. 1984. "Tinnitus: Some Thoughts about Its Origin." *Journal of Laryngology and Otology, Supplement 9*, 31–37.

Eggermont, J.J. 1990a. "On the Pathophysiology of Tinnitus; a Review and a Peripheral Model." *Hearing Research, 48*, 111–124.

Eggermont, J.J. 1990b. *The Correlative Brain: Theory and Experiment in Neural Interaction.* Berlin: Springer Verlag.

Eggermont, J.J. 1991. "Rate and Synchrony Measures of Periodicity Coding in Cat Primary Auditory Cortex." *Hearing Research, 56*, 153–167.

Eggermont, J.J. In press. "Salicylate-Induced Changes in the Spontaneous Activity in Cat Auditory Cortex."

Eggermont, J.J. and Epping, W.J.M. 1987. "Coincidence Detection in Auditory Neurons: A Possible Mechanism to Enhance Stimulus Specificity in the Grassfrog." *Hearing Research, 30*, 219–230.

Eggermont, J.J., Johannesma, P.I.M., and Aertsen, A.M.H.J. 1983. "Reverse Correlation Methods in Auditory Research." *Quarterly Review of Biophysics, 16*, 341–414.

Engel, A.K., König, P., Kreiter, A.K., and Singer, W. 1991. "Interhemispheric Synchronization of Oscillatory Neuronal Responses in Cat Visual Vortex." *Science, 252*, 1177–1179.

Epping, W.J.M. and Eggermont, J.J. 1987. "Coherent Neural Activity in the Auditory Midbrain of the Grassfrog." *Journal of Neurophysiology, 57*, 1461–1483.

Evans, E.F., Wilson, J.P., and Borerwe, T.A. 1981. "Animal Models of Tinnitus." In *Tinnitus (Ciba Foundation Symposium 85)*, p.108–138. London: Pitman Books, Ltd.

Friedman, A. and Gutnick, M.J. 1989. "Intracellular Calcium and Control of Burst Generation in Neurons of Guinea-Pig Neocortex in Vitro." *European Journal of Neuroscience, 1*, 374–381.

Frostig, R.D., Gottlieb, Y., Vaadia, E., and Abeles, M. 1983. "The Effect of Stimuli on the Activity and Functional Connectivity of Local Neuronal Groups in the Cat Auditory Cortex." *Brain Research, 272*, 211–221.

Goldstein, M.H., Hall, J.L., and Butterfield, B.O. 1967. "Single Unit Activity in the Primary Cortex of Unanesthetized Cats." *Journal of the Acoustical Society of America, 43*, 444–455.

Gray, C.M., König, P., Engel, A.K., and Singer, W. 1989. "Oscillatory Responses in Cat Visual Cortex Exhibit Intercolumnar Synchronization which Reflects Global Stimulus Properties." *Nature, 338*, 334–337.

Gray, C.M. and Singer, W. 1988. "Stimulus-Specific Neuronal Oscillations in Orientation Columns of Cat Visual Cortex." *Proceedings of the National Academy of Science USA 86*, 1698–1702.

Harrison, R.V. and Prijs, V.F. 1984. "Single Cochlear Fibre Responses in Guinea Pigs with Long-Term Endolymphatic Hydrops." *Hearing Research, 14,* 79–84.

Hudspeth, A.J. 1989. "How the Ear's Works Works." *Nature, 341,* 397–404.

Hudspeth, A.J. and Corey, D.P. 1977. "Sensitivity, Polarity, and Conductance Change in the Response of Vertebrate Hair Cells to Controlled Mechanical Stimuli." *Proceedings of the National Academy of Sciences USA, 74,* 2407–2411.

Imig, T.J. and Morel, A. 1988. "Organization of the Cat's Auditory Thalamus." In G.M. Edelman, W.E. Gall, and W.M. Cowan (Eds.), *Auditory Function. Neurobiological Basis of Hearing,* pp. 457–484. New York: J. Wiley.

Jastreboff, P.J. and Sasaki, C.T. 1986. "Salicylate-Induced Changes in Spontaneous Activity of Single Units in the Inferior Colliculus of the Guinea Pig." *Journal of the Acoustical Society of America, 80,* 1384–1391.

Javel, E. 1981. "Suppression of Auditory Nerve Responses. I. Temporal Analysis, Intensity Effects, and Suppression Contours." *Journal of the Acoustical Society of America, 69,* 1735–1745.

Javel, E., McGee, J.A., and Horst, J.W., and Farley, G.R. 1988. "Temporal Mechanisms in Auditory Stimulus Coding." In G.M. Edelman, W.E. Gall, and W.M. Cowan (Eds.), *Auditory Function. Neurobiological Basis of Hearing,* pp. 515–558. New York: J. Wiley.

Johnson, D.H. and Kiang, N.Y.-S. 1976. "Analysis of Discharges Recorded Simultaneously from Pairs of Auditory Nerve Fibers." *Biophysical Journal, 16,* 719–734.

Kiang, N.Y.-S., Watanabe, T., Thomas, E.C., and Clark, L.F. 1965. *Discharge Patterns of Single Fibers in the Cat's Auditory Nerve.* Cambridge, MA: MIT Press.

Koerber, K.C., Pfeiffer, R.R., Warr, W.B., and Kiang, N.Y.-S. 1966. "Spontaneous Spike Discharges from Single Units in the Cochlear Nucleus after Destruction of the Cochlea." *Experimental Neurology, 16,* 119–130.

Legendy, C.R. and Salcman, M. 1985. "Bursts and Re-

currences of Bursts in the Spike Trains of Spontaneously Active Striate Cortex Neurons." *Journal of Neurophysiology, 53,* 926–939.

Liberman, M.C. and Kiang, N.Y.-S. 1978. "Acoustic Trauma in Cats. Cochlear Pathology and Auditory Nerve Activity." *Acta Otolaryngologica, Supplement 358,* 1–63.

Liberman, M.C. and Oliver, M.E. 1984. "Morphometry of Intracellularly Labeled Neurons of the Auditory Nerve: Correlations with Functional Properties." *Journal of Comparative Neurology, 223,* 163–176.

Manley, G.A. and Robertson, D. 1976. "Analysis of Spontaneous Activity of Auditory Neurons in the Spiral Ganglion of the Guinea Pig Cochlea." *Journal of Physiology, 258,* 323–336.

McCormick, D.A., Connors, B.W., Lighthall, J.W., and Prince, D.A. 1985. "Comparative Electrophysiology of Pyramidal and Sparsely Spiny Stellate Neurons of the Neocortex." *Journal of Neurophysiology, 54,* 782–806.

Meyer zum Gottesberge, A.-M. 1988. "Imbalanced Calcium Homeostasis and Endolymphatic Hydrops." *Acta Otolaryngologica (Stockholm), Supplement 460,* 18–27.

Møller, A.R. 1976. "Dynamic Properties of Primary Auditory Fibers Compared with Cells in the Cochlear Nucleus." *Acta Physiologica, 98,* 157–167.

Møller, A.R. 1984. "Pathophysiology of Tinnitus." *Annals of Otology, Rhinology, and Laryngology, 93,* 39–44.

Oertel, D., Wu, S.H., and Hirsch, J.A. 1988. "Electrical Characteristics of Cells and Neuronal Circuitry in the Cochlear Nucleus Studied with Intracellular Recordings from Brain Slices." In G.M. Edelman, W.E. Gall, and W.M. Cowan (Eds.), *Auditory Function. Neurobiological Basis of Hearing,* pp. 313–336. New York: J. Wiley.

Perkel, D.H., Gerstein, G.L., and Moore, G.P. 1967. "Neuronal Spike Trains and Stochastic Processes. II. Simultaneous Spike Trains." *Biophysical Journal, 7,* 419–440.

Pernier, J. and Gerin, P. 1975. "Temporal Pattern Analysis of Spontaneous Unit Activity in the Neocortex." *Biological Cybernetics, 18,* 123–136.

Phillips, D.P. 1989. "The Neural Coding of Simple and Complex Sounds in the Auditory Cortex." In J.S. Lund (Ed.), *Sensory Processing in the Mammalian Brain,* pp. 172–203. Oxford: Oxford University Press.

Rodieck, R.W., Kiang, N.Y.-S., and Gerstein, G.L. 1962. "Some Quantitative Methods for the Study of Spontaneous Activity of Single Cells." *Biophysical Journal, 2,* 351–368.

Russell, I.J. 1971. "The Pharmacology of Efferent Synapses in the Lateral Line System of Xenopus laevis." *Journal of Experimental Biology, 54,* 643–658.

Schreiner, C.E. and Langner, G. 1988. "Coding of Temporal Patterns in the Central Auditory Nervous System." In G.M. Edelman, W.E. Gall, and W.M. Cowan (Eds.), *Auditory Function. Neurobiological Basis of Hearing,* pp. 337–361. New York: J. Wiley.

Schreiner, C.E. and Snyder, R.L. 1987. "A Physiological Animal Model of Peripheral Tinnitus." In H. Feldmann (Ed.), *Proceedings III International Tinnitus Seminar, Munster, 1987* pp. 100–106. Karlsruhe: Harsch Verlag.

Schreiner, C.E. and Urbas, J.V. 1986. "Representation of Amplitude Modulation in the Auditory Cortex of the Cat. I. The Anterior Auditory Field (AAF)." *Hearing Research, 21,* 227–241.

Sewell, W.F. 1990. "Synaptic Potentials in Afferent Fibers Innervating Hair Cells of the Lateral Line Organ in Xenopus laevis." *Hearing Research, 44,* 71–82.

Siebert, W.M. 1965. "Some Implications of the Stochastic Behavior of Primary Auditory Neurons." *Kybernetik, 2,* 206–215.

Sininger, Y., Eggermont, J.J., and King, J. In press. "Spontaneous Activity from the Peripheral Auditory System in Tinnitus."

Smith, D.R. and Smith, G.K. 1965. "A Statistical Analysis of the Continual Activity of Single Cortical Neurons in the Cat Unanaesthetized Isolated Forebrain." *Biophysical Journal, 5,* 47–74.

Smith, R.L. 1988. "Encoding the Sound Intensity by Auditory Neurons." In G.M. Edelman, W.E. Gall, and W.M. Cowan (Eds.), *Auditory Function. Neurobiological Basis of Hearing,* pp. 243–274. New York: J. Wiley.

Spoendlin, H. 1987. "Inner Ear Pathology and Tinnitus." In H. Feldmann (Ed.), *Proceedings III International Tinnitus Seminar, Munster, 1987,* pp. 42–51. Karlsruhe: Harsch Verlag.

Sterkers, O., Bernard, C., Ferrary, E., Sziklai, I., Tran Ba Huy, P., and Amiel, C. 1988. "Possible Role of Ca Ions in the Vestibular System." *Acta Otolaryngologica, Supplement 460,* 28–32.

Stypulkowski, P.H. 1990. "Mechanisms of Salicylate Ototoxicity." *Hearing Research, 46,* 113–146.

Viemeister, N.F. 1983. "Auditory Intensity Discrimination at High Frequencies in the Presence of Noise." *Science, 221,* 1206–1208.

Yin, T.C.T. and Chan, J.C.K. 1988. "Neural Mechanisms Underlying Interaural Time Sensitivity to Tones and Noise." In G.M. Edelman, W.E. Gall, and W.M. Cowan (Eds.), *Auditory Function. Neurobiological Basis of Hearing,* pp. 385–430. New York: J. Wiley.

Young, E.D. and Sachs, M.B. 1989. "Auditory Nerve Fibers Do not Discharge Independently When Responding to Broadband Noise." ARO Abstracts #136.

CHAPTER 5

MECHANISMS OF TINNITUS

HARALD FELDMANN
University of Münster

INTRODUCTION

Tinnitus is a symptom that, like deafness, can be caused by many and very different mechanisms. Forms of objective tinnitus due to vascular or muscular disorders will not be discussed here. The mechanisms producing these abnormal sounds—for example, turbulence of blood flow, opening movements of the Eustachian tube—are obvious and do not seem to offer any problem. The etiology of some types of muscular activity underlying the production of abnormal sounds, however, is not yet well understood. This, for instance, is the case in the palatal clonus and spasmodic contractions of the stapedial muscle.

This chapter deals solely with the so-called subjective tinnitus. The hypotheses that will be presented here are based on a synopsis of relevant features from the following fields of research:

1. Anatomy and physiology of the normal ear and the entire hearing system including electro-physiology and biochemistry.
2. Experimental psychoacoustic phenomena of normally hearing ears.
3. Clinical findings in tinnitus patients.
4. Psychoacoustic findings in tinnitus ears.
5. Pathology of well-defined ear diseases frequently associated with tinnitus.
6. Experimental animal models of tinnitus.

Some of the basic facts and new findings of anatomy and physiology that in the author's view are of special importance for the generation of

tinnitus shall be explained briefly for readers who might not be familiar with these details.

BASIC FACTS

Anatomical Details of the Organ of Corti

The outer hair cells of the organ of Corti (about 15,000 altogether) are arranged in three rows. Each cell carries about 100 to 120 stereocilia, which differ in length. The longest stereocilia of the outer hair cells are firmly connected to the tectorial membrane. The outer hair cells are able to perform tonic contractions as well as very fast oscillating contractions (Zenner 1986, 1988; Lim, Hahamure, and Ohashi 1989).

The inner hair cells (about 5,000) are arranged in one row. Each cell has about 60 stereocilia, which normally do not contact the tectorial membrane. Inner hair cells do not have the capability of active motion.

The inner and outer hair cells are connected to the central auditory pathways by two systems. Afferent fibers starting from the bipolar cells in the spiral ganglion lead to the cochlear nuclei in the brainstem, ipsilaterally and contralaterally. Efferent fibers reach the cochlea via the olivo-cochlear bundle.

Although the outer hair cells outnumber the inner hair cells by a ratio of three to one, it is the inner hair cells that are almost exclusively connected to the afferent system: 90 to 95 percent of the afferent fibers arise from the inner hair cells. About 20 to 30 unbranched fibers are attached to each inner hair cell. The outer hair cells are connected to only 5 to 10 percent of the afferent fibers, each fiber serving a bunch of outer hair cells along the basilar membrane at a length of 0.6 to 1 mm.

This means that information transferred from the cochlea to the central pathways almost exclusively comes from the inner hair cells. The outer hair cells, on the other hand, have a very rich efferent innervation with enormous synaptic contact areas between nerve endings and hair cell (Spoendlin 1988).

Mechanical Processes in the Cochlea

The stapes driven via the tympanic membrane and the ossicular chain by sound pressure waves carries out piston-like or tilting movements. These movements cause a dynamic displacement of the cochlear partition in the shape of a traveling wave. The amplitude of the traveling wave has a clearly defined maximum, the location of which depends on the frequency: High frequencies have their maximum near the stapes; low frequencies travel further along the cochlear partition to the apex.

The outer hair cells play an active part in this mechanical processing of sound by their active motor capacity. Slow contractions of the outer hair cells can alter the stiffness of the cochlear partition in sharply restricted areas, thus modifying the envelope of the traveling wave. The fast contractions, which respond to frequencies well above 5000 Hz (Zenner 1987) and are phase-locked to the stimulating sound, can augment the oscillations and boost the mechanical stimulation of the inner hair cells in a sharply tuned way. The active oscillations of the outer hair cells generate the otoacoustic emissions. They obviously can be monitored by efferent impulses, since the efferent fibers almost exclusively contact the outer hair cells.

The discovery that the cochlea spontaneously emits acoustic energy, usually in the form of nearly sinusoidal signals, gave rise to the expectation that the underlying active process in the cochlea might be the source of tinnitus. Investigations to prove this widely failed (Wilson 1987). Otoacoustic emis-sions are found only in ears with nearly normal hearing. If spontaneous otoacoustic emissions are present in ears with inner ear disorders, the frequencies emitted usually correspond to areas in which the hearing threshold is normal (Penner 1988, 1989; Zwicker 1987).

Subjects with loud spontaneous otoacoustic emissions do not hear these, and they do not have the sensation of tinnitus in the relevant frequency region. Patients suffering from tinnitus do not have otoacoustic emissions corresponding in frequency or pitch to their tinnitus. Observations indicating that such a correspondence might be present are rare exceptions and seem to be due to chance.

According to this concept, the outer hair cells act as mechano-amplifiers within the cochlea. They feed amplified mechanical oscillations to the inner hair cells, but they are not directly involved in the transformation of mechanical parameters into neural activity. This is the domain of the inner hair cells.

If these concepts are correct, it can be concluded that subjective tinnitus does not arise directly at the level of the outer hair cells, but the lowest level where cochlear tinnitus might originate would be the inner hair cells.

Electrical and Biochemical Aspects

The mechanical movement impinged on the organ of Corti by the traveling wave is transduced into alterations of electrical potentials and ultimately into neural activity. The intracellular compartments of the hair cells are electronegative relative to the adjacent fluids of endolymph, Corti-lymph, and perilymph. This is due to the specific concentrations of ions, especially potassium, in the different compartments.

In the cell membrane there are channels, each specialized to gate, that is, to monitor, the passage of one particular type of ion: K^+-channel, Cl-channel, Ca^{++}-channel. In the hair cells such channels are primarily localized at the apical end associated with the stereocilia and the cuticular plate, but similar channels have also been identified at the lateral walls of the cells facing the perilymphatic and Corti-lymphatic space.

Shearing movements of the stereocilia, as effected through displacement of the cochlear partition by the traveling wave, open K^+-conducting channels and allow potassium ions to pass into the cell according to the electrochemical gradient. The influx of positive charges rapidly depolarizes the intracellular potential. A simultaneous influx of calcium ions, monitored by the depolarization, regulates the calcium level. These factors, depolarization and the presence of calcium ions, release a neurotransmitter, which in turn activates synapses of nerve fibers in contact with the cell membrane. Thus a neural impulse is triggered, and a signal in which certain parameters of the physical stimulus are coded is transported towards higher levels of the auditory system for further processing. This is the predominant method of response in the inner hair cells—transforming mechanical vibrations into neural impulses.

In the outer hair cells, the depolarization is probably accompanied by the additional induction of mechanical movement in the cytoskeleton of actin. Thus the transduction process in the outer hair cell is effective in two opposite directions: Mechanical movement induces depolarization of the electrical potential, depolarization induces mechanical movement (Zenner 1987).

Such a system is adapted to perform positive feedback, and it is in principle liable to get out of control. The underlying processes, however, are highly nonlinear, reaching a state of saturation very soon. This probably is the reason for the system's not running out of control.

The efflux of potassium ions from the cytoplasm into the perilymph and Corti-lymph through channels in the lateral cell membrane is dramatically increased during the depolarization and helps to repolarize the hair cell. After completing such a cycle the cell is ready for another discharge.

It is easily conceivable that this complicated system of ion concentrations and electrical potentials, which has been outlined here only roughly, can be disturbed in such a manner that neural discharges are triggered without an acoustic stimulus, giving rise to the sensation of tinnitus, by an abnormal distribution of certain ions, defects of ion channels, defects of membranes with consequent leakage of certain ions, defects of enzymes monitoring metabolic processes, and so on. Some of these hypothetical causes of tinnitus will be discussed in more detail later.

Pattern of Neural Discharge; Place Theory Versus Periodicity Theory of Pitch Perception

The concept of the traveling wave means that the energy of sound fed into the cochlea is distributed according to frequency: Energy of low frequencies is transported to the apex of the cochlea, and energy of high frequencies is concentrated in the basal end near the stapes. Only the hair cells at the maximum of the traveling wave are stimulated in the way described above. Thus the information about the frequency of the signal is coded through the place along the basilar membrane where the maximum of displacement is located, which means it is coded through the ordinal number of the hair cells stimulated. This principle also emerges from pathological findings: The cochleae of subjects who during lifetime had high-frequency hearing losses have corresponding losses of hair cells in the basal turn.

Theories about cochlear origin of tinnitus have to take into account this basic principle, and the first approach obviously should be that tinnitus of a certain pitch is likely to originate in those elements that normally are engaged in the perception of sounds corresponding to this pitch.

This principle, called the *place theory of pitch perception*, however, is not the only way by which the auditory system identifies, discriminates, and codes frequencies. The hair cells are only stimulated in the way described above, and the impulses along the afferent nerve fibers are triggered only during that phase when the cochlear partition moves upwards. A single hair cell, due to its refractory pause, cannot respond to every movement; if it does respond, the impulse sent off is phase-locked to the signal and the upward movement of the cochlear partition. The ensemble of nerve impulses within a set of hair cells and in the corresponding afferent nerve fibers, therefore, precisely represents the frequency of the stimulating signal and shows a clear relation to the *phase* of the signal. Phenomena attributable to periodicity analysis are restricted to the lower and medium frequency range up to 3 to 5 kHz and the level of the first neuron.

Thus hair cells in the high-frequency region may take part in recording the *periodicity* of low frequencies, and a mixture of high or middle frequencies, such as a musical chord, may have a common fundamental periodicity, which is perceived as a low pitched tone, although physically this tone is not present. This is the well-known phenomenon of the missing fundamental (Schouten 1940).

In discussing the origin of tinnitus this physiological supplementary and alternative pitch perception by periodicity must not be neglected.

Central Pathways

The auditory nerve is composed of approximately 30,000 fibers with diameters ranging from 3 to 10 μm. Most fibers have a spontaneous activity with discharge rates from a few spikes per minute to about 100 per second. The arrangement of the fibers reflects a tonotopic structure, that is, certain sound frequencies are associated with certain fibers.

Compression of cranial nerves in the posterior fossa by blood vessels can cause symptoms of both hyperactivity and progressive loss of function (Møller 1987). It is known that trigeminal neuralgia and hemifacial spasm are caused by vascular compression of the fifth and the seventh cranial nerves, respectively.

The portion of the cranial nerve that is covered by central myelin (oligodendrocytes) obviously is more susceptible to vascular compression than the portion covered by peripheral myelin. In the auditory nerve, the transitional zone between these two types of myelin (Obersteiner-Redlich zone) is lo-

cated in the internal auditory meatus. Thus the entire intracranial portion of the auditory nerve is covered by central myelin and might in principle be sensitive to vascular compression.

It is not unlikely that in some cases this mechanism is the cause of tinnitus. However, tinnitus of this origin apparently is not conspicuous by any particular characteristic of pitch, pulsation, or other feature that could be used as a clue for a differential diagnosis.

All fibers of the auditory nerve end in the cochlear nucleus. Each fiber contacts between 75 and 100 cells of the nucleus. On the other hand, each cell of the cochlear nucleus has synaptic contacts with numerous fibers of the auditory nerve. This divergence-convergence principle of neuronal connection is typical for the central nervous system and builds up an extremely complex meshwork of ipsilateral and contralateral, afferent and efferent routes. In such a system any attempt to "locate" a central origin of tinnitus appears simplistic and almost impossible.

FEATURES OF TINNITUS AND THEIR PHYSIOLOGICAL COUNTERPARTS

Frequency and Frequency Spectrum

Tinnitus usually has a quality that is described by the subject as hissing, ringing, buzzing, or roaring. The physiological counterpart to this category of quality is frequency and frequency spectrum. It is common usage in the evaluation of tinnitus to have the patient match externally presented acoustic signals to the subjective sensation of tinnitus. In cases of purely tonal tinnitus this usually is accomplished in a satisfactory way.

Since tinnitus often has a very high pitch one must bear in mind that frequency judgments in this region normally are poor. The highest tone used in musical instruments, c^v, has a frequency of 4096 Hz. Frequency discrimination at two octaves above this, up to about 16,000 Hz, which is the upper limit of hearing, is by a factor 2 or 3 less exact than in the middle frequency range (Ranke

1953). In addition, patients suffering from high-pitched tinnitus often have a high-frequency hearing loss, which certainly impairs their pitch discrimination (Dauman and Cazals 1989). Therefore, test-retest reliability in matching the frequencies of audiometer tones to the pitch of tinnitus may appear poor.

In judging pitch in music, it is a common feature that octaves are confused. Although some authors feel that octave confusion is frequent in pitch matching of tinnitus (Vernon 1987), it is not very likely that this happens in a systematic way. Octave confusion is based on the fact that all sounds used in music, even single tones of an instrument, are composed of a number of frequencies, among which the relation of one to two, designating an octave, is regularly present. Pure tones of the audiometer do not have these additional components (harmonics), and there is not the least evidence of likelihood that tonal tinnitus in itself, as a rule, has this harmonic quality of a musical sound. It probably is just the fact that tinnitus usually is not composed of a spectrum of harmonics that makes frequency matching difficult. The perception of musical harmony and of musical intervals is based on the periodicity common to the components of a chord or the components forming a musical interval.

The pitch of tonal tinnitus often corresponds to frequencies where there is a hearing loss in the audiogram. From this and other evidence discussed below, it seems likely that pitch perception of tinnitus follows the place of lesion (place theory of pitch perception) rather than the periodicity of neural impulses.

Beats

If two zones are presented simultaneously to the ear, one with a frequency of 500 Hz, the other one with a frequency of 502 Hz, the sensation is not that of two tones but that of one tone with its amplitude modulated at a rate of 2 per second. This is called beating. It plays an important role in music and tuning of music instruments.

When these two tones are presented dichotically, one to the right ear, the other one to the left ear, the sensation is that the tone oscillates between right and left side, or that it circles around the head. This is due to the changing phase relation between the two tones.

These phenomena are based on phase-locked representations of the acoustic signals in the cochlea and, for phenomena of binaural hearing, in the lower stages of the auditory pathway.

It has often been attempted to produce beats with a tonal tinnitus by presenting external tones of frequencies very near to the frequency exactly matching the tinnitus. There is not convincing evidence that this ever was successful and that beating with tinnitus as one component could be produced. This is a strong proof that tinnitus originating in the cochlea or in the lower stages of the auditory system is not represented by phase-locked nerve impulses or by some sort of periodicity.

Loudness

The normal ear covers the enormous range of 13 logarithmic units of sound energy from the just audible threshold to the threshold of pain. In a first naive approach everybody is likely to presume that the distress caused by tinnitus is correlated to its loudness.

If, however, the loudness of tinnitus is measured by matching it to acoustic signals of similar quality, either in the afflicted ear or in the normal contralateral ear, the loudness thus assigned to the tinnitus is only in the range of 5 to 10 dB sensation level (SL). This, indeed, is a very low level by all standards, even if the matching was carried out in an ear with recruitment.

The mechanisms by which loudness is coded in the auditory system are not yet completely understood. It appears that the total amount of firing in the afferent fibers and the distribution among the total population of fibers carry the information about loudness. When a pure tone is presented to the ear at a low level, only one fiber, whose best frequency was hit, will respond. If the intensity of the tone is raised, other fibers will join the first one, and the number of fibers involved increases.

If in a psychoacoustic experiment one tone of a given intensity is presented to the ear, it will produce a certain subjective loudness. The same loudness is produced by two tones, or a number of tones presented simultaneously within a small interval. If, however, this interval is widened, there is a critical distance beyond which the loudness of the combined tones suddenly increases. This is called the *critical bandwidth*. In the middle and high frequency range it corresponds to about one-third octave. The critical bandwidth also plays an important role in masking procedures. It is believed that the elements along the basilar membrane, hair cells and their nervous supply, can be functionally coupled within small sections in order to fulfill certain tasks, such as in loudness coding and in masking (Fletcher 1940; Scharf 1970; Shailer, Tyler, and Coles 1981; Zwicker 1982).

The discussion of maskability elsewhere in this book will show that tinnitus in many aspects is different from the sensation caused by an external physical sound of appropriate quality, although the sensations seem to be very similar or even identical. This difference is already based on the fact that a physical acoustic signal is always represented in the auditory system by a combination of two modes of coding: the place theory and periodicity analysis. In addition, these two modes of coding are probably modulated by funneling and inhibition through the efferent fibers. Tinnitus as a pathologic excitation of isolated elements does not have this concomitant pattern of neural activity—this is the fundamental difference between physiology and pathophysiology, between hearing external acoustic signals and tinnitus.

It is very likely that this fundamental difference is also present in loudness coding. The distress caused by tinnitus may thus be based on the fact that the clues for loudness in tinnitus do not fit in the ensemble of the other neural parameters associated with tinnitus. An analogy might be found in the sensation of itching on the skin and phantom pain in a missing limb, where unusual combinations of tactile sensibility, pain, deep sensibility, and sympathetic irritations seem to be involved.

The topic representation of frequencies is maintained throughout the auditory system from the cochlea through the afferent fibers, the nuclei of the central auditory pathway up to the auditory cortex. Recently it was demonstrated that the intensity is also represented in the auditory cortex in an amplitopic organization that is intermingled with the tonotopic organization in a type of network (Pantev, Hoke, Lehnertz, Lütkenhöner, Anogianakis, and Wittkowski 1988; Hoke 1988). It is conceivable that the discrepancy between the loudness of tinnitus as measured by matching it with external acoustic signals and the subjective grading of discomfort and loudness is due to an abnormal constellation of pitch and loudness in the tonotopic-amplitopic net of the auditory cortex. It is hoped that further investigation using biomagnetic recordings will throw light on this problem (Hoke, Feldmann, Pantev, Lütkenhöner, and Lehnertz 1988).

Localization and Projection

Patients suffering from tinnitus usually can tell where the tinnitus is localized: right ear, left ear, both ears, in the head. This corresponds to the everyday situation where a normally hearing subject can locate a real sound source in the three dimensions of his or her surroundings. The ability of directional hearing and localization is bound to certain fundamental phenomena.

Only if the acoustic signals reaching both ears are coherent can they be fused to form one image. Coherence means that they must originate from the same physical process and must have essential characteristics in common, particularly a common time pattern, which may be periodical or random.

The following simple experiment will elucidate this important point. The signal of a noise generator is fed simultaneously by earphones to both ears of the subject. The sensations of both ears at once fuse to form a single image: There is only one noise. This sensation is compelling and the subject has no means whatsoever to separate the two noise signals. Now the signal of the noise generator is recorded for several minutes on the first track, after that for several minutes on the second track of a tape. Then the recordings on the two tracks are played simultaneously, one to the right ear, the other to the left ear. The tape is cut into two pieces. One is played to the right ear and simultaneously the other one is played to the left ear. Although both recordings are identical with respect to intensity and frequency spectrum, they do not fuse. The subject will hear two separate noises, one in the right ear, the other one in the left ear. This sensation is equally compelling, and the subject has no means whatsoever to fuse the two noises into one image. The noise signals on the tapes are incoherent.

The physiological process identifying this, a kind of cross correlation, is bound to a phase-locked coding of the signals. It is effective mainly in the frequency range below 1.5 kHz. The place theory of frequency analysis alone cannot account for these features (Feldmann 1965, 1988).

If the signals reaching both ears are coherent the localization of the fused image is governed by two factors: loudness and time delay.

If both signals have identical intensity and if they reach both ears absolutely simultaneously, the image is located in the middle of the head. If there is a difference in loudness between both ears of 5 to 10 dB or more, the image shifts to the ear that is hit by the louder signal.

If there is a time delay between both signals of about 10^{-4} sec or more, the signal shifts to the ear that gets the signal a little earlier. This time delay is often confused with phase shift. It is indeed identical with a defined phase shift, if only one frequency is involved, but for complex sounds, such as a noise signal, the concept of phase angle does not describe well what the essential feature really is.

In such a situation of interaural intensity difference or time delay, the subject has the compelling sensation that the sound is localized only in one ear. He has no means—except moving the head or blocking one ear—to find out whether or not the other ear is involved. A purely unilateral stimulation will produce an almost identical sensation. The addition of the attenuated or delayed signal to the other ear only slightly influences the volume of the sound image but not its localization. Audiologists use this phenomenon in Stenger's test to prove simulation of a pretended unilateral deafness.

If these well-known features of binaural processing of acoustic signals are applied to the sensation of tinnitus, the following conclusions can be drawn:

1. Tinnitus that is heard "in the right ear <u>and</u> the left ear" originates from at least two sources, which do not fuse to form a single image, although they might be similar in spectrum and intensity. They lack coherence, they are not phase-locked, and they are not linked by a common time pattern.

2. Tinnitus located "in the right ear only" (or "in the left ear only") probably is generated there. It cannot be excluded that the other ear is also involved; however, the signal generated there would have to be coherent with the first one, but softer or delayed by a time shift so that the subject would be unable to detect it. Such a constellation is very unlikely.

3. Tinnitus "in the head" might theoretically be due to the fusion of tinnitus signals coming from both peripheral organs. However, these two signals would have to be coherent. It is hardly conceivable how this coherence could be brought about by pathological processes in the right and left ear. Therefore tinnitus "in the head" probably arises at stages of the central auditory pathways where the peripheral processing of coherence has already been superseded by coding of a higher level.

4. These concepts of location of tinnitus, however, can be applied only to sensations corresponding to the low and middle frequency range, not to high-pitched sensations (above 3 to 5 kHz) where phase locking does not play a major part.

Masking

The interactions between two acoustic stimuli presented simultaneously to one ear have been studied extensively in psychoacoustic experiments in man as well as in animals using electrophysiological methods. Two phenomena that arise from such an interaction have already been discussed, namely loudness with regard to the critical bandwidth, and beats. It could be demonstrated that tinnitus with respect to these two phenomena does not behave as if it were elicited in the cochlea by an acoustical signal.

A third mode of interaction between two acoustic signals, which is of greatest interest here, is masking. Masking means that in the presence of one acoustic signal the threshold of perception of a second signal is raised.

When in a psychoacoustic experiment two stimuli of known parameters acting as masking signal and masked signal are fed into a normally hearing ear, it can precisely be predicted what the subject will hear. This is true also for the time course of the reaction, the onset, the steady state, and the post stimulus period. If, however, tinnitus is used as the signal to be masked, the outcome is unpredictable. Among the manifold reasons for this only the following may be mentioned (Feldmann 1971, 1983, 1984).

Although the masking signal can be defined exactly by its physical properties, its sensational equivalent for the individual subject is not known precisely, because the subject's hearing usually is distorted due to hearing loss, recruitment or loudness, and fatigue. Since tinnitus is the signal to be masked, the properties of this component of the psychoacoustic interaction regarding frequency spectrum, loudness, and time course are even less well-defined. Thus in the case of tinnitus, masker and maskee are ill-defined, and this partly accounts for the unpredictability of the outcome of the masking experiment. The main reason, however, is the essential fact that tinnitus in the masking experiment often does not behave as

though it were produced by an external acoustical stimulus.

In the normal psychoacoustic experiment, low frequencies are more effective maskers than high frequencies. In tinnitus imitating a pure tone, this typical frequency dependence is not present or it is even reverse in such a way that tones of higher frequencies than the pitch of the tinnitus are more effective in masking the tinnitus than tones of lower frequencies.

Normally it is impossible to mask a thermal noise by a tone. Tinnitus resembling a thermal noise or a broadband noise (particularly in Ménière's disease), however, is often easily masked by a single tone of minimal suprathreshold intensity. In these cases any tone of the whole frequency range is equally effective in masking the noise-like tinnitus.

The usual psychoacoustic experiment requires that masking signal and masked signal are presented to the same ear. The masking effect does not extend to the opposite ear, unless the stimuli are so intense that they are physically conducted across the skull. Unilateral tinnitus, however, can often be masked by soft signals applied to the opposite ear at intensities which by no means can cross the skull.

Fundamental differences between tinnitus and a sensation aroused by a physical stimulus are also evidence in the time course of the masking reaction. In the normal psychoacoustic experiment during simultaneous masking, when both signals are present, there is a steady state which can be sustained for a long time without any change occurring in the relation between masker and masked signal. With tinnitus as a masked signal there can be three different types of reactions (Feldmann 1983):

1. A steady state as in normal masking.
2. Fatigue of tinnitus.
3. Fatigue of masker.

In the normal psychoacoustic experiment, the effect of the masker extends into the post-stimulatory period for only a few milliseconds (forward masking). In masking of tinnitus we often find a prolonged after-effect of masking, the "residual inhibition", which can last for many seconds or even minutes.

Data from electrophysiological experiments with recordings from different levels of the hearing system down to the hair cells, data from direct observations of the basilar membrane, and data from experiments with suppression of otoacoustic emissions (Zwicker 1987) proved that the simultaneous phase of masking in the normal psychoacoustic situation takes place before the neural transformation, that is, at the stage of vibrations in the cochlea. The post-stimulus masking is established in or after the first synapse.

From all that is known about spontaneous acoustic emissions it can be presumed that, as a rule, subjective tinnitus is not associated with mechanical vibrations of the cochlear partition. This explains why tinnitus does not present the pattern of simultaneous masking that would be expected of a physical sound.

The external masking stimuli, on the other hand, activate vibrations of the cochlear partition with a traveling wave and a maximum of displacement sharply tuned to the frequency. These vibrations, however, do not encounter and do not compete with other physical vibrations representing the tinnitus. Thus the whole masking process of tinnitus lacks this important vibratory stage, which characterizes the steady state of simultaneous masking in the normal psychoacoustic situation. Therefore, the masking process of tinnitus can only begin at the stage where normally the post-stimulatory masking takes place, at the neural transformation or the first synapse between the inner hair cells and the afferent fibers.

This concept, based on new experimental findings, supports the theory, repeatedly put forward since 1969 (Feldmann 1969, 1971, 1987), that masking of tinnitus is primarily a process of neural inhibition: lateral inhibition involving adjacent neural elements along the cochlear partition in one ear, contralateral inhibition in the other ear, possibly mediated via the efferent system. Higher levels, of course, might as well be involved.

GENERAL HYPOTHESES ON PATHOPHYSIOLOGY OF TINNITUS

Tinnitus is a functional disorder of the auditory system that probably can originate from different lesions and at different sites. The auditory system, however, is so complex, involving highly complicated peripheral organs, a multitude of afferent and efferent pathways, and a great number of nuclei which form a meshwork capable of logistic processes of the highest order, such as habituation, recognition, memory, learning, that the aim to pinpoint a certain disorder to one structure or to assign a certain malfunction to one defined lesion is questionable. Somehow the whole system is always involved.

This is best demonstrated by the fate of patients who suffered from tinnitus following surgery for otosclerosis (Douek 1987). At the beginning, after stapedectomy, the damage—sensorineural hearing loss, vestibular dysfunction, and tinnitus—was clearly located in the peripheral organ. In order to alleviate the tinnitus, in some patients further surgery was carried out comprising a series of interventions: sealing a perilymph fistula, labyrinthectomy, excision of the cochlea, and section of the auditory nerve. After each intervention there was only short relief of tinnitus, but it recurred. In the long run no case was cured of tinnitus by the destructive surgery, including section of the auditory nerve. The "site of lesion" causing or perpetuating the functional disorder "tinnitus" must have shifted centrally step-by-step following the interventions.

In the auditory system at each level, there is a spontaneous activity of neurons with discharging rates ranging from 0 to about 100 per second for the individual unit (Kim and Molnar 1979). This is so in the absence of any external stimulus and its sensational equivalent is quietness.

The modulation of the background activity

may be an increase in the discharge rate of single fibers, a decrease, or a combination of both, forming areas of increased discharge rates surrounded by areas of inhibited spontaneous activity, or it may be a synchronization of discharges in adjacent fibers, brought about by phase-locking to the acoustic signal.

Tinnitus imitates an acoustic signal. Although at lower stages of the auditory system tinnitus does not behave like a physical acoustic stimulus in some respects, as was shown in the previous sections, at higher stages it obviously is represented in a pattern very similar to that elicited by a physical acoustic stimulus, so that a patient can be misled into taking his or her tinnitus for the image of a real sound. Therefore, at higher levels the modulation of the spontaneous activity representing the real stimulus will probably be of a similar pattern as that produced by tinnitus.

Møller (1984) put forward the idea that some forms of tinnitus could be explained by an abnormal synchronization of neural activity in auditory nerve fibers. Pathological processes that could induce such synchronization of spontaneous activity among adjacent fibers might be a partial breakdown of the myelin of individual nerve fibers, resulting in direct electrical contact between axons (ephaptic transmissions, "crosstalk" among fibers).

Such a theory could very well explain the observation that tinnitus following surgical trauma to the cochlea could not be stopped by subsequent destruction of the cochlea and section of the auditory nerve. Each step of surgery might have established a new level of trauma where the breakdown of insulation was installed.

This theory is based on the concept of periodicity pitch discrimination. However, from this point of view it is difficult to explain how the high pitch often characterizing tinnitus can be created and kept constant by such a pathological synchronization of many fibers. Fibers of the auditory nerve have a refractory period of about 1.25 msec. This means that a single fiber can discharge at a rate of maximally 800 per second. Where, then, is the pacemaker to monitor correlated discharges among adjacent fibers representing a pitch of 5,000 Hz or 10,000 Hz, which for tonal tinnitus is not uncommon (Feldmann 1988)?

In the previous sections on beats and masking, evidence was produced that could not easily be reconciled with the concept that periodicity analysis is primarily involved in determining the pitch of tinnitus.

If priority is given to the place theory, however, a very simple model of tinnitus generation is conceivable. The shearing motion of the stereocilia on top of the hair cells opens and closes potassium channels, thus triggering a depolarization of the cell, releasing a transmitter and activating afferent synapses. A defect in the stereocilia, the cuticular membrane or in the potassium channel itself, could cause a leak and a constant influx of potassium, which periodically would depolarize the cell and trigger the discharge of connected nerve fibers. Since the place of the firing hair cell would determine the pitch and not the phase-locked periodicity of the discharges, this would explain the constancy of the pitch and its close relation to the pathology of the cochlea and the site of damage. It is indeed a common finding that the pitch of tinnitus is correlated to the slope or dip of a high-frequency hearing loss in the audiogram.

This pathological excitation of one hair cell or a small group of hair cells is different from the excitation pattern caused by an appropriate acoustic stimulus in that it lacks the periodicity related to the pitch as a supplementary clue, and in that it lacks the normal background associated with a real acoustic stimulus: contribution from outer hair cells, pattern of inhibition in adjacent units, and the like.

Experiments with spontaneous and evoked acoustic emissions seem to prove that the outer half cells act through mechanical-electricomechanical transduction as an amplifier producing positive feedback. The information transmission is exclusively or predominantly performed by the inner hair cells. As in tinnitus, there are no spontaneous mechanical vibrations present (no spontaneous acoustic emissions related to tinnitus), and it can be concluded that the outer hair cells generally are not involved in the production of tinnitus by fast oscillating contractions. The lowest stage where information transmission takes place is in the inner hair cells, and, therefore, the lowest stage where tinnitus can be generated as a neural signal is in the inner hair cells. One of the conceivable modes might be a defect of the cell membrane or of an ion-channel.

Other hypotheses on the origin of tinnitus based on changes in osmolarity or other biochemical parameters in the cochlear fluids will be discussed in the sections on Ménière's disease and sudden deafness.

PATHOLOGY AND PATHOPHYSIOLOGY OF WELL-KNOWN DISEASES ASSOCIATED WITH TINNITUS

Acute Acoustic Trauma

Acute acoustic trauma causes a severe sensorineural hearing loss, which almost invariably is associated with tinnitus. In chronic acoustic trauma (noise-induced hearing loss) the symptoms are very similar, but tinnitus is not as regularly present as after the acute trauma.

The hearing loss due to an acute acoustic trauma usually is restricted to the high-frequency region and presents a dip around 4 kHz. The tinnitus is of tonal quality, and as a rule corresponds in pitch to the cut-off frequency of the pure-tone audiogram, that is, to the region between normal and damaged areas of the organ of Corti. In cases of minor damage the pitch of the tinnitus tends to coincide with the frequency of the dip. Tinnitus, indeed, seems to occur mainly in areas where the organ of Corti is only partially damaged (Spoendlin 1987).

It can be deduced from this finding that the pathology generating the tinnitus is located in this area. The striking feature in this area is the dominant damage of the outer hair cells, whereas the inner hair cells are much more resistant. Even in areas where the outer hair cells are completely disintegrated, the inner half cells often appear quite

normal. In zones of less severe damage where only slight distortions of the outer hair cells are visible, these distortions might well interfere with the monitoring and amplifying action of the outer hair cells. This would account for the hearing loss. It can generally be assumed that dysfunction of the delicate submicroscopic structures of the hair cells, such as ion-channels, by far precedes visible damages.

It has been demonstrated that under intense stimulation the stereocilia of the outer hair cells lose their stiffness (Spoendlin 1987), which at first is a reversible reaction. It is very likely that the stereocilia of the inner hair cells are distorted in a similar way, but to a lesser degree that is not demonstrable by present morphological methods.

The spontaneous activity of cochlear neurons in the region of noise-induced damage is significantly altered as compared to neurons coming from normal areas of the cochlea (Liberman and Kiang 1978). According to Spoendlin (1987) the predominant damage to the outer hair cells, and consequently a dissociation of outer and inner hair cells, is the outstanding feature of pathology in areas where abnormal activities occur, and therefore this dissociation can be assumed to be the neurophysiological expression of tinnitus.

The mechanism by which tinnitus is generated following acoustic trauma might be a correlation and synchronization of discharges (Møller 1984), or a deafferentiation of small and large diameter fibers (Tonndorf 1987). In the author's view, however, the simplest and most probable explanation is a leak in the hair cell membrane or a defect of the submicroscopical ion-channels (Feldmann 1988). Evidence in favor of this hypothesis was brought forward in the previous sections. It is further supported by the finding that the spontaneous discharge rate is increased in areas of noise induced damage. According to this hypothesis, hearing losses up to 40 to 50 dB would be due to damage of the outer hair cells; this corresponds to their contribution in boosting the vibratory excitation of the inner hair cells. Tinnitus would be generated in the damaged inner hair cells themselves.

Ménière's Disease

In Ménière's disease, sensorineural deafness and tinnitus are leading symptoms. In the early stages of the disease they are present only associated with the attacks of vertigo, and they disappear during the intervals. Later on they tend to become permanent, but fluctuating in intensity with the attacks.

The hearing disorder in Ménière's disease begins in the low frequency range; later it spreads to all frequencies resulting in a flat curve in the pure-tone audiogram. The tinnitus usually resembles a broadband or thermal noise.

The pathology of Ménière's disease is fairly well known: There is an enlargement of the endolymphatic space, endolymphatic hydrops, with Reissner's membrane bulging into the scala vestibuli. It is assumed that the attack itself is caused by a rupture of Reissner's membrane followed by a mixture of the two fluids endolymph and perilymph. This results in a breakdown of the normal electrical potentials and a potassium intoxication of the hair cells (Zenner 1987). It is remarkable that morphological alterations at the hair cells or other parts of the organ of Corti so far could not be demonstrated.

Zenner (1987) found that a potassium intoxication of the perilymph causes a contraction of the outer hair cells, which initially is reversible. This would result in a shearing movement of the stereocilia or in their decoupling from the tectorial membrane. In addition, the positive mechanical feedback could get out of control. Furthermore, a release of mechanical energy is stimulated by the potassium. These mechanisms were postulated to give rise to tinnitus in Ménière's disease.

Dulon and colleagues (Dulon, Aran, and Schacht 1987) demonstrated that small changes in the osmolarity in vitro medium induce fast contractions (hypo-osmotic solution) or elongations (hyper-osmotic solution) in isolated outer hair cells. These reactions were reversible. The authors suggest that a fluctuant change in osmolarity might be the fundamental mechanism in Ménière's disease

and that a rupture of Reissner's membrane must not necessarily be postulated to explain all the characteristic symptoms of the disease, including the responsiveness to glycerol.

Pujol (personal communication) observed that in the chronic phase of Ménière's disease no otoacoustic emissions can be evoked. After administration of glycerol (glycerol-test) and slight improvement of the threshold, otoacoustic emissions could be elicited by acoustic stimuli as in normal ears.

Based on these observations, the following comprehensive hypothesis on the pathophysiology of hearing loss and tinnitus in Ménière's disease can be put forward.

Changes in the osmolarity (hypo-osmotic) or potassium intoxication likewise induce a contraction of the outer hair cells. This interferes with their normal function to supply positive mechanical feedback to the inner hair cells and accounts for the raise of threshold. However, it does not easily explain the generation of tinnitus. In the section entitled "General Hypotheses on Pathophysiology of Tinnitus," it was maintained that the lowest stage where tinnitus as neural (mimicked) information could be produced is the inner hair cells. The stereocilia of the outer hair cells are connected to the tectorial membrane, the stereocilia of the inner hair cells do not have such an attachment. A contraction of the outer hair cells, following K$^+$-intoxication or following hypo-osmolarity will pull the tectorial membrane down towards the basilar membrane, thereby approaching, touching, or even bending the stereocilia of the inner hair cells.

This, indeed, would be the appropriate stimulus for the inner hair cells and would raise their spontaneous discharge rates. Since this would involve all the inner hair cells of the area where the contraction of the outer hair cells occurs, and since it would be an enhancement of their spontaneous activity without synchronizing or phase locking, the resulting pattern of neural stimulation would resemble a broadband or thermal noise.

The contraction of the outer hair cells due to

hypo-osmolarity or potassium intoxication would impair their ability to react to sound stimuli with phase-locked mechanical oscillations, hence the hearing loss and the finding that no otoacoustic emissions can be evoked. The osmotic influence of glycerol would temporarily correct these disturbances and lift the tectorial membrane off the inner hair cells, thus restoring the hearing capacity and relieving the tinnitus.

It is reasonable to assume that under normal conditions the presence of a real acoustic stimulus will phase lock the spontaneous activity of all sensory units in the appropriate place (following the place theory) and inhibit spontaneous activity in other areas. If this concept is correct and if tinnitus in Ménière's disease is due to a raised rate of random spontaneous activity in the inner hair cells, it is very well conceivable that any real sound fed into the cochlea could monitor this spontaneous activity just as in a normal ear, partly phase lock it, according to the periodicity analysis, and partly inhibit it. In Ménière's disease, the tinnitus usually is easily masked or inhibited by any acoustic signal that is presented slightly above threshold. This finding fits very well into the hypothesis discussed here.

Salicylate Intoxication

High doses of salicylate are known to produce reversible hearing loss and tinnitus in man, and, therefore, it has been used in animal models of tinnitus (Jastreboff, Brennan, and Sasaki 1988; Jastreboff 1990). So far no morphological pathology could be demonstrated in the cochlea after administration of salicylate, however, a significant increase of spontaneous activity of cochlear neurons was found (Schreiner and Snyder 1987).

Salicylates are antagonists to prostaglandins, which probably help to control the stiffness of the stereocilia. Perhaps it is a similar mechanism as that proposed for Ménière's disease here: contraction of the outer hair cells, pulling the tectorial membrane towards the cilia of the inner hair cells, increasing spontaneous activity. This hypothesis

would very well explain all symptoms of a salicylate intoxication, including their reversibility.

Sudden Deafness

From a clinical point of view, there is variety of conditions that may lead to the symptomatology of a unilateral sensorineural hearing loss of sudden onset, conditions which often are not diagnosed correctly, such as viral infection or VIIIth nerve tumor.

However, there seems to be one entity of idiopathic sudden deafness which resembles Ménière's disease, except that there are no attacks of vestibular disorder. It is characterized by its sudden onset, and it is often associated with tinnitus. The hearing loss may be restricted to the low frequency or to the high-frequency region, it may be mild, severe or profound, and often it is fluctuating. The etiology is assumed to be a vascular disorder, the obstruction of a small branch of the labyrinthine artery caused either by a spasm of the artery itself or by sludging of erythrocytes. Therapy with hemodilution, if applied early, often leads to full restoration of the hearing capacity, but relapses are not uncommon. On the other hand, there is a high rate of spontaneous remissions. The pitch and spectrum of the tinnitus usually reflects the hearing loss, as demonstrated in the pure-tone audiogram.

This symptomatology is highly suggestive of a similar pathophysiology as in Ménière's disease. However, since the attacks of vertigo do not occur, it is reasonable to assume that there are no ruptures of Reissner's membrane. The experimental findings of Dulon and colleagues (1987) seem to offer an explanation. A fluctuant change in the osmolarity of the endolymph or perilymph, due to a circulatory or metabolic disorder, could very well account for the clinical symptoms. A tonic contraction of outer hair cells induced by the change in osmolarity would interfere with their ability to booster the excitation of the inner hair cells by fast synchronized oscillating contractions. This would explain the hearing loss. On the other hand, the tonic contractions of the outer hair cells would pull down the tectorial membrane, which in its turn would bend the inner hair cell stereocilia, open the ion channels, and increase their rate of spontaneous activity. The good response of this type of sudden deafness to hemodilution might support this hypothesis.

REFERENCES

Dauman, R. and Cazals, Y. 1989. "Auditory Frequency Selectivity and Tinnitus." *Archives of Otolaryngology, 246,* 252–255.

Douek, E. 1987. "Tinnitus Following Surgery." In H. Feldmann (Ed.), *Proceedings III International Tinnitus Seminar, Munster, 1987,* pp. 64–69. Karlsruhe: Harsch Verlag.

Dulon, D., Aran, J.-M., and Schacht, J. 1987. "Osmotically Induced Motility of Outer Hair Cells: Implications for Meniere's Disease." *Archives of Otolaryngology, 244,* 104–107.

Feldmann, H. 1965. "Experiments of Binaural Hearing in Noise. The Central Nervous Processing of Acoustic Information." *Translations of the Beltone Institute for Hearing Research, 18,* 1–42.

Feldmann, H. 1969. "Untersuchungen zur Verdeckung subjektiver Ohrgeräusche—ein Beitrag zur Pathophysiologie des Ohrensausens." *Z. Laryng. Rhinol. Otol., 48,* 528–545.

Feldmann, H. 1971. "Homolateral and Contralateral Masking of Tinnitus by Noise Bands and Pure Tones." *Audiology, 10,* 138–144.

Feldmann, H. 1983. "Time Pattern and Related Parameters in Masking of Tinnitus." *Acta Otolaryngologica (Stockholm), 95,* 594–598.

Feldmann, H. 1984. "Tinnitus Masking Curves (Updates and Review)." *Journal of Laryngology, Supplement 9,* 157–160.

Feldmann, H. 1987. "Masking Phenomena in Tinnitus." In H. Feldmann (Ed.), *Proceedings III International Tinnitus Seminar, Munster, 1987,* pp. 224–228. Karlsruhe: Harsch Verlag.

Feldmann, H. 1988. "Pathophysiology of Tinnitus." In M. Kitahara (Ed.), *Tinnitus—Pathophysiology and Management,* pp. 7–35. Tokyo/New York: Igaku-Shoin.

Fletcher, H. 1940. "Auditory Patterns." *Rev. Modern Physics, 12,* 47–85.

Hoke, M. 1988. "SQUID-based Measuring Techniques—A Challenge for the Functional Diagnostics in Medicine." In B. Kramer (Ed.), *The Art of Measurement,* pp. 287–335. Weinheim: VICHI.

Hoke, M. Feldmann, H., Pantev, C., Lütkenhöner, B., and Lehnertz, K. 1989. "Objective Evidence of Tinnitus in Auditory Evoked Magnetic Fields." *Hearing Research, 37,* 281–286.

Jastreboff, P.J. 1990. "Phantom Auditory Perception (tinnitus): Mechanisms of Generation and Perception." *Neuroscience Research, 8,* 221–254.

Jastreboff, P.J., Brennan, J.F., and Sasaki, C.T. 1988. "An Animal Model for Tinnitus." *Laryngoscope, 98,* 280–286.

Kim, D.O. and Molnar, C.E. 1979. "A Population Study of Cochlear Nerve Fibres: Comparison of Spatial Distribution of Average-Rate and Phase-Locking Measures of Responses to Single Tones." *Journal of Neurophysiology, 42,* 16–30.

Liberman, M.C. and Kiang, N.Y.-S. 1978. "Acoustic Trauma in Cats. Cochlear Pathology and Auditory Nerve Activity." *Acta Otolaryngologica (Stockholm), Supplement 358,* 1–63.

Lim, D.J., Hahamure, Y., and Ohashi, Y. 1989. "Structural Organization of the Outer Hair Cell Wall." *Acta Otolaryngologica (Stockholm), 107,* 398–405.

Møller, A.R. 1984. "Pathophysiology of Tinnitus." *Annals of Otology, Rhinology, and Laryngology, 93,* 39–44.

Møller, A.R. 1987. "Vascular Compression of the Eighth Nerve as Cause of Tinnitus." In H. Feldmann (Ed.), *Proceedings III International Tinnitus Seminar, Munster, 1987,* pp. 340–347. Karlsruhe: Harsch Verlag.

Pantev, C., Hoke, M., Lehnertz, K., Lütkenhöner, B., Anogianakis, G., and Wittkowski, W. 1988. "Tonotopic Organization of the Human Auditory Cortex Revealed by Transient Auditory Evoked Magnetic Fields." *Electroencephalography and Clinical Neurophysiology, 69,* 160–170.

Penner, M.J. 1988. "Audible and Annoying Spontaneous Otoacoustic Emissions. A Case Study." *Archives of Otolaryngology—Head and Neck Surgery, 114,* 150–153.

Penner, M.J. 1989. "Aspirin Abolishes Tinnitus Caused by Spontaneous Otoacoustic Emissions." *Archives of Otolaryngology—Head and Neck Surgery, 115,* 871–875.

Pujol, R. 1987. Personal Communication.

Ranke, O.F. 1953. *Physiologie des Gehörs.* Berlin: Springer.

Scharf, B. 1970. "Critical Bands." In J.V. Tobias (Ed.), *Foundations of Modern Auditory Theory, Vol. 1,* pp. 157–202. New York: Academic Press.

Schouten, J.F. 1940. "The Residue Revisited." In R. Plomp and G.F. Smoorenburg (Eds.), *Frequency Analysis and Periodicity Detection in Hearing.* Leiden.

Schreiner, C.E. and Snyder, R.L. 1987. "A Physiological Animal Model of Peripheral Tinnitus." In H. Feldmann (Ed.), *Proceedings III International Tinnitus Seminar, Munster, 1987,* pp. 100–106. Karlsruhe: Harsch Verlag.

Shailer, M.J., Tyler, R.S., and Coles, R.R. 1981. "Critical Masking Bands for Sensorineural Tinnitus." *Scandinavian Audiology, 10,* 157–162.

Spoendlin, H. 1987. "Inner Ear Pathology and Tinnitus." In H. Feldmann (Ed.), *Proceedings III International Tinnitus Seminar, Munster, 1987,* pp. 42–51. Karlsruhe: Harsch Verlag.

Spoendlin, H. 1988. "Neural Anatomy of the Inner Ear." In A.F. Jahn and J. Santos-Sacchi (Eds.), *Physiology of the Ear,* pp. 201–219. New York: Raven Press.

Tonndorf, J. 1987. "The Origin of Tinnitus—A New Hypothesis: An Analogy with Pain." In H. Feldmann (Ed.), *Proceedings III International Tinnitus Seminar, Munster, 1987,* pp. 70–74.

Vernon, J.A. 1987. "Assessment of the Tinnitus Patient." In J.W.P. Hazell (Ed.), *Tinnitus,* pp. 71–95. Edinburgh: Churchill Livingstone.

Wilson, J.P. 1987. "Theory of Tinnitus Generation." In J.W.P. Hazell (Ed.), *Tinnitus,* pp. 20–45. Edinburgh: Churchill Livingstone.

Zenner, H.P. 1986. "Motile Response in Outer hair Cells." *Hearing Research, 22,* 83–90.

Zenner, H.P. 1987. "Modern Aspects of Hair Cell Biochemistry, Motility and Tinnitus." In H. Feldmann (Ed.), *Proceedings III International Tinnitus Seminar, Munster, 1987,* pp. 52–57. Karlsruhe: Harsch Verlag.

Zenner, H.P. 1988. "Motility of Outer Hair Cells as an Active, Actin-Mediated Process." *Acta Otolaryngologica (Stockholm), 105,* 39–44.

Zwicker, E. 1982. *Psychoakustik.* Berlin: Springer.

Zwicker, E. 1987. "Objective Otoacoustic Emissions and Their Uncorrelation to Tinnitus." In H. Feldmann (Ed.), *Proceedings III International Tinnitus Seminar, Munster, 1987,* pp. 75–81. Karlsruhe: Harsch Verlag.

CHAPTER 6

TINNITUS IN CHILDREN WITH HEARING LOSS

JOHN M. GRAHAM
Royal Ear Hospital, London

INTRODUCTION

Children get tinnitus, and they also suffer from tinnitus, though with the typical tolerance of childhood, they seldom complain of tinnitus.

The literature on tinnitus in children (Thomas 1938; J.T. Graham 1965; Nodar 1972; J.M. Graham 1981a,b, 1987; Nodar and Le Zak 1984; Mills and Cherry 1984; Mills, Albert, and Brain 1986; Viani 1989; J.M. Graham and Butler 1984; Goodey 1981; Kemp 1981; Glanville, Coles, and Sullivan 1971; Reich 1987) consists mainly of observations on its prevalence, severity, and timing. Thomas (1938) suggested that tinnitus was uncommon in children. Venters (1953) failed to identify any child under 15 years of age with tinnitus. Fowler and Fowler (1955) stated that children before puberty seldom mention either tinnitus or unilateral deafness. J.T. Graham (1965) related the apparent failure of prepubertal children to develop tinnitus to the various developmental stages of the adult form of the ego.

Nodar (1972) used direct questioning to identify a 15 percent incidence of tinnitus in an unselected population of school children aged 10–18. J.M. Graham (1981a,b) reported that 59 percent of 92 hearing-impaired children questioned by their class teacher in a moderately severely deaf (40 to 60 dB averaged thresholds) and 29 percent of 66 children in a severe to profoundly deaf (80 to 110 dB averaged thresholds) school population aged 12–18 had tinnitus. Nodar and Le Zak

(1983) reported a 55 percent incidence of tinnitus among 56 hearing-impaired children: 35 percent in those with severe to profound deafness; 100 percent in those with less severe or high-frequency deafness. Mills and Cherry (1984) found a 38.5 percent incidence of tinnitus in a population of 109 severely hearing-impaired children aged 5–17. Mills and colleagues (1986) questioned 93 children aged 5–17 attending routine school and community medical examinations and found that 29 percent said on direct questioning that they had noises in their ears; however, only 3 percent of children over the age of 5 attending ENT and audiology clinics said spontaneously that they had tinnitus without direct questioning, and all 13 of these children had ear disease (10 secretory otitis media, 3 sensorineural hearing loss). Viani (1989) interviewed 102 children aged 6–17 with severe to profound deafness and found a 23 percent incidence of tinnitus.

PREVALENCE OF TINNITUS COMPARED WITH THE SPONTANEOUS COMPLAINT OF TINNITUS

Although the earlier authors (Thomas 1938; Venters 1953; Fowler and Fowler 1955) assumed that children are less likely than adults either to have or to notice tinnitus, the later authors (Nodar 1972; J.M. Graham 1981a,b, 1987; Nodar and Le Zak 1984; Mills and Cherry 1984; Mills et al. 1986; Viani 1989; J.M. Graham and Butler 1984) point out that children both have tinnitus and notice it but are less likely than adults to complain spontaneously about the symptom. Mills and colleagues (1986) in particular compared the 3 percent of children from one population who volunteered tinnitus as a symptom with the 29 percent and 38.5 percent of two other groups of children who admitted to having tinnitus only on direct questioning; similarly only 3 of Viani's (1989) group of 24 children had complained spontaneously of tinnitus before her study began. This characteristic failure of children to report their tinnitus without prompting is interesting and might justify a study by a child psychologist, since the audiologists and otolaryngologists in the existing literature on this subject generally confine themselves to simple, common sense suggestions to explain the phenomenon.

PRECIPITATION OF TINNITUS
BY HEARING AIDS

Two of the studies mentioned above (J.M. Graham 1981b; Viani 1989) looked at the relationship between unilateral tinnitus and (a) the use of hearing aids and (b) asymmetrical hearing thresholds. In one study (J.M. Graham 1981b) 73 percent of 30 hearing-impaired children with unilateral aiding had tinnitus in the aided ear. In the other study (Viani 1989), conducted later and in a different part of the United Kingdom, only 3 of 24 children with tinnitus had unilateral aiding, so no conclusions could be drawn.

INFLUENCE OF NOISE

In deaf children (J.M. Graham 1981b) with intermittent tinnitus, some reported that environmental noise, the use of their hearing aids, and the high intensity pure tones presented during audiometry all provoked tinnitus. Here the mechanism of tinnitus is likely to be similar to that found in adults with noise-induced tinnitus. This form of tinnitus is also increasingly reported by children without pre-existing hearing loss as the result of "recreational noise" as the intensity of amplified

music increases in discotheques and live performances and as the use of personal stereo headphones becomes more common.

IS THERE A MECHANISM THAT
PREVENTS DEAF CHILDREN FROM
HAVING CONSTANT TINNITUS?

Apart from the special cases of venous hums, myoclonus, and noise-induced tinnitus, little of the information found in the literature suggests mechanisms for the tinnitus found in deaf children. It is likely that these mechanisms (described elsewhere in this book) are common to adults and to children. However, there is one major difference between adults and children: Adults usually have constant tinnitus while in children tinnitus is almost always intermittent. In 519 adult patients with tinnitus, Meikle and colleagues (Meikle, Schuff, and Griest 1987) reported that tinnitus was constant in 90.5 percent of cases. In contrast, the figures given for intermittent tinnitus in children are: 100 percent (Mills et al. 1986), 29 of 31 cases (Nodar and Le Zak 1984), 23 of 24 cases (Viani 1989), 46 of 48 cases (J.M. Graham 1981b), 16 of 18 cases (Reich 1987). The remainder of this chapter will therefore discuss not the mechanisms that may produce tinnitus in children, but possible mechanisms to explain why children do not have (that is, do not perceive) tinnitus as a constant symptom.

It is likely that most forms of tinnitus have a primary generator mechanism in the cochlea whether the tinnitus is constant or intermittent. This cochlear activity passes along the auditory pathway and leads to the perception of tinnitus. Children do not get constant tinnitus either because constant generation of this ascending neural activity does not occur in congenital or early acquired deafness, or because such activity, when constant, remains below the threshold for conscious perception.

A possible mechanism for the first of these explanations, the absence of the cochlear activity that would cause constant tinnitus, is that if an infant's hearing has not been lost but simply has never been present then the efferent activity that would have triggered the hair-cell generators of tinnitus in a deafened adult may never occur.

However, two phenomena make the second explanation more likely and occupy extreme ends of the quantitative spectrum of electrical activity in the auditory pathway. In silence and with an intact cochlea some spike activity continues to occur in the auditory nerve. This activity, however, averaged over the full frequency range, is too low to reach the threshold that would lead to the perception of sound: It remains a steady-state phenomenon at a subthreshold level. A model of the other extreme of a steady-state phenomenon remaining below the threshold of perception was reported by Glanville and associates (Glanville et al. 1971). They described a child and his father who both had objective high-frequency tonal tinnitus in their left ears; each subject had a notch in his audiogram in the left ear at the frequency of the tinnitus. Neither father nor child was aware of his or her own tinnitus, though the child was aware of a similar high-frequency objective tinnitus which was *intermittently* present in his opposite, right, ear. These two cases draw attention to the phenomenon that to be perceived, tinnitus in congenital hearing loss seems to need to be intermittent rather than a constant, steady-state, phenomenon. If, as seems likely, the unperceived objective tinnitus in these two cases was giving rise to some afferent activity in the ipsilateral auditory nerve, and if the cochleae in some congenitally deaf children similarly generate a raised but constant level of afferent activity, then at some level there is a barrier preventing the passage of this steady state neural activity to the level of conscious perception. The imposition and setting of this signal filter could be at a cortical level or at some level between cochlea and cortex and is likely to occur early in the development of the fetus or infant. This may be related to the maturation of the auditory system and to the development of an auditory memory.

In the cochlear nuclei of the maturing congenitally deaf baby without objective tinnitus it is possible that, although there is a constant input of a steady state of increased neural activity arising from the first order neurons in the cochlea, this activity, being constant, disrupts the maturation of the postsynaptic neurons and their immediate onward connections. Assuming that this raised steady-state input is frequency related (either pure tone or narrow band) then the failure of maturation would similarly be tonotopic and confined only to part of the cochlear nucleus. Deprivation experiments, in which the opposite steady-state phenomenon occurs (i.e., the complete cessation of any neural electrical activity), are known to produce such structural and functional postsynaptic changes in and beyond the cochlear nucleus, or its equivalent in other species, during the stages of maturation of the peripheral auditory pathway while plasticity persists. It is possible that normal maturation of these peripheral structures relies not only on the presence of peripheral input but also, to some degree, on fluctuations in this input.

In the auditory cortex, a high proportion of neurons are sensitive to temporal factors such as frequency shifts, intensity changes, and onset or cessation of neural input (Evans 1968). At a gross level, the slow vertex response from the areas of the cortex that receive projections from the primary auditory cortex is both an "on" and "off" response rather than a response to a steady state. In behavioral terms, an animal uses the non-autonomic part of its sensory nervous system more for identifying changes in its external environment than for taking notice of a steady state in this environment. Thus the plasticity of the cerebral cortex would tend to allow the raising of thresholds for any constant, steady-state, input during the maturation of a child's auditory pathway. In this way the afferent electrical activity that would, in a deafened adult, cause the conscious perception of tinnitus would not be perceived as tinnitus by a child, having been present before the stage at which a child was consciously aware of any sounds.

Reader, behold! This monster wild
Has gobbled up the infant child.
The infant child is not aware
It has been eaten by the bear (Housman, 1937)

Adaptation of the auditory cortex for specific frequencies has certainly been described, for example, in the mustached bat (Suga, Niwa, Taniguchi, and Margoliash 1987), which has a "personalized auditory cortex" in which the doppler-shifted CF processing area of an individual bat's auditory cortex (where the characteristic frequency of that bat's own voice reflected to it as a doppler-shifted echo is received), is "phenomenally overrepresented".

One further clue comes from the paper by Glanville and associates (1971). The infant child with objective tinnitus in his left ear could not hear it in that ear but *was* able to hear that tinnitus when it was recorded and presented to him through a loudspeaker. The authors concluded that this was because he could then hear the sound in his opposite, right, ear. Assuming that this was the case, then there cannot have been a blanket cortical lack of sensitivity to neural input resulting from auditory stimulation, but only to such activity coming from the left ear. This suggests that the functional barrier to perception of the sound as tinnitus was not a simple frequency-specific reduction in cortical sensitivity.

IS TINNITUS MORE COMMON IN THE BETTER-HEARING EAR?

The first study (J.M. Graham 1981b) found that in children with an asymmetrical hearing loss consisting of a threshold difference of 10 dB or more averaged over four frequencies, 81 percent had tinnitus in their better-hearing ear. The second study (Viani 1989) failed to confirm this, finding no significant relationship between unilateral tinnitus and the better or worse hearing ear.

INFLUENCE OF HEARING THRESHOLD ON TINNITUS

When children from two types of United Kingdom secondary schools were compared (J.M. Graham 1981b), partial hearing units, which contained children with less severe deafness, seemed also to contain a higher percentage of children with tinnitus (66 percent of 92 children questioned) than did schools for the deaf (29 percent of 66 children questioned) that contained pupils with more profound deafness. Unfortunately, the average hearing thresholds were only obtained for the children in each group who had tinnitus. The four-frequency averaged thresholds for the children with tinnitus in each type of school were 52.5 dB nHL and 95 dB nHL respectively. Although it is likely that this does represent the relative average hearing level of each school population, it would have been helpful both to have evidence of this and comparison of the average hearing thresholds between children with and without tinnitus in each type of school. Without these data it is still possible to speculate that the less severe the hearing loss, the more likely it is that a deaf child will have tinnitus. It should be remembered, however, that if there seemed to be a significant relationship between hearing threshold and tinnitus in deaf children, a possible additional factor could be the difficulty that profoundly deaf children have both in understanding the concept of tinnitus (Goodey 1981) and distinguishing tinnitus from other external noises that they find equally bizarre and hard to understand (Kemp 1981).

DIAGNOSIS: IS THERE A RELATIONSHIP BETWEEN PATHOLOGY AND TINNITUS IN THE CHILD POPULATION?

In the papers (J.M. Graham 1981a,b; Viani 1989) that supplied information about etiology, the pathogenicity of deafness seemed not to be related to the presence or absence of tinnitus. However, three less common forms of special tinnitus should be mentioned: These have more obvious generating mechanisms. Venous hums (J.M. Graham 1987), low-frequency, usually non-pulsatile noises, occur in children with normal hearing and can also be heard by anyone placing a stethoscope on the child's neck. These hums change in intensity with respiration and are abolished by gentle compression over the internal jugular vein in the neck. They are probably the result of turbulence in the internal jugular vein or its larger tributaries rather than coming from any part of the auditory system.

The venous system was also thought to be the origin of the high-frequency, nearly pure-tone, tinnitus described in a family by Glanville and colleagues (1971). They concluded that this tinnitus was likely to be generated by fibrous strands stretched across a non-pulsatile flow of venous blood near the ear, probably in the jugular bulb.

Palatal myoclonus should also be mentioned. This may occur in children (Hazell 1984) as well as in adults. Although the mechanism of the palatal contractions that give rise to these irregular clicks is clear, the underlying etiology is not known.

CONCLUSION

There is a short story by Oscar Wilde (son of the famous ENT surgeon) called "The Birthday of the Infanta". A grotesque hunchbacked dwarf child is found in the forest and brought to the Spanish court to amuse the 12-year-old daughter of the King of Spain. The dwarf enjoys being the center of attention and laughter but finally sees his own reflection for the first time in a mirror and dies heartbroken. The late twentieth century reader is likely to consider that the story dwells embarrassingly on the grotesque and monstrous shape of the unfortunate dwarf, and to find such negative views of congenital abnormality unacceptable; for a deaf child born into a hearing family, the conscious realization that he or she is deaf is nevertheless the cause of some distress to that child. Considering the high incidence of intermittent tinnitus in this group of children it is fortunate that the tinnitus is seldom a constant reminder of the handicap of deafness. This chapter has done no more than draw attention to this well-recognized phenomenon of intermittency in childhood tinnitus and to suggest in the broadest terms some possible mechanisms that might be the subject of experimental testing.

REFERENCES

Evans, E.F. 1968. "Cortical Representation." In A.V.S. De Reuck and J. Knight (Eds.), *Hearing Mechanisms in Vertebrates* (Ciba Foundation Symposium), pp. 272–295.

Fowler, E.P. and Fowler, E.P. Jr. 1955. "Somatopsychic and Psychosomatic Factors in Tinnitus, Deafness, and Vertigo." *Annals of Otology, Rhinology and Laryngology, 64,* 29–37.

Glanville, J.D., Coles, R.R.A., and Sullivan, B.M. 1971. "A Family with High-Tonal Objective Tinnitus." *Journal of Laryngology and Otology, 85,* 1–10.

Goodey, R.J. 1981. "Discussion: Tinnitus in Children with Hearing Loss." In *Ciba Foundation Symposium 85,* p. 184. London: Pitman.

Graham, J.M. 1981a. "Paediatric Tinnitus." In Proceedings of First International Tinnitus Seminar, New York, 1979. *Journal of Laryngology and Otology, Supplement 4,* 117–120.

Graham, J.M. 1981b. "Tinnitus in Children with Hearing Loss." In D. Evered and G. Lawrenson (Eds.), *Tinnitus* (Ciba Foundation Symposium 85, p. 172–181. London: Pitman.

Graham, J.M. and Butler, J. 1984. "Tinnitus in Children." In Proceedings of Second International Tinnitus Seminar, New York, 1983. *Journal of Laryngology and Otology, Supplement 9,* 236–241.

Graham, J.M. 1987. "Tinnitus in Hearing-Impaired Children." In J.W.P. Hazell (Ed.), *Tinnitus,* pp. 131–143. Edinburgh: Churchill Livingstone.

Graham J.T. 1965. "Tinnitus Aurium." *Acta Otolaryngologica, Supplement 202.*

Hazell, J.W.P. 1984. "Discussion on Tinnitus Masking." In Proceedings of the Second International Tinnitus Seminar, New York, 1983. *Journal of Laryngology and Otology, Supplement 9,* 253.

Housman, A.E. 1937. In L. Housman, *AEH,* p. 256.

Kemp, D.T. 1981. "Discussion: Tinnitus in Children with Hearing Loss." In *CIBA Foundation 85,* p. 184. London: Pitman.

Meikle, M., Schuff, N., and Griest, S. 1987. "Intra-Subject Variability of Tinnitus: Observations from the Tinnitus Clinic." In H. Feldmann (Ed.), *Proceedings of III International Tinnitus Seminar, Munster, 1987,* pp. 175–180. Karlsruhe: Harsch Verlag.

Mills, R.P., Albert, D.M., and Brain, C.E. 1986. "Tinnitus in Childhood." *Clinical Otolaryngology, 11,* 431–434.

Mills, R.P. and Cherry, J.R. 1984. "Subjective Tinnitus in Children with Hearing Disorders." *International Journal of Paediatric Otorhinolaryngology, 7,* 21–27.

Nodar, R.H. 1972. "Tinnitus Aurium in School-Age Children." *Journal of Auditory Research, 12,* 133–135.

Nodar, R.H. and Le Zak, M.H.W. 1984. "Pediatric Tinnitus (A Thesis Revisited)." In Proceedings of Second International Tinnitus Seminar, New York, 1983. *Journal of Laryngology and Otology, Supplement 9,* 234–235.

Reich, G. 1987. Personal Communication. In J.W.P.

Hazell (Ed.), *Tinnitus,* p. 133. Edinburgh: Churchill Livingstone.

Suga, N., Niwa, H., Taniguchi, I., and Margoliash, D. 1987. "The Personalized Auditory Cortex of the Mustached Bat: Adaptation for Echolocation." *Journal of Neurophysiology, 58,* 643–654.

Thomas, C.H. 1938. "Physical Aspects of Tinnitus." *Journal of Laryngology and Otology, 53,* 68–78.

Venters, R.S. 1953. "Tinnitus Aurium." *Proceedings of the Royal Society of Medicine, 46,* 826–829.

Viani, L.G. 1989. "Tinnitus in Children with Hearing Loss." *Journal of Laryngology and Otology, 103,* 1142–1145.

CHAPTER 7

MODELS OF TINNITUS

GENERATION, PERCEPTION, CLINICAL IMPLICATIONS

JONATHAN W.P. HAZELL

University Hospital ILOF, Middlesex Hospital Annex, London

INTRODUCTION

The information used to construct a clinical model is based on what we learn from our patients and from clinical research programs. This is the real value of such a model. Tinnitus is wholly subjective, a phantom perception (Jastreboff 1990), and those who suffer from it can only enlighten others by describing their experiences as best they can. We must not be fooled into thinking that measurements we make of what we believe are objective correlates of tinnitus (e.g., pitch/loudness/otoacoustic emissions) are measurements of the patient's perception of tinnitus. Neither are they indicators of tinnitus distress, the underlying reason for the consultation.

Models of tinnitus are important, not only for our understanding of its mechanisms but in designing strategies for helping the patient. It is obvious that a total model for tinnitus will be extremely complex. For example, it cannot be concerned only with cochlear mechanisms, although this purely otocentric approach to tinnitus has been fashionable in the past.

At the same time, any model should withstand analysis from a neurophysiological viewpoint, showing that it is consistent with animal and other research data from the auditory system. This model is based primarily on clinical observations made on over 10,000 patients who have attended our tinnitus clinics since 1977, and also on a number of research studies performed during this time (Hazell, Wood, Cooper, Stephens, Corcoran, Coles, Baskill, and Sheldrake 1985; Hazell 1981a,b; Hazell and Wood 1981; Hazell 1987a). However, the editors of this book have invited the authors to muse and be speculative about the mechanisms of tinnitus. The gentle reader should therefore be aware that parts of this chapter are indeed speculative, and unsupported as yet by research or neuroscience data.

In the tinnitus clinic environment patients are not selected on the basis of their pathophysiology, but simply because they hear a noise which appears to be coming from inside the head. In about 7 percent of cases tinnitus is the result of hearing sounds created elsewhere in the head or neck. These include vascular pulsations, palatal and intra-tympanic myoclonus, patulous eustachian tube syndrome, the jugular outflow syndrome, cervical crepitus etc. (Hazell et. al. 1985; Hazell 1981a,b; Hazell and Wood 1981; Hazell 1987a; Ward, Babin, Calcaterra, and Konrad 1975; MacKinnon 1968; Arenberg and McCreary 1971; Glanville, Coles, and Sullivan 1971; Hazell 1990a). These were previously but inappropriately referred to as "objective" tinnitus. We use the term "somatosounds" first devised at the Ciba symposium (Anon, 1981). While tinnitus refers to a perception to which there may be objective correlates, it is *by definition* wholly subjective, and the terms "objective" and "'subjective'" tinnitus must be abandoned.

Tinnitus distress does not depend on generator site. Somatosounds can be just as troublesome as tinnitus of neurophysiological origin. Regardless of the generator, tinnitus always involves the final common pathways of central auditory processing: signal detection, tinnitus perception, and evaluation (see below). Therefore the ideas that have developed about the processing of "neurophysiological" tinnitus (e.g., generated within the cochlea or auditory nerve) also apply to the perception of tinnitus resulting from objective phenomena such as vascular bruits and palatal myoclonus. Although such somatosounds in theory at least, have a pragmatic, surgical, or medical solution, in practice this does not necessarily mean that their eradication is either a straightforward or a trivial matter (Hazell 1990b), and the general mechanisms of tinnitus distress and its treatment need also to be applied in such cases.

I will concentrate on the commonest type of tinnitus, which accounts for over 85 percent of patients attending our tinnitus clinic. For these patients, clinical and research data suggests that tinnitus is generated within the auditory system, that is, at some point between the stapes footplate and the auditory cortex. In this group, patients most commonly complain of high-frequency tones or hisses in one or both ears or somewhere in the head, although in some the perceptions may be numerous and complex.

Eventually many different models will be needed to explain tinnitus arising at different locations within the auditory pathways. But until we can be confident about the exact location of the tinnitus generator in each case, we need some simple overall concepts that take account of the abnormalities of auditory function commonly found in tinnitus patients in clinical practice.

In every patient presenting with tinnitus, it is convenient to think of tinnitus as being composed of four basic components:

1. a tinnitus "generator".
2. a pathway for transmission of the tinnitus signal

3. a subconscious process of signal detection and modulation
4. a conscious episode involving tinnitus perception and evaluation.

This generator may occur in the peripheral or central nervous system, but signal detection, perception, and further cognitive activity related to tinnitus must be central. It is a crucial factor in every single case of tinnitus.

PROBLEM AND NO-PROBLEM TINNITUS

The definition of tinnitus used here is that of a sound perceived for more than five minutes at a time, in the absence of any external acoustical or electrical stimulation of the ear and not occurring immediately after exposure to loud noise. Although approximately 17 percent of the whole population have experienced tinnitus, only 7 percent visit a doctor, and a very much smaller percentage (between 1/2 percent and 1 percent) find the tinnitus continuously distressing and intrusive (Hazell 1990b; Coles 1984, 1987; MRC-IHR 1981, McFadden 1982). This means that the greater proportion of those individuals having the experience of tinnitus either do not find the sound troublesome or rapidly habituate to it.

Our clinical evaluation and audiometric measurements suggest (but cannot prove) that there is no difference in the psychoacoustical properties (as measured audiometrically) or characteristics (as described by the patient) between "problem" and "no-problem" tinnitus (Hazell et al. 1985). These descriptives would include features such as overall duration, periodicity, perceived pitch, apparent loudness, as well as audiometric measurements such as tinnitus loudness balance or tinnitus minimal masking levels, and the like. In addition, many of the patients in our retraining program change from the problem to the no-problem category without any change in the psychoacoustical properties of their tinnitus as measured in the individual patient (Hazell 1990a,b; Hazell, Jastreboff, Meerton, and Conway 1993). Indeed, the difference between these two groups does not appear to be due to changes in the underlying pathophysiology associated with the tinnitus generator and there has usually been no surgical or medical intervention that would be likely to affect the generator. However, patients have received treatment involving specific counseling, and the fitting of auditory prosthetic devices, such as hearing aids or low-level white noise generators (previously referred to as tinnitus maskers), and all but a few patients experience an improvement in their tinnitus. Later we consider what improvement means, and how it is being mediated.

Significance of Tinnitus as a Threat

Patients in the problem group have at some time evaluated their tinnitus as presenting a threat either to their life or to their life quality. To them it may signify the presence of serious pathology such as a brain tumor or impending stroke (potentially life threatening), or a loud noise which will permanently interfere with their concentration, recreational activities and sleep, or simply present as a continual annoyance ("life-quality" threatening). They may imagine they have a condition that will persist forever and for which there is no cure. Many patients believe that tinnitus is the reason that they cannot hear well, or that it may eventually result in total deafness. Many prize the quality of silence whereby they can relax in a quiet environment and be totally free from the intrusiveness of external sounds. For them tinnitus means that this desirable state can no longer be experienced; the tinnitus is a territorial intrusion into their personal, private, and previously silent environment.

Patients in the no-problem group see their tinnitus as being similar to environmental noise around them, as a sound which does not have an any special meaning or significance, and therefore does not attract their attentional focus or interfere with planned thoughts or activities. It is described as being like rain, the sea, running water, or distant church bells. The terms used to describe the tinnitus are themselves benign and may even be associated with pleasant experiences. The tinnitus

is not connected with unpleasant sequelae, or potentially fatal intracranial disease. In such patients there is often a low level of somatic anxiety and they may also have received early, appropriate, and adequate reassurance. Such patients tend to be optimists rather than pessimists (unpublished data). We will enlarge on the clinical and neurophysiological implications of tinnitus threat later in the chapter.

THE MEANING OF SILENCE

Heller and Bergman (1953) performed the classical experiment of taking 100 normally hearing young volunteers into a totally soundproofed room and asking them to describe what they heard. Nearly all identified internally generated sounds, which for some may have been somatosounds. None of these individuals was experiencing tinnitus in a normal environment, that is, in the presence of low-level environmental noise. However, this does demonstrate that tinnitus may be an almost universal experience, depending on the level of background noise present. Many people describe the "sound of silence" that can be heard in a quiet room at night, and consisting of a fairly high-frequency broadband noise heard generally within the head or in both ears. We have had patients who were profoundly distressed by this phenomenon, because of an unshakable belief that this was, or could become, TINNITUS, which they perceived as an incurable disease capable of ruining their lives.

Tinnitus Generators: A Small Abnormality Generating a Weak Signal?

The *patient's* intuitive model for tinnitus generation and perception is usually one of a powerful generator creating a loud, unpleasant, and inescapable barrage of noise. Such models are often expressed by publicity material from tinnitus support groups depicting pictures of tinnitus ears which conceal jackhammers, alarm bells, or train whistles. The not-unreasonable concept is that what we perceive is always a true reflection of the stimulus responsible for the perception. If we hear a loud sound, then something somewhere must be making a loud sound. While this is true for a simple acoustic system like the child's toy consisting of two tin cans with a piece of string stretched between them, the human auditory system is quite different in its construction and infinitely more complex. The need to develop a perceptive mechanism that can selectively pick out sounds of special significance and place them in the center of our attentional focus has resulted, as we shall see, in a powerful process of signal enhancement that can work for us or against us.

Clinical observations suggest that the tinnitus generator, far from being a powerful source of neural energy, is more likely a very weak signal generated often by a relatively small disturbance in the auditory system (Jastreboff 1990; Hazell and Jastreboff 1990; Hazell et al. 1993). This would account for the general failure of attempts to identify objective correlates of tinnitus. We do not find significant asymmetry in the ABR except in grouped data (Jastreboff, Ikner, and Hassen 1992), tinnitus is not derived from an otoacoustic emission except in rare circumstances (Penner 1989a,b; Penner and Burns 1987), it cannot be detected in auditory nerve random activity (Sininger, Eggermont, and King 1992), or (disappointingly) in magnetic evoked cortical potentials (Colding-Jorgensen, Lauritzen, Johnsen, Mikkelson, and Saermark 1992).

Despite the fact that many patients with troublesome tinnitus describe it as much louder than external sounds, loudness balance measurements consistently suggest that tinnitus is perceived as being equivalent to an external sound of less than 10 dB sensation level (SL). Frequently it may be as little as 2 or 3 dB SL, even taking into account the narrow dynamic range that may occur at the tinnitus frequency (Tyler and Stouffer 1989; Tyler and Conrad-Armes 1983; Goodwin and Johnson 1980a,b; Hulshof 1986).

Random Activity Means Silence

Møller's model of a retrocochlear tinnitus generator (Møller 1984) states that in the normal ear there is random background activity in auditory nerve fibers, in the absence of external auditory stimulation. This activity is random (or chaotic) in one afferent neuron with respect to time, and also at the same time with respect to other afferent fibers. This is the "code for silence". Synchrony of firing of afferent fibers is associated with the perception of sound. Anything in the auditory pathway that could interfere with random activity, resulting in an identifiable pattern, might be perceived as phantom auditory sensation: tinnitus.

Although the clinical observations which led to Møller's hypothesis were of pressure on the auditory nerve by arteries in the internal auditory meatus, interference with this random activity could take place anywhere in the auditory nerve, leading to signal generations finally perceived as tinnitus. Only very small variations from random (or chaotic) activity need be present to result in tinnitus detection if we postulate a powerful meaning-based central mechanism for signal detection and pattern recognition.

PERIPHERAL VERSUS CENTRAL

The common simplistic approach of trying to assign tinnitus to either a "peripheral" or a "central" site is limiting and inaccurate, and by definition there must always be a central perceptive component. At the present moment there is no test to accurately identify the site of tinnitus generation. The only case where we may state with confidence that there is NOT an endorgan component is following bilateral acoustic nerve section. Every scheme so far for assigning a site to tinnitus makes assumptions about its pathophysiology which are not yet known, and usually disregards the effects of higher centers in auditory processing, perception, evaluation, and cognitive input.

Where there is obvious pathology affecting part of the auditory tract (e.g., unilateral sensory deafness, or otosclerosis), it is tempting to place the generator at the site of known pathology, particularly when both are on the same side. In most cases it seems inevitable that such pathologies will result in irregularities or nonlinearities in the cochlea, modulating neural activity and becoming potential tinnitus generators. At the very least, such cochlear abnormalities have the potential to cause a disturbance in the "code for silence".

As we shall see later, where such nonlinearities reflect alterations in cochlear micromechanics, we might also suspect that fluctuations of efferent tone could result in modulation of these potential tinnitus signals via efferent innervation of outer hair cells (OHC), and inner hair cell (IHC) afferent nerve fibers (Hazell 1987a; Hazell and Jastreboff 1990).

Tinnitus Onset Triggers

It is interesting that tinnitus onset often postdates by some years the appearance of abnormalities in the pure-tone audiogram, that is, a high-frequency hearing loss, with which it is often associated on the basis of perceived pitch, and/or laterality. The tinnitus onset "trigger" is far more often an unrelated event such as emotional stress—for example, a bereavement, or intercurrent illness or surgery (not necessarily otosurgery). It is likely that fluctuation of mood, acute anxiety, or depression, which bring about changes in the overall state of arousal, result in the very first moment of perception of the weak signal from the tinnitus generator. This idea might help to explain why one-third of those with abnormal audiograms, even with profound deafness, experience no tinnitus at all. Clearly it is not simply a matter of what is happening in the periphery whether or not tinnitus is perceived. In the absence of an appropriate change in arousal state, tinnitus could remain undetected, despite the presence of marked nonlinearities in the periphery. However, under other circumstances of fluctuation in emotional state with arousal enhancement, these nonlinearities could give rise to the detection and perception of subsequently annoying tinnitus.

Where auditory signals result from external sounds, there is extensive signal processing before perception occurs. It is naive to think that tinnitus signals will not be subjected to the same augmentation and modulation as externally generated sound.

Indeed, it is our feeling that internally generated sounds may be subjected to special processing in the central auditory pathways, identifying them as separate entities to external sound. Detection of externally generated signals must remain the first priority and objective of the healthy auditory system. Therefore it is probable that special mechanisms exist to suppress the detection of internal noise (tinnitus) in an attempt to produce the best signal to noise ratio for external sound perception.

One possible mechanism could involve interaction between the vestibular and auditory systems. Vestibular connections with the auditory system are integrated to check the relationship between head/body movement and the change of location of external sound sources as measured by binaural phase and loudness alteration. Where head movement resulted in no such phase or loudness change (because the signal was generated within the auditory system) then a mismatch between vestibular input and binaural auditory phase and loudness information could identify that particular auditory signal as "internally generated" and actively suppress it. While this is a fanciful idea, it might account for the not uncommon clinical experience of patients whose tinnitus changes in loudness or quality with small head movement, and sometimes with eye movement. (Lovely, Cacace, Winter, and Parnes 1993; Wall, Rosenberg, and Richardson 1987).

The Role of Cochlear Tinnitus Generators

We have previously described a model for a tinnitus generator in the cochlea associated with high-frequency hearing loss (Hazell 1987a; Hazell and Jastreboff 1990). This is based on the frequent finding in our clinic of tinnitus patients with symmetrical high-frequency hearing loss due to degeneration of hair cells (principally OHC) in the basal turn of the cochlea (Soucek, Michaels, and Frohlich 1986, 1987). It is now well established that the cochlea is not simply a passive receptor of sound, but has a high energy requirement resulting in intrinsic mechanical and electrical activity, particularly in the OHC, without which much of its sensitivity and frequency selectivity is lost.

The OHC have an active role in reducing the damping of the basilar membrane (BM) to allow detection of low-energy sound close to the threshold of human hearing. It is well established that the OHC have the ability to undergo a relatively slow contractile process to about four-fifths of their maximum length (Holley and Ashmore 1988; Brownell, Imredy, and Shehata 1990; Zenner and Plinkert 1992), and by a different mechanism can perform very fast vibratory movements up to 10K/sec or more (Ashmore 1987; Brownell 1984). It is well established that this activity alters the dynamics within the cochlea, but precisely how, and what effect this may have on any tinnitus that may be generated there, is still a matter of conjecture and one which has been addressed by other authors in this book (see chapters 11, 15, and 18). Some authors suggest that the OHC transfer their fast vibratory energy directly to the BM (like tiny gymnasts bouncing on a trampoline) (Zenner, Arnold, and Gitter 1988; Plinkert, Gitter, and Zenner 1990; Ashmore 1987; Brownell, Zidanic, and Spirou 1986). Another approach suggests that OHC achieve their amplifier-like effect by changing the working point on the BM as a result of the slow contractile movement (LePage 1987, 1989; Zenner et al. 1988). The two mechanisms are not mutually exclusive (Jastreboff 1990).

The efferent system undoubtably has a role in controling cochlear function both through OHC via the medial olivocochlear bundle (MOCB), and the lateral olivocochlear bundle (LOCB) which synapses at the side of the afferent nerve fiber just below the IHC. Stimulation of the crossed efferent fibers can be performed electrically in the anesthetized laboratory animal, or in humans with low-level acoustic stimulation of the contralateral ear. With such stimulation, changes occur in 2f1-f2 distortion products (Puel and Rebillard 1990; Moulin, Collet, and Morgon 1992; Siegel, Kim, and Molnar 1982), click-evoked otoacoustic emissions (Puel and Rebillard 1990; Moulin et al. 1992; Siegel et al. 1982; Abe, Tsuiki, Ito, Endo, Suzuki, and O-Uchi 1990; Collet, Kemp, Veuillet, Duclaux, Moulin, and Morgan 1990; Ryan,

Kemp, and Hinchcliffe 1991; Maurer, Beck, Mann, and Mintert 1992), cochlear microphonics (CM) and the whole nerve action potential (CAP) (Puel and Rebillard 1990; Moulin et al. 1992; Siegel et al. 1982; Abe et al. 1990; Collet et al. 1990; Ryan et al. 1991; Maurer et al. 1992; Bonfils, Remond, and Pujol 1986; Kawase and Liberman 1992; Veuillet, Collet, Disant, and Morgan 1991; Hildesheimer, Makai, Muchnik, and Rubinstein 1990; Patuzzi and Rajan 1990; LePage 1989; Warren and Liberman, 1989a,b; Bonfils and Puel 1987; Folsom and Owsley 1987). It is clear that the efferents play an important role in modulating cochlear activity and are likely to influence the resulting patterns generated in the afferent nerve fibers. Thus, nonlinearities in the cochlea, potential tinnitus generators, and the neural signals that they generate (however weak) are also likely to be modulated by changes in efferent activity.

Clinical Considerations

The microstructure of the normally hearing human audiogram shows numerous irregularities (Kemp, 1979). Peaks of sensitivity are sometimes associated with the experience of tonal tinnitus. In very rare cases spontaneous otoacoustic emissions can be shown to be an objective correlate of annoying tinnitus (Penner, 1988, 1989a).

In the cochlear model already described (Hazell 1987a), mild to moderate degrees of high-frequency hearing loss resulting from OHC degeneration principally as a result of a normal aging process are associated with a high-frequency tonal or narrowband type of tinnitus. The frequency of the tinnitus is often found adjacent to the area of maximum hearing loss, although accurate frequency discrimination of tinnitus is not a simple task (Penner 1983). The generation of a random pattern for silence by the cochlea depends on the absence of any marked variations in cochlear activity from one part of the BM to another. Any localized alteration in the physical property of the basilar membrane or change in the activity of OHC at any point could result in an area of changed sensitivity (increased or decreased). In addition, Tonndorf has already proposed that decoupling of the hair cell stereocilia from the tectorial membrane would result in a significant increase (up to 30dB) of thermal noise in the cochlea (Tonndorf 1981).

Any of these events could result in alterations in the pattern of neural activity in afferent auditory nerve fibers which could, in turn, give rise to phantom perceptions.

The Efferent System: Possible Effects on Tinnitus Generation

The MOCB principally innervates the OHC at a ratio of 1 fiber to roughly 50 OHC. The idea that the efferent system works as a feedback loop for adjusting auditory sensitivity was first proposed by Fex (1959). Applying sound to one ear in an experimental animal increases the overall neural activity in the MOCB and this can have a frequency specific reduction of the AP in the contralateral ear (Warren and Liberman 1989a,b).

We have previously described mechanisms by which the efferent system could be involved in modulation of potential tinnitus generators, and might give rise to certain forms of tinnitus de novo (Hazell 1987a; Hazell and Jastreboff 1990). Electrical and acoustical stimulation of the COCB in animals results in an increase of CM, and a reduced AP (Wiederhold and Kiang 1970; Rajan and Johnstone 1988). This is a frequency specific effect (Igarashi, Cranford, Allen, and Alford 1979; Gifford and Guinan 1983). Efferent neurons are frequency specific, that is, have characteristic frequencies like their afferent neighbors. This implies that there is a frequency specific control mechanism for the cochlea which is mediated through the MOCB to the OHC, and also probably through modification of afferent nerve fiber activity via the LOCB. The effect via the OCB is primarily one of inhibition. Increased activity in the OCB results in a reduction of the AP and an increase in the CM.

OHC begin to degenerate from early life (Wright, Davies, Bredberg, Ulehova, and Spencer

1987), although up to 30 percent may be lost without a measurable change in the pure-tone audiogram (Bohne and Clark 1982). As part of the aging process, increasing numbers of OHC disappear, particularly in the basal turn of the cochlea.

The hypothesis is that irregularities in OHC population along the BM result in nonlinearities in micromechanical activity. This could affect both fast and slow components of OHC motility, or result in areas on the BM where OHC activity was largely absent. This results in local changes in the damping of basilar membrane activity along its length with consequent fluctuations in IHC input and afferent nerve fiber activity from point to point. By itself this could interfere with the random "code for silence", creating tinnitus.

A further possibility is that efferent feedback to the cochlea results in MOCB activity intended to "correct" such nonlinearities. Reduced OHC activity is associated with an increased auditory threshold which could itself result in a localized area of efferent dysinhibition through this feedback loop. The idea of such a feedback loop was first proposed by Fex (1959). The innervation of OHC is in the ratio of some 50 OHC to one fiber in the MOCB. Therefore, some OHC adjacent to an area of damage could be exposed to inappropriate dysinhibition by the MOCB, resulting in overactivity of normal OHC adjacent to an area of damage with an enhancement or amplification of a small frequency band within the cochlea. In other words preexisting nonlinearities within the cochlear amplifier due to (minimal) OHC degeneration could be made more marked by efferent feedback. Overall changes in efferent tone (e.g., on waking) could have a short term effect on cochlear tinnitus generators. If this mechanism proved important, then one future therapeutic approach might be a pharmacological attack to try to modulate efferent function.

Autonomic Influence on Efferent Function

The fibers of the efferent system originate in the reticular formation of the brainstem, the control center for the autonomic nervous system, and the reticular activating system that maintains conscious awareness. One of the efferent neurotransmitters has been identified as acetylcholine (Housley and Ashmore 1991; Eybalin and Altschuler 1990; Kujawa, Glattke, Fallon, and Bobbin 1992), which is also found in the parasympathetic nervous system. The frequent clinical finding that tinnitus onset and fluctuation occurs during periods of emotional lability led us several years ago to the hypothesis that the efferent system could be a pathway between the autonomic centers and the cochlea (Hazell 1987a).

Effects of Central Processing

Whatever the peripheral generator, and it is likely that many mechanisms are implicated at one or another time, it is clear that such signals are very weak compared to those generated by the high energies and broad frequency spectra of everyday environmental sounds, many of which do not reach our consciousness, or are easily and consistently ignored. In addition, tinnitus probably never wakes us from sleep (though it may be very evident immediately on waking), and is frequently easily masked by low levels of environmental sound. Nevertheless, the distressed patient's *perception* of tinnitus is of a loud and unpleasant noise constantly in the center of the attentional focus. To understand this, we need to look at the role of central auditory processing in enhancement of the tinnitus signal.

For externally generated sounds, patterns of activity in the auditory nerve reflect the pattern of frequencies arriving at the tympanic membrane, and subsequently at the cochlea, at any one time. The cochlea performs a frequency analysis of complex sounds which are encoded as action potentials (AP) in each afferent fiber of the auditory nerve, depending on its characteristic frequency. The CAP consists of information on all frequency components carried in the auditory nerve. These encoded patterns will ultimately reach the auditory subcortex in the temporal lobe, where sound

perception occurs. However, during the 300 msecs between the cochlear and acoustic nerve response and our conscious perception, much signal processing occurs. This has a profound effect on which sounds we hear, and how we hear them. This powerful mechanism also processes the signals of internally generator sounds (tinnitus generators), and plays a major part, perhaps the major part, in what tinnitus sounds like to the individual, and the effect it has as a potential complaint.

Signal Detection

Signal detection in the auditory system is the ability to identify the relevant pattern of electrical activity and extract it from other signals and unwanted background noise. Such pattern recognition starts at quite a low level in the central auditory pathways, well before conscious perception of sound occurs. An example of this would be binaural interaction at the cochlear nucleus level concerned with sound localization. It is beyond the scope of this chapter to elaborate at length on these complex processes when more extensive monographs and comprehensive textbooks should be consulted (Jastreboff 1990; Pribram 1971, 1987; Pickles 1988; Goldman-Rakic, 1988, 1989).

Theories of signal detection do have a relevance to tinnitus. The neural networks involved in identifying signal patterns allow for the enhanced detection of such signals once they have been identified and classified in terms of significance and importance (Carpenter and Grossberg 1987; Grossberg 1987). Such a process involves learning (e.g., as with constant attention to a signal such as tinnitus). This learning process is able to establish through these neuronal networks and their inherent plasticity (ability to change functionally and physically) the facilitated detection and transmission of even extremely weak signals.

Tinnitus Perception and Evaluation

Perception of sound occurs in the subcortex of the temporal lobe. The conscious act of hearing any sound involves a process of pattern matching and pattern recognition. Patterns of electrical activity reaching the subcortex must be matched with patterns stored previously in auditory memory. The absence of memory patterns means that normal audition is impossible. This is one of the reasons for the failure of cochlear implants in adult prelingually totally deaf individuals (and in whom tinnitus is a rarity). However, in a hearing person, once a memory pattern has been established, a match may be made very easily by presenting the ear with the original sound used to establish the memory (or even something similar to it). Indeed, in adult postlingually deafened subjects who receive cochlear implants, relatively crude electrical representations of speech used to stimulate the cochlear nerve may initially sound most unspeech-like, but with learning eventually become almost indistinguishable from the memories of sound pre-dating the onset of deafness. In this situation a learning process allows one auditory signal to evoke a very different memory pattern. A similar mechanism is required to understand speech where strong foreign accents are being experienced.

These are examples of plasticity in the subcortex, *and indicate that perception is far from an invariate function of stimulus*. It may also account for the persistence of identical tinnitus after acoustic nerve section, or successful surgery to relieve conductive deafness.

Cognitive Factors

Various sensory perceptions are suppressed when they are deemed uninformative. For instance, we may feel our clothes as we put them on in the morning, but during the day have no conscious awareness of the signals being transmitted by millions of sensory nerve fibers from the skin. In auditory perception, the loudness and intrusiveness of external sounds can also be altered by cognitive function. The sound of our own name being called, even quietly in a noisy environment, can have a profoundly distracting effect, whereas someone else's name passes unnoticed. The sound of a television set

through the wall is perceived as much less intrusive when it belongs to a much loved elderly relative (perhaps slightly hearing impaired!), than an unpleasant and antisocial neighbor to whom a dislike has already been taken.

Therefore, learned significance and meaning can strengthen and increase the perception of even very weak signals. This has an important role in the detection and perception of tinnitus.

The Survival Reflex and Warning Signals

In the process of evolution, we have developed the ability to detect patterns of sound of very low energy even when immersed in a background of loud environmental noise. Such an ability is essential to survival in the avoidance of predators. Successful predators make very little noise and are often visually camouflaged as well. To avoid such threats to life requires the detection of extremely small auditory and visual signals. This ability is rapidly developed by natural selection, as failure to detect predators usually results in the animal's death. It will also allow the enhanced detection of any weak signal in noise, provided it has appropriate meaning or significance.

The establishment of the survival response to such threats and warning signals involves high-level central auditory mechanisms, cognitive and learning processes, although some parts of this response may be genetically determined. The reflex may be modified by emotional state, and changes in arousal dependent on anxiety or mood swing may sensitize the response. The response may also be altered in the light of further experience and learning, or a change of environment. Despite the involvement of complex cognitive mechanisms in the establishment of the reflex, it is essential that the orienting response to such danger be immediate and invariate, and not reversed by anything but a lengthy process of relearning which factors constitute danger.

The neurophysiological basis for this mechanism is sound. Subcortical perception is influenced by extensive projections from the limbic system (concerned with emotion and learning) and from the prefrontal cortex (concerned with behavior) (Goldman-Rakic 1988, 1989; Pribram 1971, 1987). Therefore, what we perceive, how we perceive it (or whether we perceive it at all), and in what way the further process of evaluation affects our response to that perception is determined by the strong influence of these subconscious centers. At the same time these centers are learning, or being programmed by conscious experience and thought, and subsequently dictate response of the individual to all kinds of sensory information.

Tinnitus and the Survival Reflex

The enhanced perception hypothesis sees tinnitus as evoking a response similar to the survival reflex, and there is good clinical evidence for this. Where tinnitus is distressing, it is invariably identified as a threat, either to life, or to life quality. The sudden onset of noise in the head most reasonably provokes anxiety about the possibility of brain tumors, strokes, or impending madness and possible suicide. Often these fears are enhanced by early inappropriate counseling, unqualified by any further explanation for the phenomenon.

Tinnitus patients are frequently told "You'll have to have a brain scan to exclude an acoustic neuroma"; "Tinnitus is due to blockage of an artery in the ear"; "When you are totally deaf the tinnitus will disappear" (untrue) and "You're obviously distressed and need to see a psychiatrist". The belief that tinnitus is incurable is further enhanced by negative counseling, such as, "There is no cure", "Nothing can be done", "Learn to live with it". While such comments seem to be appropriate in a straightforward medical approach, and reflect the teaching about tinnitus management received by the professional person during training, they simply confirm the patient's worst fears and activate what can become an unshakable belief that tinnitus is a serious disease.

Furthermore, the exhibition of interventionist, unproven, empirical therapies ("take these tablets and come back in three weeks") further reinforces the concept that no effective treatment is avail-

able. On close questioning in our clinic, it is often seen that tinnitus *only* becomes loud, intrusive, and problematical after such interviews or experiences. In these cases, the tinnitus distress must be considered an iatrogenic illness.

Whether the weak tinnitus signal is seen as a life threat or a life-quality threat, or indeed to possess any negative qualities, the powerful signal detection and pattern enhancement mechanism (developed to detect potential predators in the wild) is able to maintain tinnitus perception in the center of the patient's attentional focus. Constant monitoring of tinnitus, either by diary keeping, or simply in an attempt to obtain reassurance that it isn't getting any worse, acts as a training and reinforcement program to ensure that tinnitus perception persists, and often becomes stronger. A similar process of (usually harmless) nonhabituation occurs in professionals (e.g., otolaryngologists, audiologists) who continually monitor their tinnitus out of academic curiosity!

This model predicts our clinical experience—that tinnitus perception habituates with time, provided that there are no negative beliefs associated with it. The eradication of these beliefs by specific counseling techniques (Hazell 1990b; Hazell et al. 1993) can on their own be enough to permanently remove tinnitus perception. As expected, tinnitus of long duration has very well established and highly facilitated signal detection and pattern extraction. In some cases it may not be possible to completely reverse these processes, even with the patient's full cooperation, and naturally many remain highly skeptical that such a process is possible at all. However, in almost all cases, even of long-standing troublesome tinnitus, we are able to remove the unpleasant secondary effects of autonomic and limbic system response, even though the tinnitus remains as a continuous, though quite benign perception.

Emotional Response to Tinnitus and Distress Mechanisms

The neurophysiological interaction of the limbic system and prefrontal cortex with auditory perception is a two-way process. Most sounds—music, laughter, alarm bells—evoke an emotional response from us, sometimes a very strong one. Some sounds are intrinsically and universally unpleasant, like chalk scratching the blackboard. Our clinical experience is that distressing tinnitus frequently results in alteration in mood, usually anxiety and depression, and that these conditions often predate tinnitus onset (House 1981; Stephens and Hallam 1985; Lindberg, Scott, Melin, and Lyttkens 1987; Harrop-Griffiths, Katon, Dobie, Sakai, and Russo 1987; Sullivan, Katon, Dobie, Sakai, Russo, and Harrop-Griffiths 1988; Halford and Anderson 1991). Other emotions may become involved in a complex interaction with tinnitus. In a study of 54 patients with unilateral deafness and severe tinnitus, we found that 41 percent had had failed otosurgery (an otherwise very rare cause of unilateral dead ear). The cause of their distress was strongly related to anger about the surgeon, and guilt about submitting to the procedure (Hazell, von Schoenberg, Meerton, and Sheldrake 1992). Behavioral therapy focused on these emotional issues was very beneficial in reducing tinnitus perception and annoyance.

Many tinnitus patients complain of hyperacusis, we have shown that this is part of a central mechanism of abnormal gain control which can be reversed by low-level white noise therapy (Hazell and Sheldrake 1992). In many cases, the environmental sounds evoking sensitivity and discomfort are remarkably similar in quality or perceived frequency to the annoying tinnitus. The sensitivity and discomfort improves (indicated by a reduction in measured loudness discomfort levels) as tinnitus perception reduces with retraining and the use of low-level white noise therapy, but only over some months (Hazell and Sheldrake 1992). It is clear that not only does tinnitus act as a warning signal, but so do other sounds in the environment similar to it. This supports the hypothesis that both the environmental hypersensitivity and the tinnitus distress are due to a shared central mechanism. In 45 percent of the patients in our study, hyperacusis was present before tinnitus developed, suggesting that preexisting abnormal gain in

the central auditory system may predispose to tinnitus perception. This could open an approach to tinnitus prevention or prophylaxis.

Eradicating Tinnitus Perception

Our multidisciplinary holistic approach to tinnitus treatment has developed over a period of years, and our techniques and earlier results are published elsewhere (Hazell 1990b; Sheldrake and Hazell 1992; Hazell 1987b; Hazell et al. 1993). It consists of a process of retraining, in which we aim to

1. alter nonlinearities in the cochlea usually identified on the audiogram and treated with appropriate hearing aids
2. interfere with signal detection and pattern matching using *low levels* of broadband white noise from portable ear-level devices
3. alter beliefs about the meaning of tinnitus and its associations by directive counseling
4. modulate autonomic and limbic system responses to tinnitus perception by behavioral techniques and occasionally antidepressants

From this model it will be clear that changing strongly held beliefs about the negative properties of tinnitus is essential to the success of any strategy. In addition, we use low-level white noise generators (previously referred to as tinnitus maskers) to reduce the detection of weak tinnitus signals. As predicted by neuroscience, to be effective these devices should emit broad spectrum white noise, and be used at a sensation level just above threshold for extended periods of time. It is important to be aware that making tinnitus inaudible by so-called "masking devices" is counterproductive in this retraining process, where it is important to be able to detect the object about which retraining is taking place. Our expectation is now to remove the perception of tinnitus totally and permanently in about 30 percent of cases, although this process can take twelve to eighteen months, depending on the duration of tinnitus and the strength of the individual's negative beliefs. In all cases, it appears possible over this time to remove the unpleasant secondary autonomic responses associated with tinnitus perception.

We also have a number of patients (>10) who have used masking devices continuously from the early days of our tinnitus clinic (Hazell and Wood 1981) as a means of obliterating tinnitus perception, quite literally as maskers. Such devices have been worn at high output levels for more than fifteen years in some cases. Although no more than age-related changes in hearing have occurred, on removing the masker the tinnitus remains at its original intensity level, and with the same annoyance as before. None had received any counseling in the significance of tinnitus meaning or belief. We are now entering these patients into a retraining program with low-level white noise therapy and directive counseling with early good effects in the reduction of tinnitus annoyance levels. These initial findings support the hypothesis that beliefs about tinnitus and its meaning are extremely powerful factors in potentiating detection and perception of the tinnitus signal.

These models have been developed in an attempt to understand the mechanisms involved in tinnitus distress, and have proved instrumental in directing our retraining program for dealing with tinnitus. In a simplified form, the models are extensively used in the retraining of our patients about the mechanisms of tinnitus and in particular in reinforcing its benign nature.

I am most grateful to Dr. Rena Graham for (among many things) her critical reading of this manuscript. J.W.P. Hazell is supported by grant no 621-089 from the Royal National Institute for Deaf People, London, U.K.

REFERENCES

Abe, T., Tsuiki, T., Ito, S., Endo, Y., Suzuki, K., and O-Uchi, T. 1990. "Suppression of Evoked Otoacoustic Emissions by Contralateral Noise Exposure in Humans." *Nippon Jibiinkoka Gakkai Kaiho, 93*,1890–1897.

Anon. 1981. "Definition and classification of tinnitus." *Ciba Foundation Symposium 1981,* 300–302.

Arenberg, I.K. and McCreary, H.S. 1971. "Objective Tinnitus Aurium and Dural Arteriovenous Malformations of the Posterior Fossa." *Annals of Otology, Rhinology and Laryngology, 80,* 111–120.

Ashmore, J.F. 1984. "A Fast Motile Response in Guinea-Pig Outer Hair Cells: The Cellular Basis of the Cochlear Amplifier." *Journal of Physiology, 388,* 323–347.

Bohne, B.A. and Clark, W.W. 1982. "Growth of Hearing Loss and Cochlear Lesion with Increasing Duration of Noise Exposure." In R.P. Hamernik, D. Henderson, and R. Salvi (Eds.), *New Perspectives on Noise-Induced Hearing Loss,* pp. 283–302. New York: Raven Press.

Bonfils, P. and Puel, J.-L. 1987. "Functional Properties of the Crossed Part of the Medial Olivo-cochlear Bundle." *Hearing Research, 28,* 125–130.

Bonfils, P., Remond, M., and Pujol, R. 1986. "Efferent Tracts and Cochlear Frequency Selectivity." *Hearing Research, 24,* 277–283.

Brownell, W.E. 1984. "Microscopic Observation of Cochlear Hair Cell Motility." *Scanning Electron Microscope, 3,* 1401–1406.

Brownell, W.E., Zidanic, M., and Spirou, G.A. 1986. Standing Currents and Their Modulation in the Cochlea. In R.A. Altschuler, R.P. Bobbin, and D.W. Hoffman (Eds.), *Neurobiology of Hearing: The Cochlea,* pp. 91–107. New York: Raven Press.

Brownell, W.E., Imredy, J.P., and Shehata, W.E. 1990. "Slow Passive Length Changes in Isolated Outer Hair Cells." (Abstract) Association for Research in Otolaryngology, p. 28.

Carpenter, G.A. and Grossberg, S. 1987. "Neural Dynamics of Category Learning and Recognition: Attention, Memory Consolidation, and Amnesia." In S. Grossberg (Ed.), *The Adaptive Brain I: Cognition, Learning, Reinforcement, and Rhythm,* pp. 239–286. Amsterdam: Elsevier Science Publishers B.V.

Colding-Jorgensen, E., Lauritzen, M., Johnsen, N.J., Mikkelsen, K.B. and Saermark, K. 1992. "On the Auditory Evoked Magnetic P200 Peak as an Objective Measure of Tinnitus." In J.-M. Aran and R. Dauman (Eds.), *Proceedings of the Fourth International Tinnitus Seminar, Bordeaux, France, 1991,* pp. 321–326. Amsterdam/New York: Kugler Publications.

Coles, R.R. 1984. "Epidemiology of Tinnitus: (1) Prevalence." *Journal of Laryngology and Otology, Supplement, 9,* 7–15.

Coles, R.R.A. 1987. "Epidemiology of Tinnitus." In J.W.P. Hazell (Ed.), *Tinnitus*, pp. 46–70. Edinburgh: Churchill Livingstone.

Collet, L., Kemp, D.T., Veuillet, E., Duclaux, R., Moulin, A., and Morgan, A. 1990. "Effect of Contralateral Auditory Stimuli on Active Cochlear Micro-mechanical Properties in Humans." *Hearing Research, 43,* 251–262.

Eybalin, M. and Altschuler, R.A. 1990. "Immuno-electron Microscopic Localization of Neurotransmitters in the Cochlea." *Journal of Electron Microscope Technology, 15,* 209–224.

Fex, J. 1959. "Augmentation of the Cochlear Microphonics by Stimulation of Efferent Fibres to Cochlea." *Acta Otolaryngologica, 50,* 540–541.

Folsom, R.C. and Owsley, R.M. 1987. "N1 Action Potentials in Humans; Influence of Stimultaneous Contralateral Stimulation." *Acta Otolaryngologica (Stockholm) 103,* 262–265.

Gifford, M.L. and Guinan, J.J. 1983. "Effects of Crossed-Olivocochlear-Bundle Stimulation on Cat Auditory Nerve Fiber Responses to Tones." *Journal of the Acoustical Society of America, 74,* 115–123.

Glanville, J.D., Coles, R.R., and Sullivan, B.M. 1971. "A Family with High-Tonal Objective Tinnitus." *Journal of Laryngology and Otology, 85,* 1–10.

Goldman-Rakic, P.S. 1988. "Topography of Cognition: Parallel Distributed Networks in Primate Association Cortex." *Annual Review of Neuroscience, 11,* 137–156.

Goldman-Rakic, P.S. 1989. "Circuitry of Primate Prefrontal Cortex and Regulation of Behavior by Representational Memory." In *Handbook of Physiology, Vol V: The Nervous System - Higher Functions of the Brain*, pp. 373–417. Bethesda, MD: American Physiological Society.

Goodwin, P.E. and Johnson, R.M. 1980b. "The Loudness of Tinnitus." *Acta Otolaryngologica (Stockholm) 90,* 353–359.

Goodwin, P.E. and Johnson, R.M. 1980a. "A Comparison of Reaction Times to Tinnitus and Nontinnitus Frequencies." *Ear and Hearing, 1,* 148–155.

Grossberg, S. 1987. "The Adaptive Self-Organization of Serial Order in Behavior: Speech, Language, and Motor Control." In S. Grossberg (Ed.), *The Adaptive Brain II: Vision, Speech, Language, and Motor Control*, p. 313–400. Amsterdam: Elsevier Science Publishers B.V.

Halford, J.B. and Anderson, S.D. 1991. "Anxiety and Depression in Tinnitus Sufferers." *Journal of Psychosomatic Research, 35,* 383–390.

Harrop-Griffiths, J., Katon, W., Dobie, R., Sakai, C., and Russo, J. 1987. "Chronic Tinnitus: Association with Psychiatric Diagnoses." *Journal of Psychosomatic Research, 31,* 613–621.

Hazell, J.W. 1981a. "A Tinnitus Synthesizer Physiological Considerations." *Journal of Laryngology and Otology, Supplement,* 187-195.

Hazell, J.W. 1981b. "Patterns of Tinnitus: Medical Audiologic Findings." *Journal of Laryngology and Otology, Supplement,* 39–47.

Hazell, J.W.P. 1987a. "A Cochlear Model for Tinnitus." In H. Feldmann (Ed.), *Proceedings III International Tinnitus Seminar, Munster, 1987,* pp. 121–128. Karlsruhe: Harsch Verlag.

Hazell, J.W.P. 1987b. "Tinnitus Masking—Is It Better than Counselling Alone?" In H. Feldmann (Ed.), *Proceedings III International Tinnitus Seminar, Munster, 1987,* pp. 239–250. Karlsruhe: Harsch Verlag.

Hazell, J.W. 1990a. "Tinnitus. II: Surgical Management of Conditions Associated with Tinnitus and Somatosounds." *Journal of Otolaryngology, 19,* 6–10.

Hazell, J.W. 1990b. "Tinnitus. III: The practical management of sensorineural tinnitus." *Journal of Otolaryngology, 19,* 11–18.

Hazell, J.W. and Jastreboff, P.J. 1990. "Tinnitus. I: Auditory Mechanisms: A Model for Tinnitus and Hearing Impairment." *Journal of Otolaryngology 19,* 1–5.

Hazell, J.W.P., Jastreboff, P.J., Meerton, L.E., and Conway, M.J. 1993. "Electrical Tinnitus Suppression: Frequency Dependence of the Effects." *Audiology, 32,* 68–77.

Hazell, J.W.P. and Sheldrake, J.B. 1992. "Hyperacusis and Tinnitus." In J.M. Aran and R. Dauman (Eds.), *Proceedings of the Fourth International Tinnitus Seminar, Bordeaux, 1991,* pp. 245–248. Amsterdam/New York: Kugler Publications.

Hazell, J.W., von Schoenberg, L.J, Meerton, L.J and Sheldrake, J.B. 1992. "Tinnitus and the Unilateral Dead Ear." In *Proceedings of the Fourth International Tinnitus Seminar, Bordeaux, 1991,* pp. 261–264. Amsterdam/New York: Kugler Publications.

Hazell, J.W. and Wood, S. 1981. "Tinnitus Masking—A Significant Contribution to Tinnitus Management." *British Journal of Audiology, 15,* 223–230.

Hazell, J.W., Wood, S.M., Cooper, H.R., Stephens,

S.D., Corcoran, A.L., Coles, R.R., Baskill, J.L., and Sheldrake, J.B. 1985. "A Clinical Study of Tinnitus Maskers." *British Journal of Audiology, 19,* 65–146.

Heller, M.F. and Bergman, M. 1953. "Tinnitus in Normally Hearing Persons." *Annals of Otology, 62,* 73–83.

Hildesheimer, M., Makai, E., Muchnik, C., and Rubinstein, M. 1990. "The Influence of the Efferent System on Acoustic Overstimulation." *Hearing Research, 43*(2–3), 263–267.

Holley, M.C. and Ashmore, J.F. 19488. "A Cytoskeletal Spring in Cochlear Outer Hair Cells." Nature, 355, 635–637.

House, P.R. 1981. "Personality of the Tinnitus Patient." *Ciba Foundation Symposium 1981, 85,* 193–203.

Housley, G.D. and Ashmore, J.F. 1991. "Direct Measurement of the Action of Acetylcholine on Isolated Outer Hair Cells of the Guinea Pig Cochlea." *Proceedings of the Royal Society of London [Biology], 244,* 161–167.

Hulshof, J.H. 1986. "The Loudness of Tinnitus." *Acta Otolaryngologica (Stockholm) 102,* 40–43.

Igarashi, M., Cranford, J.L., Allen, E.A., and Alford, B.R. 1979. "Behavioral Auditory Function after Transection of Crossed Olivo-Cochlear Bundle in the Cat. V. Pure-Tone Intensity Discrimination." *Acta Otolaryngologica 87,* 429–433.

Jastreboff, P.J. 1990. "Phantom Auditory Perception (Tinnitus): Mechanisms of Generation and Perception." *Neuroscience Research, 8,* 221–254.

Jastreboff, P.J., Ikner, C.L. and Hassen, A. 1992. "An Approach to the Objective Evaluation of Tinnitus in Humans." In J.M. Aran and R. Dauman (Eds.), *Proceedings of the Fourth International Tinnitus Seminar, Bordeaux, 1991,* pp. 331–339. Amsterdam/New York: Kugler Publications.

Kawase, T. and Liberman, M.C. 1992. "Efferent-Mediated Anti-Masking?: Contralateral Noise Enhances Auditory Nerve Response to a Tone in Noise Complex." Abstracts 15th Midwinter Research Meeting: ARO (Abstract).

Kemp, D.T. 1979. "Evidence of Mechanical Nonlinearity and Frequency Selective Wave Amplification in the Cochlea." *Archives of Otorhinolaryngology, 224,* 37–45.

Kujawa, S.G., Glattke, T.J., Fallon, M., and Bobbin, R.P. 1992. "Intracochlear Application of Acetylcholine Alters Sound-Induced Mechanical Events within the Cochlear Partition." *Hearing Research, 61,* 106–116.

LePage, E.L. 1987. "Frequency-Dependent Self-Induced Bias of the Basilar Membrane and Its Potential for Controlling Sensitivity and Tuning in the Mammalian Cochlea." *Journal of the Acoustical Society of America, 82,* 139–154.

LePage, E.L. 1989. "Functional Role of the Olivo-Cochlear Bundle: A Motor Unit Control System in the Mammalian Cochlea." *Hearing Research, 38,* 177–198.

Lindberg, P., Scott, B., Melin, L., and Lyttkens, L. 1987. "Long-Term Effects of Psychological Treatment of Tinnitus." *Scandinavian Audiology, 16,* 167–172.

Lovely, T.J., Cacace, A.T., Winter, D.F., and Parnes, S.M. 1993. "Characteristics of Two Patients with Gaze Evoked Tinnitus." Abstracts 16th midwinter meeting: ARO, 6. (Abstract)

MacKinnon, D.M. 1968. "Objective Tinnitus Due to Palatal Myoclonus." *Journal of Laryngology and Otology, 82,* 369–374.

Maurer, J., Beck, A., Mann, W., and Mintert, R. 1992. "Changes in Otoacoustic Emissions with Simultaneous Acoustic Stimulation of the Contralateral Ear in Normal Probands and Patients with Unilateral Acoustic Neurinoma." *Laryngorhinootologie 71,* 69–73.

McFadden, D. 1982. *Tinnitus: Facts, Theories, and Treatments,* pp. 1–150. Washington, DC: National Academy Press.

Medical Research Council's Institute of Hearing Research. 1981. "Epidemiology of Tinnitus." *Ciba Foundation Symposium 1981, 85,* 16–34.

Møller, A.R. 1984. "Pathophysiology of Tinnitus." *Annals of Otology, Rhinology, and Laryngology, 93,* 39–44.

Moulin, A., Collet, L., and Morgon, A. 1992. "Influence of Spontaneous Otoacoustic Emissions (SOAE) on Acoustic Distortion Product Input/Output Functions: Does the Medial Efferent System Act Differently in the Vicinity of an SOAE?" *Acta Otolaryngologica (Stockholm) 112,* 210–214.

Patuzzi, R. and Rajan, R. 1990. "Does Electrical Stimulation of the Crossed Olivo-Cochlear Bundle Produce Movement of the Organ of Corti?" *Hearing Research, 45,* 15–32.

Penner, M.J. 1983. "Variability in Matches to Subjective Tinnitus." *Journal of Speech and Hearing Research, 26,* 263–267.

Penner, M.J. 1988. "Audible and Annoying Spontaneous Otoacoustic Emissions. A Case Study." *Archives of Otolaryngology—Head and Neck Surgery, 114,* 150–153.

Penner, M.J. 1989a. "An Estimate of the Prevalence of Tinnitus Caused by Spontaneous Otoacoustic Emissions." (UnPub).

Penner, M.J. 1989b. "Aspirin Abolishes Tinnitus Caused by Spontaneous Otoacoustic Emissions. A Case Study." *Archives of Otolaryngology—Head and Neck Surgery, 115,* 871–875.

Penner, M.J. and Burns, E.M. 1987. "The Dissociation of SOAEs and Tinnitus." *Journal of Speech and Hearing Research, 30,* 396–403.

Pickles, J.O. 1988. "Sensorineural Hearing Loss." In *An Introduction to the Physiology of Hearing,* pp. 297–320. London: Academic Press.

Plinkert, P.K., Gitter, A.H., and Zenner, H.P. 1990. "Tinnitus Associated Spontaneous Otoacoustic Emissions. Active Outer Hair Cell Movements as Common Origin?" *Acta Otolaryngologica (Stockholm) 110,* 342–347.

Pribram, K.H. 1971. *Languages of the Brain—Experimental Paradoxes and Principles in Neurophysiology,* pp. 1–432. Englewood Cliffs, NJ: Prentice Hall.

Pribram, K.H. 1987. "Holography and Brain Function." In G. Adelman (Ed.), *Encyclopedia of Neuroscience,* pp. 499–500. Boston: Birkhauser.

Puel, J.L. and Rebillard, G. 1990. "Effect of Contralateral Sound Stimulation on the Distortion Product 2F1-F2: Evidence That the Medial Efferent System Is Involved." *Journal of the Acoustical Society of America, 87,* 1630–1635.

Rajan, R. and Johnstone, B.M. 1988. "Electrical Stimulation of Cochlear Efferents at the Round Window Reduces Auditory Desensitization in Guinea Pigs. I. Dependence on Electrical Stimulation Parameters." *Hearing Resources, 36,* 53–73.

Ryan, S., Kemp, D.T., and Hinchcliffe, R. 1991. "The Influence of Contralateral Acoustic Stimulation on Click Evoked Emissions in Humans." *British Journal of Audiology, 25,* 391–397.

Sheldrake, J.B and Hazell, J.W. 1992. "Maskers v. Hearing Aids in the Prosthetic Management of Tinnitus." In J.M. Aran and R. Dauman (Eds.), *Proceedings of the Fourth International Tinnitus Seminar, Bordeaux, 1991,* pp. 395–399. Amsterdam/New York: Kugler Publications.

Siegel, J.H., Kim, D.O., and Molnar, C.E. 1982. "Effects of Altering Organ of Corti on Cochlear Distor-

tion Products f2-f1, and 2f1-f2." *Journal of Neurophysiology, 47,* 303–328.

Sininger, Y.S., Eggermont, J.J., and King, A.J. 1992. Spontaneous Activity from the Peripheral Auditory System in Tinnitus." In J.M. Aran and R. Dauman (Eds.), *Proceedings of the Fourth International Tinnitus Seminar, Bordeaux, 1991,* pp. 341–345. Amsterdam/New York: Kugler Publications.

Soucek, S., Michaels, L., and Frohlich, A. 1986. "Evidence for Hair Cell Degeneration as the Primary Lesion in Hearing Loss of the Elderly." *Journal of Otolaryngology, 15,* 175–183.

Soucek, S., Michaels, L., and Frohlich, A. 1987. "Pathological Changes in the Organ of Corti in Presbyacusis as Revealed by Microslicing and Staining." *Acta Otolaryngologica (Stockholm), 436,* 93–102.

Stephens, S.D. and Hallam, R.S. 1985. "The Crown-Crisp Experiential Index in Patients Complaining of Tinnitus." *British Journal of Audiology, 19,* 151–158.

Sullivan, M.D., Katon, W., Dobie, R., Sakai, C., Russo, J., and Harrop-Griffiths, J. 1988. "Disabling Tinnitus. Association with Affective Disorder." *General Hospital Psychiatry, 10,* 285–291.

Tonndorf, J. 1981. "Stereociliary Dysfunction, A Case of Sensory Hearing Loss, Recruitment, Poor Speech Discrimination and Tinnitus." *Acta Otolaryngologica (Stockholm) 91,* 469–479.

Tyler, R.S. and Conrad-Armes, D. 1983. "The Determination of Tinnitus Loudness Considering the Effects of Recruitment." *Journal of Speech and Hearing Research, 26,* 59–72.

Tyler, R.S. and Stouffer, J.L. 1989. "A Review of Tinnitus Loudness." *Hearing Journal, 42,* 52–57.

Veuillet, E., Collet, L., Disant, F., and Morgan, A. 1991. "Tinnitus and Medial Cochlear Efferent System." In J.-M. Aran and R. Dauman (Eds.), *Proceedings of the Fourth International Tinnitus Seminar,* pp. 205–209. New York: Kugler.

Wall, M., Rosenberg, M., and Richardson, D. 1987. "Gaze-Evoked Tinnitus." *Neurology 37,* 1034–1036.

Ward, P.H., Babin, R., Calcaterra, T.C., and Konrad, H.R. 1975. "Operative Treatment of Surgical Lesions with Objective Tinnitus." *Annals of Otology, Rhinology, and Laryngology, 84,* 473–482.

Warren, E.H. III and Liberman, M.C. 1989a. "Effects of Contralateral Sound on Auditory-Nerve Responses. I. Contributions of Cochlear Efferents." *Hearing Research, 37,* 89–104.

Warren, E.H. III and Liberman, M.C. 1989b. "Effect of

Contralateral Sound on Auditory-Nerve Responses. II. Dependence on Stimulus Variables." *Hearing Research, 37,* 105–122.

Wiederhold, M.L. and Kiang, N.Y-S. 1970. "Effects of Electric Stimulation of the Crossed Olivocochlear Bundle on Single Auditory-Nerve Fibers in the Cat." *Journal of the Acoustical Society of America, 48,* 950–965.

Wright, A., Davies, A., Bredberg, G., Ulehova, L., and Spencer, H. 1987. "Haircell Distributions in the Normal Human Cochlea." *Acta Otolaryngologica, Supplement, 444,* 1–48.

Zenner, H.P., Arnold, W., and Gitter, A.H. 1988. "Outer Hair Cells as Fast and Slow Cochlear Amplifiers with a Bidirectional Transduction Cycle." *Acta Otolaryngologica (Stockholm), 105,* 457–462.

Zenner, H.P. and Plinkert, P.K. 1992. AC and DC Motility of Mammalian Auditory Sensory Cells—A New Concept in Hearing Physiology." *Otolaryngol Pol, 46,* 333–349.

Zenner, H.P., Zimmermann, R., and Gitter, A.H. 1988. "Active Movements of the Cuticular Plate Induce Sensory Hair Motion in Mammalian Outer Hair Cells." *Hearing Research, 34,* 233–239.

CHAPTER 8

TINNITUS AS A PHANTOM PERCEPTION
THEORIES AND CLINICAL IMPLICATIONS

PAWEL J. JASTREBOFF
University of Maryland School of Medicine

DEFINITION OF TINNITUS

The word "tinnitus" bears different meaning to different people. Everybody agrees that there is no one, simple entity that can be labeled as tinnitus, but the agreement ends here. A clear definition of tinnitus is needed for a meaningful investigation of this phenomenon. It will be argued that the presently dominant definitions are not sufficiently specific and do not reflect the physiological basis of tinnitus. Furthermore, by including somato-sounds, which have a totally different physiological basis and require diverse treatment, under the label of tinnitus, the present definitions may misdirect research and clinical efforts. Consequently, a new definition of tinnitus is proposed.

Formally, tinnitus is defined by the American National Standards Institute as the sensation of sound without external stimulation (ANSI 1969). Another, prevalent description defines tinnitus as the conscious experience of sound originating in the head (McFadden 1982). Both definitions encompass auditory hallucinations related to schizophrenia, a variety of somatosounds such as palatal myoclonus, hyperpatency of the eustachian tube, temporomandibular joint disease, emissions, and bruits of vascular origin (Champlin, Muller, and Mitchell 1990; Harris, Brismar, and Cronqvist 1979; Hazell 1990; Hentzer 1968; McFadden 1982), tinnitus related to spontaneous otoacoustic emissions (Penner 1989, 1990), as well as tinnitus

resulting from dysfunctions of the cochlea or auditory nerve (Jastreboff 1990; Møller 1984). One option is to accept the general definition of tinnitus as any sound generated within the head, without regard for the underlying mechanism(s) of its origin, and to categorize the different tinnitus symptoms into a number of subclasses.

In the past, a number of dual divisions such as subjective/objective and peripheral/central tinnitus, were proposed (McFadden 1982), but these categories were not defined in a sufficiently specific manner and they were not mutually exclusive. Furthermore, the definition should reasonably stand the test of time. This problem is particularly visible in the case of the most common division into "subjective" and "objective" tinnitus. Due to the rapid progress of our knowledge about the functioning of the auditory system and measurement techniques, some cases of tinnitus previously categorized as "subjective" can now be measured as otoacoustic emission and therefore become "objective." Assuming future progress in the field, we might expect that we will finally be able to detect either physical or neural correlates for all tinnitus cases, thus eliminating its present "subjective" aspect.

In creating the definition of tinnitus, one possibility is to define a number of mutually exclusive types of tinnitus with clear delineation of their boundaries. As a result, one might propose, for example, Eustachian tube-tinnitus, palatal-tinnitus, stapedial-tinnitus, 8 kHz hearing loss-tinnitus, Ménière's-tinnitus, VIII nerve-tinnitus, acoustic neuroma-tinnitus, cochlear nuclei-tinnitus, vascular compression-tinnitus, otoacoustic emission-tinnitus, cortical-tinnitus, caffeine-tinnitus, salt-tinnitus, efferent system-tinnitus, hyperacusis-tinnitus, OHC-tinnitus, IHC-tinnitus, pain-tinnitus, presbyacusis-tinnitus, and so on. This approach, however, would create complex, hierarchic, multilevel definitions, redefined frequently, as we increase our knowledge of the functioning of the auditory system and the brain.

Another approach to define tinnitus is to restrict the word "tinnitus" to one, perhaps unique, form of this disorder, and to label other sounds originating in the head by terms relating to the mechanism of their origin. In keeping with this approach, I would like to propose a definition of tinnitus as: *The perception of a sound that results exclusively from the activity within the nervous system without any corresponding mechanical, vibratory activity within the cochlea.* If there is a vibratory component in the cochlea that can be related to the perception of sound, it will be categorized as "somatosound" with further specification reflecting its origin. This definition is based on the following reasoning.

Psychoacoustical evaluation of the vast majority of tinnitus cases shows that the perception of tinnitus differs significantly from the perception of external sound: Masking depends only a little on the frequency of masker; contralateral masking is usually as effective as ipsilateral; it is impossible to observe beats with external tones of frequency close to tinnitus pitch; tinnitus does not exhibit habituation; and residual inhibition is observed in some patients after masking of tinnitus. All these observations suggest that the perception of tinnitus results from an abnormal activity within the neuronal auditory pathways and does not result simplistically from the passive transmission of an extra sound generated in the cochlea. More elaborate analysis of these observations resulted in the proposal that the perception of tinnitus results from the presence of neuronal ac-

tivity, which cannot be induced by any combination of external sounds (Jastreboff 1990).

By inverting this reasoning, one can expect that in cases of sound perception resulting from a vibration within the cochlea, as is the case of spontaneous otoacoustic emission (SOAE), masking of this perception should be similar to masking of the external sound. Recent work has revealed that this indeed is the case, and that masking of SOAE-related tinnitus is similar to masking of external sound with the frequency corresponding to one of the frequencies of SOAE (Penner, personal communication).

This definition would also stress the differences in the clinical approach for treating somatosounds versus tinnitus. In the case of somatosounds originating outside the cochlea, the treatment can be aimed at eliminating mechanical vibrations, which are the source of sound perception. If it is of muscular origin, such as palatal myoclonus, hyperpatency of the eustachian tube, or rhythmic contraction of middle ear muscles, the remedy might involve muscle relaxants or surgery (Hazell 1990). If it is caused by the chronic partial opening of the Eustachian tube, resulting in hearing of the air flow, then restricted, small cauterization of Eustachian tube walls might be a solution (Hazell, 1990). If the patient is hearing blood flow due to partial obstruction of an artery, its clearing might be the solution (Champlin et al. 1990). Finally, if SOAE is perceived, then salicylate administration might bring relief (Penner and Coles 1992) by attenuating active processes in the cochlea (Kujawa, Fallon, and Bobbin 1992; McFadden and Plattsmier 1984; Penner and Coles 1992; Wier, Pasanen, and McFadden 1988). This last case is of particular interest since salicylates are very well known for their ability to induce or aggravate tinnitus (Flower, Moncada, and Vane 1980)!

The proposed definition has a number of theoretical and practical consequences. As defined, *tinnitus is equivalent to phantom auditory sensation,* without excluding auditory hallucinations, which are a landmark for schizophrenia (Cloninger, Martin, Guze, and Clayton 1985; Heilbrun, Diller, Fleming, and Slade 1986). The typical tendency is to segregate totally schizophrenic and tinnitus patients on the basis of different approaches used for treatment of schizophrenia and tinnitus. Nevertheless, there are a number of reasons supporting the proposed approach. First, there is no clear distinction between "central" and "cortical" tinnitus in the classical definition and hallucinations, except for the complexity of perceived sound. According to the proposed definition, "hearing voices" just indicates that abnormal cortical activity, reflected in other schizophrenia-related abnormalities, causes excitation of the cortical area involved in speech perception. There is no fundamental difference if the speech-processing area is excited due to electrical stimulation of appropriate cortical area or due to an abnormal pattern of cortical excitation, including cortical speech areas. Moreover, complex auditory (Berrios 1991; Hammeke, McQuillen, and Cohen 1983; Klostermann, Vieregge, and Kömpf 1992) or visual (Schultz and Melzack 1991) hallucinations might occur without any psychiatric disorder. On the other hand, many schizophrenics experience tinnitus, perceived as *a noise* coming from *inside* their ears, at the initial stage of schizophrenia. In about 15 to 20 percent of the cases, tinnitus diminishes and auditory hallucinations, perceived as *a voice* talking to them from *outside*, emerge instead. In such cases, after successful pharmacological treatment, hallucinations vanish and tinnitus reappears again (Zhou, personal communication). This reciprocal relationship indicates the existence of a correlation between classical tinnitus and hallucinations.

Another important aspect of the definition *disregards whatever is responsible for the abnormal activity* within the auditory system. This perception can be due to abnormal synchronization of the auditory nerve activity (Møller 1984), imbalanced activity of type I and type II afferent fibers in the auditory nerve (Tonndorf 1987), discordant damage to OHC and IHC systems (Jastreboff 1990), or central abnormalities (Hammeke et al. 1983; Hazell and Jastreboff 1992; Jastreboff 1990; Møller 1992). The final result is the same—perception of a sound without corresponding me-

chanical vibrations in the cochlea. The approach to the patient can be different, just as patients with breathing problems resulting from asthma need to be treated differently from those resulting from pneumonia.

The proposed definition also *disregards tinnitus duration*. The episodes of tinnitus can be very short or tinnitus can be continuous. The presently accepted criterion of five minutes duration is arbitrary, and does not have any clear theoretical or clinical basis or relevance. From the point of view of all proposed theories of tinnitus, the factor of time is not relevant. On the other hand, from the patient's point of view, the annoyance of tinnitus is most definitely related to its duration, but it is only one of many parameters, and whether tinnitus is perceived for more or less than five minutes has no relevance. To be of clinical importance, the duration would have to be much longer and tinnitus perceived systematically. Anyhow, for the majority of clinically relevant cases, tinnitus is continuous, with perhaps some modulation of its presence and intensity.

Another important feature of the proposed definition is that it directs attention to the *processes occurring within the nervous system* rather than relating tinnitus to any particular location. The processing of any type of information (including tinnitus-related activity) within the nervous system occurs at several interconnected levels, and involves pattern recognition, memory, interconnection with other systems, including limbic and autonomic nervous systems. Furthermore, all these processes are highly changeable and subject to plasticity, reflected at the behavioral level in creating new associations, reflexes, and memories.

In the following part of this chapter the analysis will be restricted to tinnitus as defined above.

TINNITUS VERSUS OTHER TYPES OF PHANTOM PERCEPTION

The phenomenon of phantom perception provokes questions dealing both with the philosophy of perception and with everyday clinical problems. Probably the best recognized subtypes of phantom perception are phantom limb and phantom pain (Melzack 1989, 1990, 1992; Wyant 1979). Setting aside philosophical aspects of the problem, the fundamental question remains if phantom sensation, as perceived by a patient, differs from their perception of the external world. Melzak, in a series of elegant papers (1989, 1990, 1992), presents convincing data supporting the theory that

> The experience of a phantom limb has the quality of reality because it is produced by the same brain processes that underline the experience of the body when intact; neural networks in the brain generate all the qualities of experience that are felt to originate in the body, so that inputs from the body may trigger or modulate the output of the networks, but are not essential for any of the qualities of experience.

Furthermore, he argues that similar mechanisms are involved in phantom seeing and hearing, including tinnitus (Melzack 1992; Schultz and Melzack 1991).

The theory that the proper functioning of a system is assured by the balance of two converse and, at the same time, complementary subsystems, is well-established and has been related to a variety of situations (Konorski 1948; Melzack and Wall 1965; Pribram 1971), including the generation of tinnitus (Tonndorf 1987). In this chapter an hypothesis based on the theory of the balance of two subsystems is presented, encompassing a variety of different types of tinnitus, according to present classifications. Furthermore, relevant clinical correlates are indicated.

TINNITUS GENERATION

Imbalanced Activity of Type I and Type II Auditory Nerve Fibers

A theory of tinnitus was presented recently which argued that the emergence of tinnitus results from the interaction and contribution of all the auditory

pathway centers and various parts of the central nervous system (Jastreboff 1990). Nevertheless, it is reasonable to indicate the primary source presumably responsible for initiating the process of tinnitus emergence. Clinical data point to the cochlea or the auditory nerve as a localization of such a source in most cases (McFadden 1982). The following hypothesis will be argued: *Tinnitus can be initiated by the imbalanced activity between type I and type II of the VIII nerve afferent fibers.*

This hypothesis is not assumed to cover all tinnitus cases. Tinnitus is a symptom of many etiologies and might be based on a number of different mechanisms, some of which will be discussed in this chapter. Nevertheless, this hypothesis might be a common basis for several seemingly different mechanisms of tinnitus.

The primary version of this hypothesis has been put forward by Tonndorf (1987), who based his proposal on the analogy with pain perception. He maintained similarity between somatosensory and the VIII nerve type I fibers, and between thin Aδ and C with auditory type II fibers as both invoking Melzak's gate theory of pain (Tonndorf 1987). However, there are a number of discrepancies between Melzak's and Tonndorf's theories.

Melzak's proposal is based on the counteraction of two different sensory systems, pain and somatosensory, which interact at the spinal level, and through the mechanism of presynaptic inhibition, a flow of information coming from fibers involved in pain perception is attenuated by activity evoked by tactile stimulation (Melzack and Wall 1965). Noteworthy, pain-related activity is normally present and perceived when pain stimulus occurs, and is represented by activity within C and A fibers. Furthermore, combining pain and somatosensory information is crucial for localizing the source of pain stimulus. Using this theory as a reference, according to Tonndorf, activity within type II fibers should be treated as a "tinnitus-pain" and in type I fibers as modulating tinnitus "somatosensory" activity. The evident implications from Tonndorf's theory would be that: 1) tinnitus-related activity is continuously present, since all available data indicate that OHC are active and involved in the transduction of sound; 2) continuous activity of type I fibers is needed to attenuate tinnitus signal—otherwise we would perceive tinnitus all the time; 3) by increasing activity in type I fibers (by sound) we should be able to eliminate tinnitus, but due to tonotopic organization of the IHC and OHC systems we should observe sharp tuning curves of masking, and the pure tone, with frequency clearly distant from perceived pitch of tinnitus, should not be effective; 4) damage of OHC with IHC reasonably intact, which is typically the case, should not result in tinnitus since then we are decreasing activity in type II fibers; 5) tinnitus should be always present in totally deaf people since total damage of hair cell systems results in degeneration of type I but not type II fibers (Pujol, Rebillard, Puel, Lenoir, Eybalin, and Recasens 1991); 6) it is reasonable to expect the perception of tinnitus as noise, but never as a single tone, since type II fibers span a significant distance along the basilar membrane, up to several mm, and make contact with number of OHC cells covering the frequency range of an octave (Liberman and Brown 1986).

Practical observations are not consistent with these implications predicted from the Tonndorf theory: For example, 1) flat masking curves are contrary to the predicted clear tuning; 2) there are frequent cases of totally deaf or people with severe hearing loss who do not have tinnitus, contrary to the expectation that all these people should have tinnitus; 3) the relationship of tinnitus occurrence with hearing loss typically involves more damage to the OHC than the IHC system, which according to Tonndorf's theory should even help in attenuating the natural tendency of the system to result in tinnitus; 4) there are a number of cases when tinnitus is perceived as pure-tone or narrowband noise. Even though Tonndorf points out that his theory is not expected to cover all possible types of tinnitus and might be applicable to some cases, nevertheless observations do not confirm the predictions based on his theory in most cases.

Although the presented proposal has some similarity to Tonndorf's theory by discussing the role of type I and type II fibers, it is substantially different in other aspects. Furthermore, it can be applied to variety of situations, the simplest of which is the discordant damage to OHC and IHC systems.

Discordant Dysfunction of OHC and IHC Systems.

Large, myelinated, afferent type I fibers innervate exclusively IHC whereas thin, unmyelinated type II fibers innervate exclusively OHC (Pujol and Lenoir 1986). Apparently, if one hair cell system is destroyed while the other is functional this will result in lack of activity in the fibers innervating damaged cells, with preserved activity originating in the other hair cell system. This will create an ultimate difference in the activity of type I and II fibers.

Recently, a hypothesis was proposed claiming that tinnitus appears when there is a discordant damage or temporal dysfunction of IHC and OHC (Jastreboff 1990; Stypulkowski 1989). This hypothesis is based on the following reasoning. In the majority of cases, an ototoxic agent (either a drug or white noise) causes damage to the basilar membrane starting from the basal, high-frequency part of the membrane and gradually progresses to the apical, low-frequency end. Furthermore, the OHC are damaged first, with the IHC more resistant to injury (Conlee, Gill, McCandless, and Creel 1989; Hunter-Duvar, Suzuki, and Mount 1982; Liberman and Dodds 1984a,b, 1987; Saunders and Flock 1985; Stypulkowski 1989). As a result, if we analyze the morphology of the basilar membrane, proceeding from basal end, we will encounter an area with totally missing OHC and IHC, followed by a region of a partially damaged IHC and absent OHC, followed by an area of normal IHC and partially damaged OHC, and finally with both hair cells systems intact. The region with IHC at least partially intact and OHC absent or heavily damaged is of particular interest. The damage to the OHC system will change the mechanical properties of the organ of Corti due to the disintegration of the mechanical coupling normally carried by OHC and their cilia.

In the simplest scenario, this might lead to the local collapse of the tectorial membrane, decreasing the distance between cilia of the still functional IHC, with a possibility of physical contact of the cilia with the tectorial membrane. This might result in tonic depolarization of IHC yielding abnormal activity in afferent fibers (Jastreboff 1990, 1992; Stypulkowski 1989).

Involvement of the Efferent Systems.   This primary hypothesis can be further expanded to entail more complex mechanisms of tinnitus, including the involvement of the efferent system (Hazell 1987; Jastreboff 1990). The position of the basilar membrane seems to be adjusted to provide an optimal working point for transduction by modulating the length of the OHC, controlled by the activity of the efferent system (LePage 1987, 1989; Zenner, Zimmerman, and Gitter 1988). Activity of type II afferent fibers innervating OHC might provide information characterizing their working point on transduction characteristics, and presumably, after including information from IHC, the position of the basilar membrane. This information, after being processed by the brainstem, modulates the activity within the efferent system, which in turn adjusts the length of OHC at a given point on the basilar membrane. Through this loop, permanent or temporary dysfunction of OHC at a part of the basilar membrane will yield decreased activity within a portion of efferent fibers, innervating this part of the basilar membrane. Data with the effects of electrical stimulation of the efferent system, contralateral sound stimulation on cochlear potentials, and on otoacoustic emissions indicate that increased activity within the efferent system attenuates active processes within the cochlea. Conversely, decreased activity might increase negative dampening exerted by OHC action, and decrease the inhibition on type I afferents coming from IHC. Both actions should result in enhancement of the activity from the functioning IHC.

For the generation of tinnitus, it is of significance that an efferent fiber branches profoundly in the cochlea, reaching as many as 100 OHC over a distance of up to 3 mm of basilar membrane of the cat (Liberman and Brown 1986). Therefore, decreasing the activity in a group of fibers will cause a release from inhibition of OHC and IHC not only from the damaged area, but from the neighboring normal portion of the basilar membrane. This anomalous decrease in efferent activity might result in the local increase of afferent discharges in type I fibers, which after further processing, including the edge effect, might be perceived as tinnitus.

Note that in the above hypothesis only the enhancement of the activity within type I fibers is postulated, without any requirement for magnifying the mechanical vibration of the basilar membrane. If the actual mechanical vibration were occurring on the basilar membrane, it should be easily masked by tone or narrowband noise with frequencies close to a frequency corresponding to the position on the basilar membrane, with clear tuning. The majority of tinnitus cases exhibit flat characteristics of masking. Furthermore, they should appear as SOAE, which, as has been shown, is not the frequent case (Penner 1990), and they should be eliminated by aspirin (Penner 1989; Penner and Coles 1992). Another common observation that tinnitus is particularly pronounced when the patient is in a quiet environment (Heller and Bergman 1953) argues against the possibility of tinnitus being a result of mechanical overamplification of external sounds by an underdamped, oscillating area of the basilar membrane. These observations further stress the possibility of a significant role played by disinhibition of afferent activity mediated by the lateral efferent system in tinnitus generation.

Damage of the VIII Nerve.   In 1984 Møller proposed a hypothesis relating tinnitus to crosstalk between VIII nerve fibers, occurring when myelin, which covers type I fibers, is partially damaged, for example, as a result of contact with an abnormally positioned vessel on the nerve (A.R. Møller 1984, 1987, 1992; M.B. Møller 1987). He argued that the nervous system should adapt continuously to changes in mean spontaneous activity of the auditory nerve fibers, but should not be able to cope with abnormal synchronization of adjoining fibers. This proposal has been further advanced by Eggermont (1990) (see chapter 4), who stressed the importance of an abnormal synchronization of spontaneous activity within the auditory nerve and the presence of abnormal temporal patterns consisting of short bursts of high-frequency activity. Computer modeling of ion influx to hair cells suggested that this abnormal activity might result from increased calcium influx into hair cells (Eggermont 1990).

Besides Møller's hypothesis, there is another complementary possibility explaining tinnitus resulting from partial damage to or severence of the VIII nerve. Type I and type II afferent fibers feature distinctively different morphological and physiological properties (Brown, Berglund, Kiang, and Ryugo 1988; Brown, Liberman, Benson, and Ryugo 1988; Eybalin and Altschuler 1990; Liberman 1988; Liberman and Brown 1986; Ryan, Keithley, Wang, and Schwartz 1990). An important observation is that damage to the IHC system results in degeneration of type I fibers, while damage of the OHC system is not followed by degeneration of type II fibers (Pujol et al. 1991). Therefore, damage to OHC and IHC systems will have a different impact on the survival or degeneration of type I and type II fibers. Furthermore, lack of myelin on type II fibers enhances the possibility of these fibers being more susceptible to mechanical or biochemical damage. This differentiated resistance to damage might result in an imbalanced population of surviving fibers in situations as described by Møller, yielding an imbalanced activity of type I and type II fibers. Therefore, tinnitus might be generated even without the presence of abnormal synchronous activity within the auditory nerve, but instead results from decreased or absent activity in type II afferent fibers.

The hypothesis of imbalanced activity in type I and type II afferents as an essence of tinnitus generation can explain a number of tinnitus puzzles and point out a new approach for clinical evaluation of patients. One common clinical observation is finding that the estimated pitch of tinnitus usually correlates with the slope of the audiogram (Hazell 1987). On the basis of the proposed theory, this is exactly what should be happening. The slope of the audiogram corresponds to the area on the basilar membrane where transition occurs from heavily damaged hair cell systems, at higher frequencies, through the area of partially damaged IHC and OHC, to relatively normal OHC and IHC. Hence this is exactly the area where one can expect to find a portion of the basilar membrane with functional IHC and damaged OHC, resulting in an imbalanced activity within the two types of afferent fibers. If the damage of hair cell systems is relatively smooth, we should expect the pitch of tinnitus to be close to the high-frequency part of the slope, since in this area we should have the heaviest damage of OHC and still some functional IHC. This again is a frequent clinical finding in our practice.

Another puzzle is the occurrence of tinnitus in patients who have no apparent hearing loss, while at the same time some patients with severe hearing loss have no tinnitus at all. It is a common clinical observation that the audiogram is not a predictor of the presence or extent of tinnitus and that it is possible to have patients with or without tinnitus but with the same audiogram. This is in apparent contradiction to the general findings that the presence of hearing loss is correlated with the presence of tinnitus (Hazell, Wood, Cooper, Stephens, Corcoran, Coles, Baskill, and Sheldrake 1985; McFadden 1982).

To explain these findings it is necessary to recall that the audiogram represents mainly the functional integrity of the IHC, and that diffuse damage of the OHC system, even as large as 30 percent, might not have significant impact on the hearing threshold (Bohne and Clark 1982; Hamernik, Patterson, Turrentine, and Ahroon 1989; Salvi, Perry, Hamernik, and Henderson 1982). Furthermore, it has been shown that exposure to the same noise, or to ototoxic drugs, results in dissimilar patterns of cochlear damage in different subjects (Davis,

Ahroon, and Hamernik 1989; Hunter-Duvar et al. 1982; Liberman and Mulroy 1982). If it is essential for tinnitus generation to have imbalanced activity within the subpopulations of the afferent fibers, then tinnitus might not appear if the patient has a hearing loss with symmetrical damage of the OHC and IHC systems. On the other hand, another patient with the same audiogram might have tinnitus if there is a difference in the dysfunction of the OHC and IHC systems. Finally, patients without hearing loss, as assessed by audiogram, might have local damage of the OHC system, causing imbalanced activity of type I and type II fibers and tinnitus.

This reasoning has a profound effect on the process of clinical evaluation of tinnitus patients. Since the audiogram does not represent the functional status of the OHC system along the basilar membrane, therefore it should be used only in combination with other measurements, which will allow for an independent evaluation of OHC to estimate the potential source of tinnitus within the cochlea. Fortunately, methods have been developed recently for evaluating cochlear emissions and distortion products. These can be used for determining the status of OHC (Bonfis, Uziel, and Pujol 1988; Harris, Lonsbury-Martin, Stagner, Coats, and Martin 1989; Kemp 1979; Kemp, Bray, Alexander, and Brown 1986; Kemp and Brown 1983; Lonsbury-Martin, Martin, Probst, and Coats 1987; Martin, Lonsbury-Martin, Probst, Scheinin and Coats 1987; Probst, Coats, Martin, and Lonsbury-Martin 1986; Probst, Lonsbury-Martin, Martin, and Coats 1987; Wier et al. 1988; Wilson 1980; Zurek, Clark, and Kim 1982), whereas traditional audiometry might be used to estimate the integrity of the IHC system. By comparison of these results, it is possible to determine the area(s) on the basilar membrane with discordant damage of OHC and IHC systems. Unfortunately, a method for directly assessing activity within type II fibers is still to be developed.

The discussed hypothesis proposes a mechanism of sound-induced temporary tinnitus, which is frequently reported after exposure to loud sound (George and Kemp 1989; Kemp and Plaisted 1986; McFadden 1982). The first morphological changes observed in the cochlea that has been exposed to intense sound is the bending of OHC stereocilia and local decoupling of OHC from the tectorial membrane, without necessarily damaging stereocilia of IHC (Hazell et al. 1985; Liberman 1987; Liberman and Dodds 1984a,b, 1987). This will preclude stimulation of OHC by sound and create the imbalance in type I and type II fibers, resulting in tinnitus. The finding that tinnitus induced in this manner disappears after several hours is consistent with morphological observations that if sound is not too intense the stereocilia return to the normal state within several hours. Exposure to very loud sound might result in permanent local damage of OHC and permanent tinnitus, providing that there are still some functional IHC in the affected area of basilar membrane. Interestingly, a comparison of sound-induced tinnitus with chronic tinnitus indicated that both kinds may arise from the same auditory processes (George and Kemp 1989).

The method of choice to induce tinnitus in humans without side effects is salicylate administration (Flower et al. 1980; McFadden 1982; Mongan, Kelly, Nies, Porter, and Paulus 1973), with loudness of salicylate-induced tinnitus being dose-dependent in humans (Day, Graham, Bieri, Brown, Cairns, Harris, Hounsell, Platt-Hepworth, Reeve, Sambrook, and Smith 1989) and animals (Jastreboff and Brennan 1992). Salicylate has been reported to abolish SOAE (Long and Tubis 1988; Martin, Lonsbury-Martin, Probst, and Coats 1988; McFadden and Plattsmier 1984) and attenuate active processes in the cochlea (Ashmore 1989; Brownell, Shehata, and Imredy 1990; Puel, Bledsoe, Bobbin, Ceasar, and Fallon 1989; Puel, Bobbin, and Fallon 1988; Shehata, Brownell, Cousillas, and Imredy 1990). These results indicate that salicylate predominantly affects the OHC system: a hypothesis that is further supported by evaluation of cochlear potentials (Puel, Bobbin, and Fallon 1990; Stypulkowski 1990), observed morphologic changes and decrease of turgor of the OHC (Brownell et al. 1990; Dieler, Shehata-Dieler, and Brownell 1991; Shehata, Brownell, and Dieler 1991), and changes in membrane properties (Ashmore 1989; Shehata et al. 1990) after exposing OHC to salicylate. Importantly, the concentration of salicylate administered corresponded to the amount measured in the perilymph of animals that exhibited behavioral changes associated with tinnitus (Jastreboff, Brennan, and Sasaki 1988a,b; Jastreboff, Hansen, Sasaki, and Sasaki 1986). A detailed discussion of the putative mechanisms of salicylate-induced tinnitus is presented elsewhere (Jastreboff 1990, 1992; Stypulkowski 1990). At this point, it is relevant to note that salicylate creates imbalanced activity in type I and type II fibers by predominantly affecting the OHC system, and partially deactivating action of those cells.

In summary, the proposed hypothesis postulates that it is irrelevant whether the imbalance in activity of type I and type II afferent fibers results from discordant damage of OHC versus IHC, noise-induced deactivation of predominantly OHC, salicylate, ionic imbalance, differential damage of type I and type II afferent fibers—the outcome of imbalanced activity yields tinnitus.

Calcium Homeostasis

The homeostasis of calcium extra- and intracellular concentration is of pivotal importance for sound transduction (Aitkin 1986; Dulon, Aran, and Schacht 1988; Ferrary, Tran Ba Huy, Roinel, Bernard, and Amiel 1988; Flock, Flock, and Ulfendahl 1986; Hudspeth 1985; Hudspeth and Corey 1977; Ikeda and Morizono 1989; Sand, Ozawa, Hagiwara 1975; Sterkers, Bernard, Ferrary, Sziklai, Tran Ba Huy, and Amiel 1988; Ulfendahl 1987; Zenner, Zimmerman, and Schmitt 1985). Calcium has been shown to influence: 1) position of the tectorial membrane (Kronester-Frei 1979); 2) hair cells' calcium-dependent potassium channels (Corey and Hudspeth 1979; Hudspeth 1983, 1986; Hudspeth and Corey 1977; Sand et al. 1975; Valli and Zucca 1976); 3) transduction properties of hair cell cilia (Orman and Flock, 1983); 4) slow motile properties of OHC (Flock et al. 1986; Jabboury, Frye, Holmes, Fraschini, and Hortobagyi 1989; Ulfendahl 1987; Zenner et al. 1988; Zenner et al. 1985); and 5) release of neurotransmitter from hair cells (Dallos

1981; Sterkers et al. 1988). It has been argued that a decrease of perilymphatic free calcium might facilitate tinnitus and that drug-induced tinnitus can be attenuated by providing the subject with an extragenous calcium supplement (Jastreboff 1990; Jastreboff, Nguyen, Brennan, and Sasaki 1992). Furthermore, L-type calcium channel blockers are effective in alleviating drug-induced tinnitus (Jastreboff and Brennan 1988; Jastreboff, Brennan, and Sasaki 1991; Jastreboff et al. 1992). A detailed discussion of the involvement of calcium in tinnitus generation has been published recently (Jastreboff 1990; Jastreboff et al. 1992), and in this chapter only points relevant to the proposed hypothesis are discussed.

Based on the available data, it has been suggested that spontaneous and evoked activity in the auditory nerve are controlled by entwined, but independent, mechanisms that are furthermore influenced by calcium levels in opposite directions (Drescher and Drescher 1987a,b). Recently, this hypothesis has been investigated in detail, with data predominantly collected from hair cells and vestibular afferents innervating the semicircular canal (Guth, Aubert, Ricci, and Norris 1991). Although these results cannot be transferred directly for the cochlea, they offer an interesting platform for future investigations. The authors present strong data supporting the hypothesis that, at least in their model, spontaneous and evoked activity is controlled by different, although complementary, processes. Moreover, different pools of calcium are involved in neurotransmitter release related to spontaneous and evoked activity. At the moment we are lacking similar data based on cochlear hair cells and cochlear afferents; nevertheless it seems reasonable to postulate that similar differentiation should exist for cochlear hair cells.

The presented hypothesis of calcium and neurotransmitter release dysfunction does not require an assumption of imbalanced activity between type I and type II fibers, and indeed might represent different mechanisms of tinnitus generation than the one discussed previously in this chapter. Nevertheless, well-established differences in the synaptic connections and receptors on the OHC and IHC systems (Puel, Ladrech, Chabert, Pujol, and Eybalin 1991; Pujol 1992; Pujol and Lenoir 1986) indicate the possibility that OHC and IHC are diversely affected by ionic calcium imbalance in the cochlea, as well as differential neurotransmitter release.

Other Hypotheses

There are a number of other potential hypotheses of tinnitus generation, which have been discussed elsewhere (Jastreboff 1990). Clearly, we have different mechanisms of tinnitus generation occurring in different patients. One recent theory involving the hypothesis of dysfunction in spontaneous neurotransmitter release resulting in tinnitus is of particular interest. Pujol proposed that there are two types of glutamate receptors on the afferent type I fibers: N-methyl-D-asparate (NMDA) type, and non-NMDA, with NMDA receptors activated only by high-intensity sounds. He further proposed that abnormal activity of NMDA receptors will result in epileptic-like discharges in the afferent fibers and tinnitus (Puel et al. 1991; Pujol 1992). Interestingly, such an activity has been observed in the external nucleus of the inferior colliculus in rats after injection of salicylate in doses shown to evoke behavioral manifestation of tinnitus (Jastreboff and Chen 1993).

Disregarding the physiological basis of generation of an abnormal activity within the auditory pathways, this signal undergoes multistage processing within the nervous system. Analysis of this stage in tinnitus emergence is crucial in understanding the phenomenon of tinnitus and has profound clinical implications.

PROCESSING OF TINNITUS SIGNALS

Neuronal Activity Related to Tinnitus

Tinnitus exhibits a number of characteristics which indicate that neuronal activity, the perception of which results in tinnitus, is abnormal. Most noticeable is the observation that tinnitus, contrary to

masking of external sounds, can be masked by a wide range of frequencies, and that frequently contralateral masking is as effective as ipsilateral. Moreover, maskability of tinnitus does not depend on its loudness in the same manner as in the case of external sounds and can be abnormally low or high (Feldmann 1971; McFadden 1982; Penner 1983, 1986, 1987, 1988; Penner and Bilger 1989; Tyler and Conrad-Armes 1984; Vernon 1987). Sometimes it is impossible to mask tinnitus no matter how intense the masker (Vernon and Meikle 1981). Furthermore, tinnitus does not exhibit phase-related phenomena (Feldmann 1988). Analysis of these data resulted in the proposal that "tinnitus results from the perception of abnormal activity within the auditory pathways which cannot be evoked by any combination of external sounds" (Jastreboff 1990).

One such situation occurs when neighboring fibers fire in a highly synchronized manner (Eggermont 1990; Møller 1984). Increase of the synchronization of the activity occurs under the normal condition, parallel with the increase of sound intensity, but with sound stimulation, it never is totally synchronous. Total synchrony occurs when the auditory nerve is stimulated by electrical current. Interestingly, the perception induced by electrical stimulation, even with a simple sine wave, is complex, resembling some type of tinnitus, and the patient is unable to match it to any combination of external sounds (Hazell, Jastreboff, Meerton, and Conway 1993). Convergence of the activity from several fibers firing in synchronous manner should have a powerful excitatory impact on the target cell, and even when relatively weak, it still should be difficult to mask by sound-evoked activity. This may explain why it is so difficult to mask some cases of tinnitus in spite of its relatively low loudness.

It is important to note that synchronism in activity can be delineated as happening when probability of firing increases or decreases simultaneously for several fibers within a certain time window. The time window may last a few ms or longer and the main conclusion presented above will be still valid. Such a situation might occur with the synchronization of short bursts of high-frequency activity. The presence of such a short burst has been proposed previously as being associated with tinnitus (Eggermont 1990; Evans and Borerwe 1982; Pujol 1992) and recently has been shown in external nucleus of inferior colliculus of rats, after salicylate doses which induce behavioral manifestation of tinnitus (Jastreboff and Chen 1993).

Abnormal activity within the auditory pathways is undergoing extensive multistage processing before being perceived as tinnitus. It is possible to distinguish stages of detection, perception, and evaluation. The appreciation of physiological processes occurring during these stages has a profound impact on theories of tinnitus and on practical diagnosis and treatment of tinnitus (Jastreboff 1990; Jastreboff and Hazell 1993). The first stage consists of detection of tinnitus-related signals from the continuous noise of the spontaneous and sound-evoked activity.

Detection

The auditory system is extremely efficient in detecting signals immersed in a background of other, frequently louder sounds. This process of detection is based on the pattern recognition principle (Jastreboff 1990). It can be inferred from loudness matching that, most commonly, the tinnitus-related signal is weak, usually within 10 to 15 dB above the threshold of hearing for tinnitus pitch. At the same time, this weak signal can be extremely difficult to mask. It has been hypothesized that this and other unique psychoacoustical features of tinnitus are reflections of the fact that tinnitus is a consequence of abnormal activity within the nervous system, defined as "neuronal activity which cannot be induced by any combination of external sounds" (Jastreboff 1990). One implication of this hypothesis is that the abnormal pattern will be easily extracted from the background spontaneous activity, since the nervous system has particularly sensitive mechanisms for detecting new, never previously experienced signals.

Another important aspect of this hypothesis is that detection of tinnitus occurs on the basis of pattern recognition, carried on by neuronal assemblies in a manner related to neuronal networks or holographic neuronal networks (Carpenter and Grossberg 1987; Freeman, Yao, and Burke 1988; Grossberg 1987; Lippmann 1989; Pribram 1971, 1987; Sejnowski, Koth, and Churchland 1988; Waibel 1989). This implies that even incomplete or weaker patterns similar to the original one will evoke nearly the same perception. Therefore, if a tinnitus generator is partially attenuated by a treatment, the perception of tinnitus may be modulated to a much smaller extent.

Perception

Once detected by subcortical auditory centers, sensory signals undergo the process of classification, categorization, and evaluation of their meaning and significance. Signals that do not offer significant information are quickly habituated. We are not aware of the presence of the majority of sensory signals reaching us, except when we are focusing our attention on them. Only signals that are new, or through experience have been associated with an emotional state, or have been associated with bringing significant information (for example, somebody's name), or are selected by focusing attention on them, are reaching the stage of conscious perception. Of particular importance are signals that are associated with survival and indicate a threat to life or its quality.

Detection of this last class of signals is particularly well developed and is strongly imprinted in centers involved in pattern recognition. Furthermore, learning the significance of these signals occurs very quickly, frequently in one association, but their extinction is extremely slow. These features have an obvious advantage for survival—the sound of a predator's step should be learned preferably in one trial (there may not be a second chance), and its pattern should be remembered. Even weak, distorted patterns have to induce very quick reflexive activities of fight or flight.

Commonly, tinnitus induces a feeling of threat to life and its quality: Patients report that when they experience tinnitus they think that they are going deaf, have a brain tumor, are becoming crazy; that tinnitus will only get worse; that nothing can be done to eliminate tinnitus—it will persist for years and as result they will not be able to cope with the situation, they will lose their jobs, families, and perhaps their lives as well. Unfortunately, the core of their anxiety is enhanced by their first encounter with medical professionals who confirm their worries that tinnitus is permanent, can get worse, and nothing can be done to alleviate it. The impact of this "negative counseling" is usually profound and enhances the detection of the tinnitus signal and the negative impact of tinnitus on the patient's life.

Detection of the tinnitus pattern is enhanced by associating it with threat, which in turn enhances the feeling of danger, which in turn further enhances tinnitus detection. A vicious circle is created and the patient has no way out of it. In this cycle the limbic system (emotion) and prefrontal cortex (controlling connection of several sensory, associative and emotional systems sustaining reflex behavior) are involved together with auditory pathways (Jastreboff 1990). Of significance is the fact that a large part of this process occurs outside the patient's awareness and is only partially controlled by conscious thinking. Therefore, although cognitive therapy can make the patient aware of this cycle and be of some help, it is usually not sufficient to break this cycle and to initiate the process of habituation of the perception of the tinnitus pattern.

This cycle can be effectively broken by retraining the centers involved in tinnitus detection and evaluation by using auditory low-level white noise over a period of time. Of crucial importance are postulates resulting from behavioral training theory that 1) during this process tinnitus should not be masked but should be perceived by the patient, and 2) this retraining process requires a substantial amount of time, measured in months, to occur (Jastreboff 1990).

CLINICAL IMPLICATIONS

The presented theories of tinnitus generation and processing of tinnitus signal have a number of clinical implications (Jastreboff 1990; Jastreboff and Hazell 1993). The hypothesis of tinnitus resulting from unbalanced activity of a subpopulation of nerve fibers and neurons implies difficulty in restoring such a balance and suggests that simply decreasing activity of the auditory nerve or subcortical centers by a drug would be effective only on rare occasions. There is still a possibility of a pharmacological approach, but it has to be highly selective to restore balance and act on a well-defined subpopulation of receptors. Furthermore, the drug therapy has to be adjusted to individual patients. This will be possible once detailed knowledge describing tinnitus-related modulation of the neuronal activity and the physiological basis of these changes are achieved. Presently, there is no drug that has been shown to be consistently helpful for significant portion of tinnitus patients.

Nevertheless, there is a possibility of alleviating aggravations induced by tinnitus using behavioral retraining of association of the perception of tinnitus with the emotional state and autonomic nervous system responses. Clinical implementation of neurophysiological analysis of the processing of tinnitus within the nervous system is presented in this section using the protocol to evaluate and treat patients in our Tinnitus Center in Baltimore as a framework.

The general approach to patients is based on an implication of this analysis, which predicts that modification of tinnitus perception and evaluation is an essential part of any treatment, and at the moment is the most effective and quickest method of tinnitus alleviation. Consequently, our approach to patients involves behavioral retraining of the connections between the auditory and limbic systems, and might require reversal of abnormal gain and high detectability of the tinnitus pattern occurring within the auditory pathways. These goals can be achieved by a technique of interfering with tinnitus perception by using external wearable white noise generators or amplified environmental sounds. It has to be stressed that although we are using devices that others are using for masking tinnitus (and therefore devices known as maskers), by definition we are not attempting to mask tinnitus. According to our theory masking tinnitus is counterproductive.

The most frequent cases consist of some high-frequency hearing loss, aberration of distortion product measures (if possible to record) in the range of perceived tinnitus pitch, and frequently abnormally low loudness discomfort levels. Typically it is difficult to associate any particular, current medical problem with tinnitus. Frequently the previous attempts to treat tinnitus with a variety of medications and other methods have failed, and the patient has visited a number of specialists seeking help, only to be told that "nothing can be done" and "he, or she, will have to learn to live with it."

Having in mind the significance of mutual interaction between perceptual (auditory system) and emotional (limbic system) and behavior-sustaining (prefrontal cortex) parts, reversal of the effects of negative counseling and the misconceptions that the patient has about his or her tinnitus, is of crucial importance. Proper counseling, including a clear explanation of the physiology of hearing and present knowledge about tinnitus generation and perception, is the first and essential part of any treatment. Attention is paid to discussing the patient's particular mechanism of tinnitus as diagnosed on the basis of medical examination, interview, and audiometric tests.

General medical, otolaryngological, and audiological evaluations serve to detect other problems in addition to tinnitus, as well as determine the presence of somatosounds. Once these other problems (defined in this chapter as auditory phantom perception) have been taken care of, the next step in the typical case involves recommending a prosthetic device to induce and proceed with behavioral retraining of the connection within the auditory system and interaction between the auditory and limbic systems.

In our approach, two types of prosthetic devices are used for treating tinnitus patients: maskers and hearing aids. The primary criterion is obviously the patient's main complaint—either tinnitus or a hearing problem. If a hearing problem is the main complaint, the choice is obvious, particularly in view that both maskers and hearing aids are equally effective if fitted to the proper group of patients (Hazell et al. 1985; Hazell, Sheldrake, and Meerton 1987; Sheldrake and Hazell 1992). Similarly, if the patient has normal hearing, a masker would be appropriate. If the main complaint is tinnitus and hearing loss is present, the most frequent case, the choice is more complex and the decision should be based on a number of factors.

The theory of tinnitus presented above proposes that in many cases tinnitus contains a central component of abnormally high gain within the nervous system resulting from prolonged decreased sensory input from a given subpopulation of VIII nerve fibers of type II. This increase might further result in an abnormally efficient detection of the tinnitus pattern. The theory predicts that by providing auditory pathways with a prolonged low-level signal through still-functioning fibers, it should be possible to reverse this process and effectively alleviate tinnitus. This reasoning has twofold clinical implications. First, external sound should be close to white noise. Although other sounds will be effective as well, white noise provides stimulation in all frequencies and through this to all parts of the basilar membrane. Again, it has to be stressed that this noise, by definition, is not aimed at masking tinnitus, which will be counterproductive. As such, focusing on any particular frequency will not provide stimulation of other areas of the basilar membrane and consequently will limit the amount of fibers stimulated within the auditory nerve.

Second, hearing aids should be equally effective, providing that environmental auditory background contains a wide range of frequencies and the patient is using a hearing aid like a white noise generator, that is, several hours per day, and particularly while the level of background sound is low. This is diametrically opposite to the typical recommendation of hearing aid use, when the patient is advised to use the hearing aid mainly to improve speech recognition, and put it aside while alone in quiet environment.

Sometimes combination devices, composed of a hearing aid and a white noise generator, are used for treating patients with profound hearing loss that prevents effective use of white noise generators where tinnitus is a significant problem. In such cases, a hearing aid alone will not be sufficient, since the level of even amplified background noise will not be sufficient to provide enough background for retraining the connection within the auditory pathways.

One of the implications of proposed theory of tinnitus is seeing hyperacusis as a reflection of an abnormally increased gain within auditory pathways, which could facilitate or be responsible for tinnitus (Jastreboff 1990; Jastreboff and Hazell 1993). From this perspective, hyperacusis without tinnitus represents a pre-tinnitus state. Desensitization procedures with low level, gradually increased white noise can not only restore normal tolerance to loud sounds (Hazell and Sheldrake 1992; Jastreboff 1990; Jastreboff and Hazell 1993), but could prevent future emergence of tinnitus as well. Moreover, if tinnitus and hyperacusis are present concurrently, it is possible to expect that a reversal of abnormally high gain within the auditory system will result in the decrease of tinnitus. Consequently, the treatment of patients with tinnitus and hyperacusis should first of all include strong aspects of restoration of the normal sensitivity to sound. The technique with low-level white noise is preferable, starting with a level of sounds lower than those used for other patients and only gradually increasing sound intensity.

Another important aspect implied from the presented theory is that since the process of retraining involves plastic changes of the synaptic connection and therefore is a lengthy one, followup visits are of fundamental importance for the successful outcome of the treatment. Sometimes it is neces-

sary to modify some aspect of the protocol. In addition, followup visits provide the patient with the opportunity to discuss any new questions or complaints, which further facilitates the habituation process of tinnitus perception.

The primary goal is to habituate tinnitus perception and to reach the state where the patient is not aware of tinnitus presence except when consciously focusing his or her attention on tinnitus. The presented theory predicts, and results from many centers confirm, that once this stage is achieved there is no need for regular use of noise generators or hearing aids for tinnitus control. When, and if, tinnitus becomes burdensome again, it is sufficient to repeat the procedure for a much shorter period of time to reach the state of tinnitus habituation. A retrospective analysis of patients who were followed up for up to ten years revealed that gradually an increased proportion of these patients were unable to perceive their tinnitus, indicating that during this time most probably the tinnitus pattern is no longer detectable. Noteworthy, this is a very slow process measured in years, and cannot be used for achieving clinically significant results.

CONCLUSIONS AND FURTHER GOALS

Tinnitus presents a significant challenge, both from basic science and clinical points of view. At the same time, it offers a unique model to study the mechanisms of different forms of phantom perception, such as phantom pain, phantom limb, phantom taste, and the effectiveness of various clinical approaches in their alleviation. This chapter attempts to outline an approach to the tinnitus phenomenon from the point of view of neuroscience, including its new definition. The neuroscience-based analysis yields the hypothesis of involvement of several levels of the nervous system in the emergence of conscious tinnitus perception, thereby dismissing the traditional approach, which focuses on one particular level as a source of tinnitus. This proposal has profound theoretical and clinical implications for the study of tinnitus and shows the method of relieving patients from tinnitus by initiating and facilitating the process of tinnitus habituation.

Presently tinnitus can be controlled but not cured. To achieve a cure it will be necessary to suppress the tinnitus generator, thereby eliminating or strongly suppressing the abnormal activity that is the source of tinnitus perception. This is a difficult task that can be achieved through better understanding of the neurophysiological basis of tinnitus generation and by creating mechanism-based methods for tinnitus alleviation. Even if only partial suppression of generators, or processes enhancing tinnitus signal can be achieved, this should significantly speed up the behavioral retraining and provide a higher rate of success. Importantly, the retraining will continue to be an essential part of any treatment, which is short of total elimination of tinnitus perception.

This work was supported by the National Institute of Health, National Institute on Deafness and other Communication Disorders grants RO1 DC00299 and RO1 DC00445.

REFERENCES

Aitkin, L. 1986. "Brainstem Lesions and Sound Localization." In *The Auditory Midbrain: Structure and Function in the Central Auditory Pathway*, pp. 24–30. Clifton, NJ: Humana Press.

American National Standards Institute Specifications for Audiometers, S3.6. 1969. New York: ANSI.

Ashmore, J.F. 1989. "Effect of Salicylate on a Rapid Charge Movement in Outer Hair Cells Isolated from the Guinea-Pig Cochlea." *Journal of Physiology, 412*, 46P.

Berrios, G.E. 1991. "Musical Hallucinations: A Statistical Analysis of 46 Cases." *Psychopathology, 24*, 356–360.

Bohne, B.A., Clark, W.W. 1982. "Growth of Hearing Loss and Cochlear Lesion with Increasing Duration of Noise Exposure." In R.P. Hamernik, D. Henderson, and R. Salvi (Eds.), *New Perspectives on Noise-induced Hearing Loss*, pp. 283–302. New York: Raven Press.

Bonfis, P., Uziel, A., Pujol, R. 1988. "Evoked Otoacoustic Emission from Adults and Infants: Clinical Applications." *Acta Otolaryngologica, 105*, 445–449.

Brown, M.C., Berglund, A.M., Kiang, N.Y.-S., and Ryugo, D.K. 1988. "Central Trajectories of Type II Spiral Ganglion Neurons." *Journal of Comparative Neurology, 278*, 581–590.

Brown, M.C., Liberman, M.C., Benson, T.E., and Ryugo, D.K. 1988. "Brainstem Branches from Olivocochlear Axons in Cats and Rodents." *Journal of Comparative Neurology, 278*, 591–603.

Brownell, W.E., Shehata, W.E., and Imredy, J.P. 1990. "Slow Electrically and Chemically Evoked Volume Changes in Guinea Pig Outer Hair Cells." In N. Akkas (Ed.), *Biomechanics of Active Movement and Deformation of Cells*, p. 493–498. Berlin: Springer-Verlag.

Carpenter, G.A. and Grossberg, S. 1987. "Neural Dynamics of Category Learning and Recognition: Attention, Memory Consolidation, and Amnesia." In S. Grossberg (Ed.), *The Adaptive Brain I: Cognition, Learning, Reinforcement, and Rhythm*, pp. 239–286. Amsterdam: Elsevier Science Publisher B.V.

Champlin, C.A., Muller, S.P., and Mitchell, S.A. 1990. "Acoustic Measurements of Objective Tinnitus." *Journal of Speech and Hearing Research, 33*, 816–821.

Cloninger, C.R., Martin, R.L., Guze, S.B., and Clayton, P.J. 1985. "Diagnosis and Prognosis in Schizophrenia." *Archives of General Psychiatry, 42*, 15–25.

Conlee, J.W., Gill, S.S., McCandless, P.T., and Creel, D.J. 1989. "Differential Susceptibility to Gentamicin Ototoxicity between Albino and Pigmented Guinea Pigs." *Hearing Research, 41*, 43–52.

Corey, D.P., and Hudspeth, A.J. 1979. "Ionic Basis of the Receptor Potential in a Vertebrate Hair Cell." *Nature, 281*, 675–677.

Dallos, P. 1981. "Cochlear Physiology." *Annual Review of Psychology, 32*, 153–190.

Davis, R.I., Ahroon, W.A., and Hamernik, R.P. 1989. "The Relation among Hearing Loss, Sensory Cell Loss and Tuning Characteristics in the Chinchilla." *Hearing Research, 41*, 1–14.

Day, R.O., Graham, G.G., Bieri, D., Brown, M., Cairns, D., Harris, G., Hounsell, J., Platt-Hepworth, S., Reeve, R., Sambrook, P.N., and Smith, J. 1989. "Concentration-Response Relationships for Salicylate-induced Ototoxicity in Normal Volunteers." *British Journal of Clinical Pharmacology, 28*, 695–702.

Dieler, R., Shehata-Dieler, W.E., and Brownell, W.E.

1991. "Concomitant Salicylate-induced Alterations of Outer Hair Cell Subsurface Cisternae and Electromotility." *Journal of Neurocytology, 20,* 637–653.

Drescher, D.G. and Drescher, M.J. 1987a. "Calcium and Magnesium Dependence of Spontaneous and Evoked Afferent Neural Activity in the Lateral-line Organ of Xenopus laevis." *Comparative Biochemistry and Physiology, 87,* 305–310.

Drescher, D.G., and Drescher, M.J. 1987b. "Spontaneous Neural Activity of a Mechanoreceptive System Is Undiminished by Replacement of External Calcium with Equimolar Magnesium in the Presence of EGTA." *Life Sciences, 40,* 1371–1377.

Dulon, D., Aran J.-M., and Schacht, J. 1988. "Potassium-Depolarization Induced Motility in Isolated Outer Hair Cells by an Osmotic Mechanism." *Hearing Research, 32,* 123–130.

Eggermont, J.J. 1990. "On the Pathophysiology of Tinnitus: A Review and a Peripheral Model." *Hearing Research, 48,* 111–124.

Evans, E.F. and Borerwe, T.A. 1982. "Ototoxic Effects of Salicylates on the Responses of Single Cochlear Nerve Fibres and on Cochlear Potentials." *British Journal of Audiology, 16,* 101–108.

Eybalin, M. and Altschuler, R.A. 1990. "Immuno-electron Microscopic Localization of Neurotransmitters in the Cochlea." *Journal of Electron Microscope Technology, 15,* 209–224.

Feldmann, H. 1971. "Homolateral and Contralateral Masking of Tinnitus by Noisebands and by Pure Tones." *Audiology (Basel), 10,* 138–144.

Feldmann, H. 1988. "Pathophysiology of Tinnitus." In M. Kitahara (Ed.), *Tinnitus: Pathophysiology and Management,* pp. 7–35. Tokyo: Igaku-Shoin.

Ferrary, E., Tran Ba Huy, P., Roinel, N., Bernard C., and Amiel, C. 1988. "Calcium and the Inner Ear Fluids." *Acta Otolaryngologica Supplement (Stockholm), 460,* 13–17.

Flock, A., Flock, B., and Ulfendahl, M. 1986. "Mechanisms of Movement in Outer Hair Cells and a Possible Structural Basis." *Archives of Otorhinolaryngology, 243,* 83–90.

Flower, R.J., Moncada, S., and Vane, J.R. 1980. "Analgesic-Antipyretics and Anti-inflammatory Agents." In A.G. Gilman, L.S. Goodman, and A. Gilman (Eds.), *The Pharmacological Basis of Therapeutics.* pp. 682–728. New York: Macmillan.

Freeman, W.J., Yao, Y., and Burke, B. 1988. "Central

Pattern Generating and Recognizing in Olfactory Bulb: A Correlation Learning Rule." *Neural Networks, 1,* 277–288.

George, R.N. and Kemp, S. 1989. "Investigation of Tinnitus Induced by Sound and Its Relationship to Ongoing Tinnitus." *Journal of Speech and Hearing Research, 32,* 366–372.

Grossberg, S. 1987. "The Adaptive Self-organization of Serial Order in Behavior: Speech, Language, and Motor Control." In S. Grossberg (Ed.), *The Adaptive Brain II: Vision, Speech, Language, and Motor Control,* pp. 313–400. Amsterdam: Elsevier Science Publishers B.V.

Guth, P.S., Aubert, A., Ricci, A.J., and Norris C.H. 1991. "Differential Modulation of Spontaneous and Evoked Neurotransmitter Release from Hair Cells: Some Novel Hypotheses." *Hearing Research, 56,* 69–78.

Hamernik, R.P., Patterson, J.H., Turrentine, G.A., and Ahroon, W.A. 1989. "The Quantitative Relation between Sensory Cell Loss and Hearing Thresholds." *Hearing Research, 38,* 199–212.

Hammeke, T.A., McQuillen, M.P., and Cohen, B.A. 1983. "Musical Hallucinations Associated with Acquired Deafness." *Journal of Neurology, Neurosurgery and Psychiatry, 46,* 570–572.

Harris, F.P., Lonsbury-Martin, B.L., Stagner, B.B., Coats, A.C., and Martin, G.K. 1989. "Acoustic Distortion Product in Humans: Systematic Changes in Amplitude as a Function of f_2/f_1 Ratio." *Journal of the Acoustic Society of America, 85,* 220–229.

Harris, S., Brismar, J., and Cronqvist, S. 1979. "Pulsatile Tinnitus and Therapeutic Embolization." *Acta Otolaryngologica (Stockholm), 88,* 220–226.

Hazell, J.W. 1990. "Tinnitus. II: Surgical Management of Conditions Associated with Tinnitus and Somatosounds." *Journal of Otolaryngology, 19,* 6–10.

Hazell, J.W., Wood, S.M., Cooper, H.R., Stephens, S.D., Corcoran, A.L., Coles, R.R., Baskill, J.L., and Sheldrake, J.B. 1985. "A Clinical Study of Tinnitus Maskers." *British Journal of Audiology, 19,* 65–146.

Hazell, J.W.P. 1987. "A Cochlear Model for Tinnitus." In H. Feldmann (Ed.), *Proceedings III International Tinnitus Seminar, Muenster, 1987,* pp. 121–128. Karlsruhe: Harsch Verlag.

Hazell, J.W.P. and Jastreboff, P.J. 1992. "Central Mechanisms of Tinnitus." *Audiology in Europe,* p. 22. Academic conference: Cambridge, UK, September 21–24, 1992.

Hazell, J.W.P., Jastreboff, P.J., Meerton, L.E., and Conway, M.J. 1993. "Electrical Tinnitus Suppression: Frequency Dependence of Effects." *Audiology, 32,* 68–77.

Hazell, J.W.P. and Sheldrake, J.B. 1992. "Hyperacusis and Tinnitus." In J.-M. Aran and R. Dauman (Eds.), *Proceedings of the Fourth International Tinnitus Seminar, Bordeaux, 1991,* pp. 245–248. Amsterdam: Kugler Publications.

Hazell, J.W.P., Sheldrake, J.B., and Meerton, L.J. 1987. "Tinnitus Masking—Is It Better than Counseling Alone?" In H. Feldmann (Ed.), *Proceedings III International Tinnitus Seminar, Muenster, 1987,* pp. 239–250. Karlsruhe: Harsch Verlag.

Heilbrun, A.B. Jr., Diller, R., Fleming, R., and Slade, L. 1986. "Strategies of Disattention and Auditory Hallucinations in Schizophrenics." *Journal of Nervous and Mental Disorders, 174,* 265–73.

Heller, M.F. and Bergman, M. 1953. "Tinnitus in Normally Hearing Persons." *Annals of Otology, 62,* 73–93.

Hentzer, E. 1968. "Objective Tinnitus of the Vascular Type. A Follow-up Study." *Acta Otolaryngologica (Stockholm), 66,* 273–281.

Hudspeth, A.J. 1983. "Mechanoelectrical Transduction by Hair Cells in the Acousticolateralis Sensory System." *Annual Review of Neuroscience, 6,* 187–215.

Hudspeth, A.J. 1985. "The Cellular Basis of Hearing: The Biophysics of Hair Cells." *Science, 230,* 745–752.

Hudspeth, A.J. 1986. "The Ionic Channels of a Vertebrate Hair Cell." *Hearing Research, 22,* 21–27.

Hudspeth, A.J. and Corey, D.P. 1977. "Sensitivity, Polarity and Conductance in the Response of Vertebrate Hair Cells to Controlled Mechanical Stimuli." *Proceedings of the National Academy of Science, USA, 74,* 2407–2411.

Hunter-Duvar, I.M., Suzuki, M., and Mount, R.J. 1982. "Anatomical Changes in the Organ of Corti after Acoustic Stimulation." In R.P. Hamernik, D. Henderson, and D. Salvi (Eds.), *New Perspectives on Noise-Induced Hearing Loss,* pp. 3–22. New York: Raven Press.

Ikeda, K. and Morizono, T. 1989. "Electrochemical Profile for Calcium Ions in the Stria Vascularis: Cellular Model of Calcium Transport Mechanism." *Hearing Research, 40,* 111–116.

Jabboury, K., Frye, D., Holmes, F.A., Fraschini, G., and Hortobagyi, G. 1989. "Phase II Evaluation of Gallium Nitrate by Continuous Infusion in Breast Cancer." *Investigating New Drugs, 7,* 225–229.

Jastreboff, P.J. 1990. "Phantom Auditory Perception (Tinnitus): Mechanisms of Generation and Perception." *Neuroscience Research, 8,* 221–254.

Jastreboff, P.J. 1992. "Appropriateness of Salicylate-based Models of Tinnitus." In J.-M. Aran and R. Dauman (Eds.), *Proceedings of the Fourth International Tinnitus Seminar, Bordeaux, 1991,* pp. 309–313. Amsterdam: Kugler Publications.

Jastreboff, P.J. and Brennan, J.F. 1988. "Specific Effects of Nimodipine on the Auditory System." *Annals of the New York Academy of Sciences, 522,* 716–718.

Jastreboff, P.J. and Brennan, J.F. 1992. "The Psychoacoustical Characteristics of Tinnitus in Rats." In J.-M. Aran and R. Dauman (Eds.), *Proceedings of the Fourth International Tinnitus Seminar, Bordeaux, 1991,* pp. 305–308. Amsterdam: Kugler Publications.

Jastreboff, P.J., Brennan, J.F., and Sasaki, C.T. 1988b. "Pigmentation, Anesthesia, Behavioral Factors and Salicylate Uptake." *Archives of Otolaryngology—Head and Neck Surgery, 114,* 186–191.

Jastreboff, P.J., Brennan, J.F., and Sasaki, C.T. 1988a. "Phantom Auditory Sensation in Rats: An Animal Model for Tinnitus." *Behavioral Neuroscience, 102,* 811–822.

Jastreboff, P.J., Brennan, J.F., and Sasaki, C.T. 1991. "Quinine-induced Tinnitus in Rats." *Archives of Otolaryngology—Head and Neck Surgery, 117,* 1162–1166.

Jastreboff, P.J. and Chen, G.-D. 1993. "Salicylate-induced Modification of the Spontaneous Activity in the Inferior Colliculus in Rats." *Association for Research in Otolaryngology, 16,* 40.

Jastreboff, P.J., Hansen, R., Sasaki, P.G., and Sasaki, C.T. 1986. "Differential Uptake of Salicylate in Serum, CSF and Perilymph." *Archives of Otolaryngology—Head and Neck Surgery, 112,* 1050–1083.

Jastreboff, P.J. and Hazell, J.W.P. 1993. "A Neurophysiological Approach to Tinnitus: Clinical Implications." *British Journal of Audiology, 27,* 7–17.

Jastreboff, P.J., Nguyen, O., Brennan, J.F., and Sasaki, C.T. 1992. "Calcium and Calcium Channel Involvement in Tinnitus." In J.-M. Aran and R. Dauman (Eds.), *Proceedings of the Fourth International Tinnitus Seminar, Bordeaux, 1991,* pp. 109–114. Amsterdam: Kugler Publications.

Kemp, D.T. 1979. "Evidence of Mechanical Non-linearity and Frequency Selective Wave Amplification in the Cochlea." *Archives of Otorhinolaryngology, 224,* 37–45.

Kemp, D.T., Bray, P., Alexander, L., and Brown, A.M. 1986. "Acoustic Emission Cochleography—Practical Aspects." *Scandinavian Audiology (Supplement), 25,* 71–95.

Kemp, D.T., and Brown, A.M. 1983. "A Comparison of Mechanical Nonlinearities in Cochleae of Man and Gerbil from Ear Canal Measurements." In R. Klinke and R. Hartmann (Eds.), *Hearing—Physiological Bases and Psychophysics* pp. 82–88. New York: Springer Verlag.

Kemp, S. and Plaisted, I.D. 1986. "Tinnitus Induced by Tones." *Journal of Speech and Hearing Research, 29,* 65–70.

Klostermann, W., Vieregge, P., and Kömpf, D. 1992. "Musical Pseudo-hallucination in Acquired Hearing Loss." *Fortschritte Neurologie-Psychiatrie, 60,* 262–273.

Konorski, J. 1948. *Conditioned Reflexes and Neuronal Organization.* Cambridge: Cambridge University Press.

Kronester-Frei, A. 1979. "The Effect of Changes in Endolymphatic Ion Concentrations on the Tectorial Membrane." *Hearing Research, 1,* 81–94.

Kujawa, S.G., Fallon, M., and Bobbin, R.P. 1992. "Intracochlear Salicylate Reduces Low-intensity Acoustic and Cochlear Microphonic Distortion Products." *Hearing Research, 64,* 73–80.

LePage, E.L. 1987. "Frequency-dependent Self-induced Bias of the Basilar Membrane and Its Potential for Controlling Sensitivity and Tuning in the Mammalian Cochlea." *Journal of the Acoustical Society of America, 82,* 139–154.

LePage, E.L. 1989. "Functional Role of the Olivo-cochlear Bundle: A Motor Unit Control System in the Mammalian Cochlea." *Hearing Research, 38,* 177–198.

Liberman, M.C. 1987. "Chronic Ultrastructural Changes in Acoustic Trauma: Serial-section Reconstruction of Stereocilia and Cuticular Plates." *Hearing Research, 26,* 65–88.

Liberman, M.C. 1988. "Response Properties of Cochlear Efferent Neurons: Monaural vs. Binaural Stimulation and the Effects of Noise." *Journal of Neurophysiology, 60,* 1779–1798.

Liberman, M.C. and Brown, M.C. 1986. "Physiology and Anatomy of Single Olivocochlear Neurons in the Cat." *Hearing Research, 24,* 17–36.

Liberman, M.C. and Dodds, L.W. 1984a. "Single-neuron Labeling and Chronic Cochlear Pathology. II. Stereocilia Damage and Alteration of Spontaneous Discharge Rates." *Hearing Research, 16,* 43–53.

Liberman, M.C. and Dodds, L.W. 1984b. "Single-neuron Labeling and Chronic Cochlear Pathology. III. Stereocilia Damage and Alteration of Threshold Tuning Curves." *Hearing Research, 16,* 55–74.

Liberman, M.C. and Dodds, L.W. 1987. "Acute Ultrastructural Changes in Acoustic Trauma: Serial-section Reconstruction of Stereocilia and Cuticular Plates." *Hearing Research, 26,* 45–64.

Liberman, M.C. and Mulroy, M.J. 1982. "Acute and Chronic Effects of Acoustic Trauma: Cochlear Pathology and Auditory Nerve Pathophysiology." In R.P. Hamernik, D. Henderson, and R. Salvi (Eds.), *New Perspectives on Noise-Induced Hearing Loss,* pp. 105–136. New York: Raven Press.

Lippmann, R.P. 1989. "Review of Neural Networks for Speech Recognition." *Neural Computation, 1,* 1–38.

Long, G.R. and Tubis, A. 1988. "Modification of Spontaneous and Evoked Otoacoustic Emissions and Associated Psychoacoustic Microstructure by Aspirin Consumption." *Journal of the Acoustical Society of America, 84,* 1343–1353.

Lonsbury-Martin, B.L., Martin, G.K., Probst, R., and Coats, A.C. 1987. "Acoustic Distortion Products in Rabbit Ear Canal. I. Basic Features and Physiological Vulnerability." *Hearing Research, 28,* 173–189.

Martin, G.K., Lonsbury-Martin, B.L., Probst, R., and Coats, A.C. 1988. "Spontaneous Otoacoustic Emissions in a Nonhuman Primate. I. Basic Features and Relations to Other Emissions." *Hearing Research, 33,* 49–68.

Martin, G.K., Lonsbury-Martin, B.L., Probst, R., Scheinin, S.A., and Coats, A.C. 1987. "Acoustic Distortion Products in Rabbit Ear Canal. II. Sites of Origin Revealed by Suppression Contours and Pure-tone Exposures." *Hearing Research, 28,* 191–208.

McFadden, D. 1982. *Tinnitus: Facts, Theories, and Treatments,* pp. 1–150. Washington, DC: National Academy Press.

McFadden, D. and Plattsmier, H.S. 1984. "Aspirin Abolishes Spontaneous Oto-acoustic Emissions." *Journal of the Acoustical Society of America, 76,* 443–448.

Melzack, R. 1989. "Phantom Limbs, the Self and the Brain (The D.O. Hebb Memorial Lecture)." *Canadian Psychology/Psychologie Canadienne, 30,* 1–16.

Melzack, R. 1990. "Phantom Limbs and the Concept of a Neuromatrix." *Trends in Neuroscience, 13,* 88–92.

Melzack, R. 1992. "Phantom Limbs." *Scientific American, 266,* 120–126.

Melzack, R. and Wall, P.D. 1965. "Pain Mechanisms: A New Theory." *Science, 150,* 971–979.

Møller, A.R. 1984. "Pathophysiology of Tinnitus." *Annals of Otology, Rhinology and Laryngology, 93,* 39–44.

Møller, A.R. 1987. "Can Injury to the Auditory Nerve Cause Tinnitus?" In H. Feldmann (Ed.), *Proceedings III International Tinnitus Seminar, Muenster, 1987.* pp. 58–63. Karlsruhe: Harsch Verlag.

Møller, A.R. 1992. "Central Neurophysiological Processes in Tinnitus." In J.-M. Aran and R. Dauman (Eds.), *Proceedings of the Fourth International Tinnitus Seminar, Bordeaux, 1991,* pp. 165–179. Amsterdam: Kugler & Ghedini.

Møller, M.B. 1987. "Vascular Compression of the Eighth Nerve as Cause of Tinnitus." In H. Feldmann (Ed.), *Proceedings III International Tinnitus Seminar, Muenster, 1987,* pp. 340–347. Karlsruhe: Harsch Verlag.

Mongan, E., Kelly, P., Nies, K., Porter, W.W., and Paulus, H.E. 1973. "Tinnitus as an Indication of Therapeutic Serum Salicylate Levels." *JAMA, 226,* 141–145.

Orman, S. and Flock, A. 1983. "Active Control of Sensory Hair Mechanics Implied by Susceptibility to Media that Induce Contraction in Muscle." *Hearing Research, 11,* 261–266.

Penner, M.J. 1983. "The Annoyance of Tinnitus and the Noise Required to Mask it." *Journal of Speech and Hearing Research, 26,* 73–76.

Penner, M.J. 1986. "Tinnitus as a Source of Internal Noise." *Journal of Speech and Hearing Research, 29,* 400–406.

Penner, M.J. 1987. "Masking of Tinnitus and Central Masking." *Journal of Speech and Hearing Research, 30,* 147–152.

Penner, M.J. 1988. "The Effect of Continuous Monaural Noise on Loudness Matches to Tinnitus." *Journal of Speech and Hearing Research, 31,* 98–102.

Penner, M.J. 1989. "Aspirin Abolishes Tinnitus Caused by Spontaneous Otoacoustic Emissions. A Case Study." *Archives of Otolaryngology—Head and Neck Surgery, 115,* 871–875.

Penner, M.J. 1990. "An Estimate of the Prevalence of Tinnitus Caused by Spontaneous Otoacoustic Emissions." *Archives of Otolaryngology—Head and Neck Surgery, 116,* 418–423.

Penner, M.J. 1992. "Linking Spontaneous Otoacoustic Emissions and Tinnitus." *British Journal of Audiology, 26,* 115–123.

Penner, M.J. and Bilger, R.C. 1989. "Adaptation and the Masking of Tinnitus." *Journal of Speech and Hearing Research, 32,* 339–346.

Penner, M.J. and Coles, R.R. 1992. "Indications for Aspirin as a Palliative for Tinnitus Caused by SOAEs: A Case Study." *British Journal of Audiology, 26,* 91–96.

Pribram, K.H. 1971. *Languages of the Brain—Experimental Paradoxes and Principles in Neurophysiology,* pp. 1–432. Englewood Cliffs, NJ: Prentice Hall.

Pribram, K.H. 1987. "Holography and Brain Function." In G. Adelman (Ed.), *Encyclopedia of Neuroscience,* pp. 499–500. Boston: Birkhauser.

Probst, R., Coats, A.C., Martin, G.K., and Lonsbury-Martin, B.L. 1986. "Spontaneous, Click-, and Toneburst-evoked Otoacoustic Emissions from Normal Ears." *Hearing Research, 21,* 261–275.

Probst, R., Lonsbury-Martin, B.L., Martin, G.K., and Coats, A.C. 1987. "Otoacoustic Emissions in Ears with Hearing Loss." *American Journal of Otolaryngology, 8,* 73–81.

Puel, J.-L., Bledsoe, S.C. Jr., Bobbin, R.P., Ceasar, G., and Fallon, M. 1989. "Comparative Actions of Salicylate on the Amphibian Lateral Line and Guinea Pig Cochlea." *Comparative Biochemistry and Physiology, 93C,* 73–80.

Puel, J.-L., Bobbin, R.P., and Fallon, M. 1988. "The Active Process Is Affected First by Intense Sound Exposure." *Hearing Research, 37,* 53–64.

Puel, J.-L., Bobbin, R.P., and Fallon, M. 1990. "Salicylate, Mefenamate, Meclofenamate, and Quinine on Cochlear Potentials." *Archives of Otolaryngology—Head and Neck Surgery, 102,* 66–73.

Puel, J.-L., Ladrech, S., Chabert, R., Pujol, R., and Eybalin, M. 1991. "Electrophysiological Evidence for the Presence of NMDA Receptors in the Guinea Pig Cochlea." *Hearing Research, 51,* 255–264.

Pujol, R. 1992. "Neuropharmacology of the Cochlea

and Tinnitus." In J.-M. Aran and R. Dauman (Eds.), *Proceedings of the Fourth International Tinnitus Seminar, Bordeaux, 1991*, pp. 103–107. Amsterdam: Kugler Publications.

Pujol, R. and Lenoir, M. 1986. "The Four Types of Synapses in the Organ of Corti." In R.A. Altschuler, D.W. Hoffman, and R.P. Bobbin (Eds.), *The Cochlea*, pp. 161–172. New York: Raven Press.

Pujol, R., Rebillard, G., Puel, J.-L., Lenoir, M., Eybalin, M., and Recasens, M. 1991. "Glutamate Neurotoxicity in the Cochlea: A Possible Consequence of Ischaemic or Anoxic Conditions Occurring in Ageing." *Acta Otolaryngologica, Supplement (Stockholm), 476*, 32–36.

Ryan, A.F., Keithley, E.M., Wang, X.Z., and Schwartz, I.R. 1990. "Collaterals from Lateral and Medial Olivocochlear Efferent Neurons Innervate Different Regions of the Cochlear Nucleus and Adjacent Brainstem." *Journal of Comparative Neurology, 300*, 572–582.

Salvi, R., Perry, J., Hamernik, R.P., and Henderson, D. 1982. "Relationship between Cochlear Pathologies and Auditory Nerve and Behavioral Responses following Acoustic Trauma." In R.P. Hamernik, D. Henderson, and R. Salvi (Eds.), *New Perspectives on Noise-Induced Hearing Loss*, pp. 165–188. New York: Raven Press.

Sand, O., Ozawa, S., and Hagiwara, S. 1975. "Electrical and Mechanical Stimulation of Hair Cells in the Mudpuppy." *Journal of Comparative Physiology, A 102*, 13–26.

Saunders, J.C. and Flock, A. 1985. "Changes in the Cochlear Hair-Cell Stereocilia Stiffness following Overstimulation." *Association for Research in Otolaryngology, 8*, 51.

Schultz, G. and Melzack, R. 1991. "The Charles Bonnet Syndrome: 'Phantom Visual Images'." *Perception, 20*, 809–825.

Sejnowski, T.J., Koch, C., and Churchland, P.S. 1988. "Computational Neuroscience." *Science, 241*, 1299–1306.

Shehata, W.E., Brownell, W.E., Cousillas, H., and Imredy, J.P. 1990. "Salicylate Alters Membrane Conductance of Outer Hair Cells and Diminishes Rapid Electromotile Responses." *Association for Research in Otolaryngology, 13*, 252–253.

Shehata, W.E., Brownell, W.E., and Dieler, R. 1991. "Effects of Salicylate on Shape, Electromotility and

Membrane Characteristics of Isolated Outer Hair Cells from Guinea Pig Cochlea." *Acta Otolaryngologica (Stockholm), 111*, 707–718.

Sheldrake, J.B. and Hazell, J.W.P. 1992. "Maskers versus Hearing Aids in the Prosthetic Management of Tinnitus." In J.-M. Aran and R. Dauman (Eds.), *Proceedings of the Fourth International Tinnitus Seminar, Bordeaux, 1991*, pp. 395–399. Amsterdam: Kugler Publications.

Sterkers, O., Bernard, C., Ferrary, E., Sziklai, I., Tran Ba Huy, P., and Amiel, C. 1988. "Possible Role of Ca Ions in the Vestibular System." *Acta Otolaryngologica Supplement (Stockholm), 460*, 28–32.

Stypulkowski, P.H. 1989. *Physiological Mechanisms of Salicylate Ototoxicity (Ph.D. thesis)*, pp. 1–176. Storrs, CT: University of Connecticut.

Stypulkowski, P.H. 1990. "Mechanisms of Salicylate Ototoxicity." *Hearing Research, 46*, 113–145.

Tonndorf, J. 1987. "The Analogy between Tinnitus and Pain: A Suggestion for a Physiological Basis of Chronic Tinnitus." *Hearing Research, 28*, 271–275.

Tyler, R.S. and Conrad-Armes, D. 1984. "Masking of Tinnitus Compared to Masking of Pure Tones." *Journal of Speech and Hearing Research, 27*, 106–111.

Ulfendahl, M. 1987. "Motility in Auditory Sensory Cells." *Acta Physiologica Scandinavica, 130*, 521–527.

Valli, P. and Zucca, G. 1976. "The Origin of Slow Potentials in Semicircular Canals of the Frog." *Acta Otolaryngologica (Stockholm), 81*, 395–405.

Vernon, J. 1987. "Assessment of the Tinnitus Patient." In J.W.P. Hazell (Ed.), *Tinnitus*, pp. 71–95. Edinburgh: Churchill Livingstone.

Vernon, J. and Meikle, M.B. 1981. "Tinnitus Masking: Unresolved Problems." In D. Evered and G. Lawrenson (Eds.), *Ciba Foundation Symposium 85, Tinnitus*, pp. 239–256. London: Pitman.

Waibel, A. 1989. "Modular Construction of Time-delay Neural Networks for Speech Recognition." *Neural Computation, 1*, 39–46.

Wier, C.C., Pasanen, E.G., and McFadden, D. 1988. "Partial Dissociation of Spontaneous Otoacoustic Emissions and Distortion Products during Aspirin Use in Humans." *Journal of the Acoustical Society of America, 84*, 230–237.

Wilson, J.P. 1980. "The Combination Tone $2f_1$-f_2, in Psychophysics and Ear-canal Recording." In G. van den Brink and F.A. Bilsen (Eds.), *Psychophysical, Physiological, and Behavioral Studies in Hearing,* pp. 43–52. Delft: Delft University Press.

Wyant, G.M. 1979. "Chronic Pain Syndromes and Their Treatment. II. Trigger Points." *Canadian Anaesthesiological Society Journal, 26,* 216–219.

Zenner, H.P., Zimmermann, R., and Gitter A.H. 1988. "Active Movements of the Cuticular Plate Induce Sensory Hair Motion in Mammalian Outer Hair Cells." *Hearing Research, 34,* 233–239.

Zenner, H.P., Zimmermann, U., and Schmitt, U. 1985. "Reversible Contraction of Isolated Mammalian Cochlear Hair Cells." *Hearing Research, 18,* 127–133.

Zurek, P.M., Clark, W.W., and Kim, D.O. 1982. "The Behavior of Acoustic Distortion Products in the Ear Canals of Chinchillas with Normal or Damaged Ears." *Journal of the Acoustical Society of America, 72,* 774–780.

CHAPTER 9

TINNITUS AND SPONTANEOUS ACTIVITY IN THE AUDITORY SYSTEM

MASAAKI KITAHARA
HIROYA KITANO
MIKIO SUZUKI
KAZUTOMO KITAJIMA
Shiga University of Medical Science

INTRODUCTION

Tinnitus is defined as the conscious experience of sound that does not originate outside the body. Although it is difficult to separate tinnitus and elementary auditory hallucination, tinnitus is usually differentiated from this psychological phenomenon that may be caused by the disturbance of imagination. The pathophysiology of tinnitus is, therefore, thought to be an increase in the spontaneous rate of firing of the central auditory fibers, which stimulates the auditory cortex. Of course, the awareness, the loudness, and the annoyance of tinnitus is strongly influenced by the psychological status of the subject as well.

In the primary auditory fibers, tinnitus originates from the increase in the spontaneous rate of firing. Objective tinnitus can be explained by this change in the primary auditory fibers, which may be caused by the convulsion or spasm of intratympanic muscles or palatopharyngeal muscles. Decoupling of the stereocilia, a possible sequence of noise exposure or administration of certain ototoxic drugs, and/or the increase of potassium concentration in the scala tympany (a possible cause of Ménière's disease) can also be considered as producers of tinnitus, as these factors increase the spontaneous rate of firing of the primary auditory fibers.

Over the years, in order to investigate the nature of altered neural activity of the primary fibers underlying tinnitus, stimuli that are known to produce tinnitus in humans, such as salicylate, kanamycin, and noise, have been administered to animals. Although the increase in the spontaneous rate of firing of the primary auditory fibers was observed by exposure to noise (Schmiedt, Zwislocki, and Hamernik 1980), most studies tended to find an opposite result with acute pathology. For example, the depression in the spontaneous rate of firing was observed by the administration of kanamycin (Kiang, Moxon, and Levine 1970; Schmiedt et al. 1980) and also exposure to noise (Liberman and Kiang 1978; Salvi, Hamernik, and Henderson 1978). Dallos and Harris (1978) failed to find a change in a spontaneous rate of firing after administration of kanamycin.

In 1981, Evans, Wilson, and Borerwe reported that the administration of salicylate induced no change in spontaneous firing in the low rate of fibers, but induced an increasing rate of spontaneous firing in the mean rate of fibers. In 1984, Prijs and Harrison studied two guinea pigs with endolymphatic hydrops. In this study, 5 percent of the neural units showed a spontaneous bursting activity which the authors suggested might be related to tinnitus. These varied results led us to the suggestion that tinnitus may possibly be caused either by the increase or by the decrease in the spontaneous rate of firing in the primary auditory fibers.

However, at the same time, these outcomes raised the following questions: Although it is understandable that a decrease in the spontaneous rate of firing is caused in primary auditory fibers, is it ever possible to find an increase in the spontaneous rate of firing even when there is careful observation? Does the fact that an application of certain types of stimuli does not cause a change in the spontaneous rate of firing imply that tinnitus is not induced by the application of these same stimuli? With these questions in mind, the effect of anoxia on the spontaneous rate of firing of the cochlear single units was examined in normal guinea pigs and those previously administered with salicylate. Anoxia is thought to increase hearing thresholds and decrease neural activity in the primary auditory fibers. Salicylate is well known for producing tinnitus in humans, but it is uncertain whether or not it affects the spontaneous rate of firing of the primary auditory fibers in animals.

MATERIAL AND METHODS

Eighteen young mature guinea pigs weighting approximately 400g each were used in this examination. After being anesthetized with sodium pentobarbital and tubocramine chloride, tracheotomies were performed. Following this, the animals were respirated artificially. Posterior craniotomies were performed to gain access to the cochlear nerve. An electrode, with a resistance of about 25 megohms, was placed in the cochlear nerve of each animal, and a reference tungsten electrode was placed on the neck muscle. Single fiber responses were monitored extracellularly and recorded after amplification. The records were analyzed with a SANEI 7T-18 signal processor. Anoxia was applied by stopping the respirator. Five of the animals were injected with 350mg/Kg i.p. of sodium salicylate 60 minutes prior to the application of anoxia.

RESULTS

Figure 9-1 shows the alternation in the spontaneous rate of firing in a cochlear neuron of a guinea pig where anoxia was applied. The spontaneous rate of firing was stable under normal respiration (a), but the rate was increased following the application of anoxia (b). Immediately after the rate increased to a peak, the rate was decreased (c) and spikes disappeared.

Figure 9-2 shows the spontaneous rate of firing of 19 cochlear neurons in cases where a statistically significant increase was demonstrated in the rate while anoxia was applied. The vertical axis

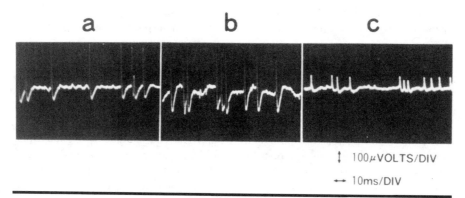

100μVOLTS/DIV

10ms/DIV

FIGURE 9-1. Spontaneous firing in a cochlear neuron of a guinea pig where anoxia was applied: (a) under normal respiration, (b) following the application of anoxia, (c) immediately after the rate increased to a peak.

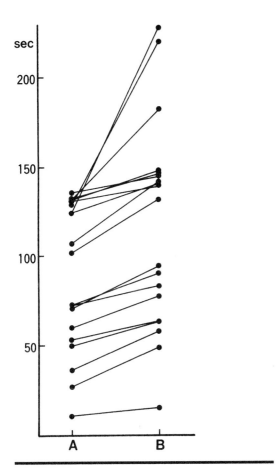

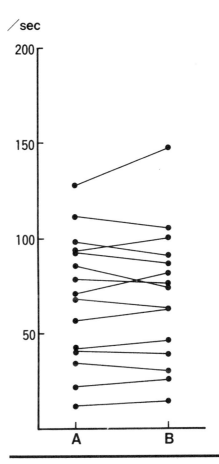

FIGURE 9-2.   Spontaneous rate of firing of 19 cochlear neurons in cases where a significant increase was demonstrated in the rate while anoxia was applied. The vertical axis indicates the average number of spontaneous discharges per second during normal respiration (A) and during anoxia (B).

FIGURE 9-3.   Spontaneous rate of 15 cochlear neurons per second in cases where a significant increase was not observed in the rate when anoxia was applied. The vertical axis indicates the average number of spontaneous discharges per second during normal respiration (A) and during anoxia (B).

indicates the average number of spontaneous discharges per second (A) during normal respiration and (B) during anoxia. Figure 9-3 shows the spontaneous rate of 15 cochlear neurons per second in cases where a statistically significant increase was not demonstrated in the rate while anoxia was applied. The average spontaneous rate of firing during normal respiration in this group (69/sec) was significantly lower than that of the former group (90/sec).

Figure 9-4 shows an alternation of the spontaneous rate of firing of a cochlear neuron in a guinea pig where anoxia was applied 60 minutes after an intraperitoneal injection of 500mg/Kg of sodium salicylate. A remarkable increase of the spontaneous rate of firing was observed after a short pause following the application of anoxia.

Figure 9-5 shows an alternation of the spontaneous rate of firing of 5 cochlear neurons of guinea pigs where anoxia was applied 60 minutes

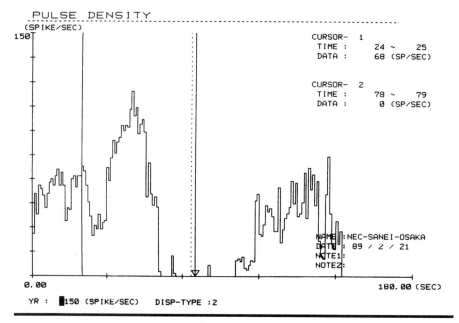

FIGURE 9-4.   Spontaneous rate of firing of a cochlear neuron in a guinea pig where anoxia was applied 60 minutes after an intraperitoneal injection of sodium salicylate. The solid line indicates the application of anoxia; the dotted line represents the beginning of respiration.

after an intraperitoneal injection of sodium salicylate. In all cases, remarkable increases were seen in the spontaneous rate of firing (B) following the application of anoxia. The average spontaneous rate (A) after administration of salicylate and before the application of anoxia, was 54/sec. The rate was even lower than that of the neurons shown in Figure 9-3A which did not increase the spontaneous rate after the application of anoxia.

COMMENTS

It is generally accepted that the reduction of the spontaneous rate of firing of the primary auditory fibers can be a cause of tinnitus; the phenomenon was often proven in animals by the application of tinnitus producers such as kanamycin or exposure to noise. This hypothesis is supported by the following experimental facts: In 1977, the 2-deoxyglucose technique offered a way to monitor the metabolic activity of the central nervous system (Sokoloff, Reivich, Kennedy, DesRosier, Patlak, Pettigrew, Sakutrada, and Skinohara 1977). In 1980, Sasaki, Kauer, and Babitz observed changes in the activity in a guinea pig's auditory pathway using an autoradiographic method of brainmapping after cochlear ablations. They found heightened activity in the central auditory pathways following ablations. This activity was thought to be a cause of tinnitus. According to Young and Voigt (1981), inhibitory interaction between neurons in the auditory system initiates from the level of the dorsal cochlear nucleus and is found in all higher centers. In the case of cochlear ablations, interneurons which act in an inhibitory way in the cochlear nucleus are supplied with a decreased input from their efferents. Thus, the abnormally large spontaneous activity caused in the central auditory pathway by the loss of the inhibition is thought to be an origin of tinnitus. It is,

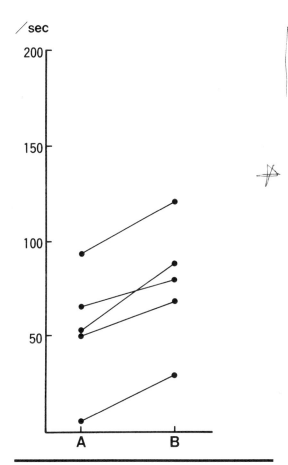

FIGURE 9-5. (B) Spontaneous rate of firing of 5 cochlear neurons of a guinea pig where anoxia was applied (A) 60 minutes after an intraperitoneal injection of sodium salicylate.

of normal electrical activity in the peripheral auditory fibers induces abnormal activity in the central auditory pathway. This abnormal activity will be continuously held by the successive loss of central inhibition. From a clinical point of view, similar assumptions were proposed by House (1981): He suggested that tinnitus appearing to start as a symptom of an end-organ, such as Ménière's disease or traumatic labyrinthitis, could be retained as a memory in the brainstem.

In a second experiment, an additional application of anoxia increased the spontaneous rate of firing of the primary auditory fibers even when the spontaneous rate was not increased after administration of salicylates. This finding implies that predisposition to tinnitus is possible, even in primary fibers with normal rates of spontaneous firing. These conditions would manifest tinnitus with mild triggers. This is considered to be an ordinary pattern in the occurrence of tinnitus in humans (Coles 1981).

REFERENCES

Coles, R.R.A. 1981. "Discussion following Animal Models of Tinnitus." In Ciba Foundation Symposium 85, Tinnitus, p. 131. London: The Pitman Press.

Dallos, P. and Harris, D. 1978. "Properties of Auditory Nerve Responses in Absences of Outer Hair Cells." *Journal of Neurophysiology, 41,* 365–383.

Evans, E.F., Wilson, J.P., and Borerwe, T.A. "Animal Models of Tinnitus." In Ciba Foundation Symposium 85, Tinnitus, pp. 108–129. London: The Pitman Press.

House, J.W. 1981. "Discussion following Animal Models of Tinnitus." In Ciba Foundation Symposium 85, Tinnitus, p. 137. London: The Pitman Press.

Kiang, N.Y.-S., Moxon, E.C., and Levine, R.A. 1970. "Auditory Nerve Activity in Cats with Normal and Abnormal Cochleas." In G.E.W. Wolstenholme and J. Knight (Eds.), *Sensorineural Hearing Loss.* London: Churchill.

Liberman, M.C. and Kiang, N.Y.-S. 1978. "Acoustic Trauma in Cats." *Acta Otolaryngologica Supplement 358,* 1–63.

Prijs, V.P. and Harrison R.V. 1984. "Eighth Nerve Re-

however, difficult to explain the occurrence of tinnitus simply by the loss of central inhibition due to lack of input from the peripheral organs because total deafness is not always accompanied by tinnitus. In this study, a temporary increase in the spontaneous rate of firing of the primary auditory fibers could be observed even in cases where stimulants such as anoxia (which reduces and stops the spontaneous rate of firing) were applied. It is easier to understand the supposition that the neural hyperactivity shown prior to the cessation sponses in Guinea Pigs with Long Term Endolymphatic Hydrops." *Revue de Laryngologie-Otologie-Rhinologie, 105, Supplement 2,* 229–235.

Salvi, R.J., Hamernik, R.P., and Henderson, D. 1978. "Discharge Patterns in the Cochlear Nucleus of the Chinchilla following Noise Induced Asymptotic Threshold Shift." *Experimental Brain Research, 32,* 301–320.

Sasaki, C.T., Kauer, J.S., and Babitz, L. 1980. "Differential (14C) 2-deoxyglucose Uptake after Deafferentiation of the Mammalian Auditory Pathway- A Model for Examining Tinnitus." *Brain Research, 194,* 511–516.

Schmiedt, R.A., Zwislocki, J.J., and Hamernik, R.P. 1980. "Effects of Hair Cell Lesions on Response of Cochlear Nerve Fibers." *Journal of Neurophysiology, 43,* 16–30.

Sokoloff, L., Reivich, M., Kennedy, C., DesRosier, M.H., Patlak, C.S., Pettigrew, K.D., Sakutrada, O., and Skinohara, M. 1977. "The (14C) Deoxyglucose Method for the Measurement of Local Glucose Utilization." *Journal of Neurochemistry, 28,* 897–916.

Young, E.D. and Voigt, H.F. 1981. "The Internal Organization of the Dorsal Cochlear Nucleus in Neural Mechanisms of Hearing." In J. Syka and L. Aitkin (Eds.), pp. 127–133. New York: Plenum Press.

CHAPTER 10

NEURAL MECHANISMS OF TINNITUS

THE PATHOLOGICAL ENSEMBLE SPONTANEOUS ACTIVITY OF THE AUDITORY SYSTEM

THOMAS LENARZ
Medical University of Hannover

CHRISTOPH SCHREINER
University of California–San Francisco

RUSSELL L. SNYDER
University of California–San Francisco

ARNE ERNST
University of Tübingen

INTRODUCTION

The cochlea is an extremely sensitive receptor system specialized for receiving and transducing sound as outlined in more detail in chapter 18 by Zenner and Ernst. Tinnitus can be linked to damage of this system in the majority of cases (e.g., Lenarz 1992). All the most common etiologies for sensory hearing loss (noise trauma, presbyacusis, otosclerosis, degenerative loss of the sensory cells, Ménière's disease, ototoxic drugs) are associated with tinnitus. And a variety of physiologic mechanisms have been proposed to account for both the loss of sensation and the induction of a pathological sensation (tinnitus) for each of these etiologies (see chapter 18). Since the symptoms of tinnitus from different mechanisms are generally quite similar, it is conceivable that various forms of cochlear damage might result in a *common* neurophysiological correlate of tinnitus located central to those lesions. At present, there are two major stumbling blocks that limit examination of

the mechanism underlying tinnitus: One is the lack of a valid animal model and the other is the inaccessibility of many neural structures in humans. Several hypotheses on neural origin of tinnitus have been proposed (Feldmann 1988). However, these hypotheses are of limited value since they were not based on, nor were they tested against, objective neurophysiological observations in humans or animals.

In this paper some underlying neurophysiological mechanisms of tinnitus are first hypothesized and critically reviewed. Then, in a second step, an experimental approach is outlined that may lead to an objectively verifiable and mechanistically more accurate neurophysiological model of tinnitus.

COMMON NEUROPHYSIOLOGICAL CORRELATES OF TINNITUS

Tinnitus is a functional disorder of the auditory system which, it appears, can be induced or modulated by activity at different locations (Figures 10-1 and

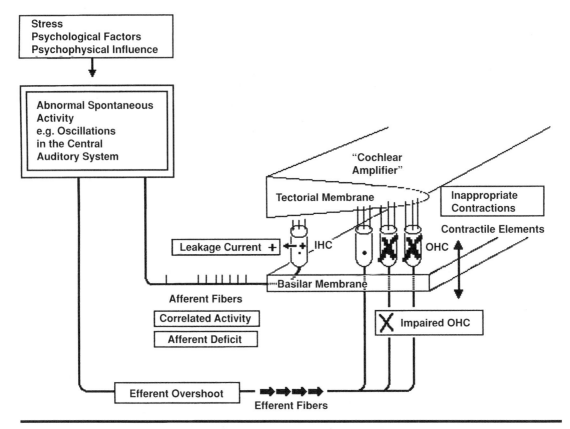

FIGURE 10-1.   Schematic view of the auditory system. The mechanisms of tinnitus induction are marked with rectangular frame, those of tinnitus generation and maintenance with a double frame.

10-2) in the auditory system. Due to the complex structure and functional organization of the auditory system, it seems worthwhile to consider whether tinnitus can be localized to any single structure or pathological mechanism. Oliveira and colleagues (Oliveira, Schuknecht, and Glynn 1990), for example, failed to establish any specific histopathological correlate of tinnitus within the cochlea.

Given the absence of a clear single localized cause of tinnitus, it is seems reasonable to consider that the generation and representation of tinnitus involves several structures which might be widely distributed over the whole auditory system. The

most striking argument against a defined localization of a tinnitus generator, especially a peripheral generator, is based on the results of ablative and destructive surgery. Douek (1987), reported on patients who developed tinnitus after stapedectomy, concluded that the primary damage was definitely localized in the cochlea, but different destructive surgical approaches (including labyrinthectomy or neurectomy) failed to improve or abolish tinnitus permanently. Ronis (1981), House and Brackmann (1981), and Wigand and colleagues (Wigand, Hellweg, and Berg 1982) have reported results on tinnitus following surgery on or sectioning of the eighth nerve. After some initial improvement, the

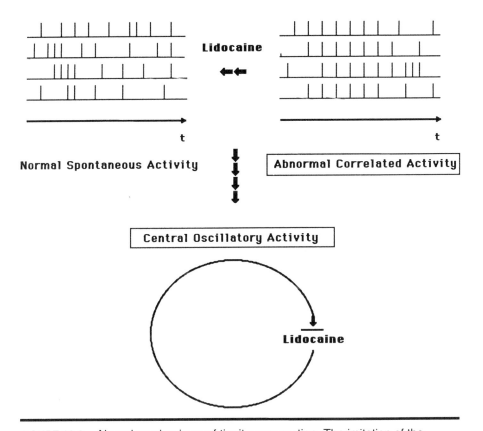

FIGURE 10-2. Neural mechanisms of tinnitus generation. The imitation of the physiological sound encoding and recognition process can be induced by cochlear as well as neural disorders. It is represented by the correlated neural activity of neighboring nerve fibers. The altered input to the central auditory system results in oscillatory activity. Both pathophysiological conditions can be reversed to normal activity with lidocaine i.v.

tinnitus referred to the affected ear recurred in the large majority of the patients, despite a complete loss of hearing on that side. These results indicate, again, that although peripheral input or damage may induce tinnitus, it is not necessary to maintain the sensation of tinnitus.

These results support the following hypotheses regarding tinnitus:

1. Tinnitus is a perceptual consequence of an altered spontaneous activity within the auditory system;
2. The *induction* of tinnitus usually involves pathologies of peripheral auditory structures that result in altered spontaneous inputs to the central auditory system in certain frequency domains;
3. The *manifestation and maintenance* of tinnitus involves central auditory structures that are not necessarily impaired;
4. Abnormal spontaneous inputs to central stations result in an altered functional state of similar characteristics in most tinnitus cases.

Under these hypotheses, tinnitus is the consequence of the spontaneous activity within some or all central auditory pathways. Normally, the stochastic spontaneous discharge pattern of the auditory nerve, and presumably the central auditory system, does not result in a percept. The rate and temporal pattern of this activity is modulated by acoustic stimulation of the cochlea and is dependent on the stimulus characteristics (e.g., Kiang, Moxon, and Levine 1970). In the case of tinnitus, the rate and/or stochastic temporal pattern of spontaneous activity may be altered (not maintained) by the pathology, and thus produces activity which simulates the presence of an acoustic signal without effective acoustic input. This pathological "signal" is processed by the same central auditory structures and physiological mechanisms as any normal driven activity (Evans, Wilson, and Borerwe 1981; Salvi and Ahroon 1983; Jacobson, Ahmad, Moran, Newman, Tepley, and Wharton 1991).

In the following sections, several models of altered peripheral activity will be reviewed, followed by the proposal of a neural tinnitus model based on the ensemble spontaneous activity of the central auditory pathways.

Cochlear Damage of Different Etiology and Locations as a Precondition of Tinnitus

In most cases of tinnitus, the transduction process seems to be impaired at the level of the cochlea, caused by a variety of underlying pathologic physiological mechanisms (see chapter 18) (Figure 10-1). Feldmann (1988) proposed a simple cochlear model for the generation of tinnitus which relies on clinical and psychoacoustic properties of cochlear tinnitus. Most lesions of the cochlea lead to damage of outer hair cells (OHCs), and OHCs have been hypothesized to act as mechanical elements with an inherent motor force to actively amplify the traveling wave (Zenner 1986; Zenner and Ernst 1992). Sounds thought to be generated by OHC activity (i.e., spontaneous otoacoustic emissions, or SOAEs), however, are not directly responsible for tinnitus generation, since there is little or no correlation between

SOAEs and tinnitus (Zwicker 1987; Probst 1990). It is argued that the precondition for the transfer of SOAEs along the cochlear partition towards the middle ear is disturbed in most cases of tinnitus that exhibit a cochlear hearing loss in the high frequency range. It is also argued that in some cases of cochlear motor tinnitus, the hypermobility of outer hair cells cannot produce an SOAE due to the uncoupling of the OHCs from adjacent structures mechanically isolating them. These arguments offer an explanation for tinnitus without an SOAE, however, they can not explain the fact that most SOAEs produce no sensation. Most patients with continuous high amplitude SOAEs are completely unaware of them (Zurek, 1981).

Nevertheless, the pathological stimulation or impairment of a few inner hair cells (IHCs) located at the maximum of hearing loss can possibly explain the generation of altered spontaneous activity that can be considered to be a tinnitus correlate or contributes to the central generation of a tinnitus percept. IHCs are responsible for the afferent signal transfer. Ion channel disorders can become a source of leakage currents which in turn continuously generate a depolarization and transmitter depletion of the synapse (for review, see chapter 18). At least several pathophysiological mechanisms (e.g., Eggermont 1990; Hazell 1987) may induce a regular discharge pattern of the afferent nerve fiber (see next section) with the one essential difference, compared to an acoustic stimulus, that there is no mechanoelectrical transduction taking place in the cochlea. However, this hypothesis requires an impairment of IHCs which have been shown to be rather resistant to damage when challenged in contrast to OHCs (e.g., Lim 1986). Moreover, this model does not explain the presence of tinnitus in patients who are without OHCs, cochleas, or auditory nerves. In any case, all disorders of outer and inner hair cells may result in an alteration of transmitter release at the IHC synapse, and thus fulfill the hypothesized requirement of altered spontaneous inputs to central auditory structures.

The Impact of the Efferent System

The micromechanics of the cochlea are controlled by the auditory system and other inputs from the CNS via the efferent system in a feedback loop (Siegel and Kim 1982). The efferent nerve fibers originate in the superior olivary complex and are arranged in the crossed olivocochlear bundle (COCB), which terminates predominantly at the OHCs, and an uncrossed bundle to the afferent fibers of the IHCs. In a silent environment, the afferent input is small or nonexistent. The efferent system modulates OHC activity to provide an optimum operation point for the amplification of the traveling wave and thus to increase the afferent input. It is hypothesized that the same holds true for pathological conditions with a lack of OHCs at circumscribed areas. The COCB stimulates the remaining OHCs at the site of the damage in order to increase the afferent input. The few intact hair cells are therefore hyperactive (Figure 10-1). They lead to a stimulation of the IHCs and may give rise to a "cochlear" tinnitus (Hazell 1987). Accordingly, in a noisy environment, the afferent input is increased by the acoustic stimulation, which will lead to a reduced efferent overstimulation of the OHCs. This is followed subsequently by a reduction in tinnitus. The above described model can serve as an interpretation of the masking phenomenon. The main objection against the model, however, is the fact that an increase in spontaneous otoacoustic emissions, as should be expected from the elevated OHC activity, is not found in most of the tinnitus cases (Zwicker 1987). In addition, the model does not explain tinnitus in patients without OHCs, cochleas, or auditory nerves.

The Gate Control Theory

Chronic tinnitus of cochlear origin can cause a sensorineural deafferentiation. Tonndorf (1987) proposed a gate control theory of tinnitus analogous to that proposed for chronic pain (Melzack and Wall 1965). The gate control theory implies the joint action of two different fiber systems in the production of subjective sensations. The input from one of the fiber systems "gates" the input of the other onto the relay neurons in the brainstem/ spinal cord and regulates the transmission of information towards the higher levels of the CNS. Balanced input from both afferent systems is necessary to produce a normal stimulus-related sensation. The balance of input from the afferent IHC and OHC fibers, respectively, to the brainstem gate seems to be unilaterally shifted when one or the other hair cell subsystem is damaged. Damage to the OHC afferent fibers, for example, might open the gate to IHC input and produce the abnormal sensation of tinnitus. The balance of activity in the two systems could also be modulated by the efferent system. However, no data exist in support of this direct analogy with pain control systems and this theoretical framework has not been completely verified for pain.

Correlated Spontaneous Activity in the Auditory Nerve as a Model of Tinnitus

An impairment of the auditory nerve itself may result directly in altered auditory nerve activity, altering the input to the central auditory system and resulting in tinnitus (M. Møller 1987). The underlying mechanisms may be damaged by a number of mechanisms, including an acoustic neuroma, a vascular compression of the auditory nerve, demyelinating diseases, or the like. Jannetta (1987) reported an improvement of neurotological symptoms—including tinnitus—after vascular decompression of the auditory nerve. Møller (1984) has hypothesized that vascular compression produces an abnormal correlation or synchronization of the spontaneous discharge pattern of several auditory nerve fibers. This correlated activity might imitate the physiological synchronization produced by an acoustic stimulus and result in tinnitus. The pulsations of an arterial loop, such as a branch of the anterior inferior cerebellar artery, or pressure from a tumor might induce a breakdown or thinning of the myelin sheaths of nerve fibers, commonly at the root entry zone. The loss of electrical isolation might in turn lead to ephaptic transmission of or crosstalk of discharges between fibers (Eggermont 1990). This hypothesis cannot explain the failure of destructive surgical methods to relief tinnitus symptoms. Surgical section of the auditory nerve should produce complete degeneration of all auditory nerve fibers and remove all correlated input from the periphery. Another limitation of this theory is the fact that neural damage is uncommon and one of the least probable causes of tinnitus.

An additional mechanism which might lead to correlated spontaneous activity in the auditory nerve fibers is proposed by Eggermont (1990) (also see chapter 4). Under nonpathological conditions, spontaneous activity in each of the afferent fibers innervating a single inner hair cell is completely independent. The detection of a signal within the stochastic spontaneous firing process can be reliably and rapidly achieved by the comparison of the temporal firing pattern of at least two fibers. The common pathological finding in different animal models in which pathologies are induced that may cause tinnitus in humans—noise trauma, salicylate intoxication, or endolymphatic hydrops—is not a change of the firing *rate*. In some conditions, the firing rate increased, in other conditions it decreased. The common finding is, rather, an abnormal *temporal pattern* in the spontaneous firing activity of individual neurons or in the temporal correlations of different fibers. The abnormal synchrony of nerve fiber activity originating from one single hair cell or several hair cells can be achieved through a synchronization of the various synapse activations by a spontaneous excess influx of potassium ions or calcium ions. These leakage currents result in a transient hair cell depolarization and cause a synchronous transmitter release at all hair cell synapses. This model can explain the tinnitus found in cochlear lesions, for example, induced by noise trauma or ototoxic drugs. Based on the short spike intervals found in auditory nerve fibers in animals under these conditions (Evans et al. 1981; Liberman and Kiang, 1978) this model explains the correlation in activ-

ity of neighboring nerve fibers that is theoretically required for the generation of tinnitus.

The correlation model is promising because it can be related to both physiological and pathophysiological data from animal experiments and to common pathological conditions in patients. For verification it requires the recording of ensemble spontaneous activity from the auditory nerve and other locations along the auditory pathways (Schreiner and Snyder, 1987). One problem with this model, again, is that it does not explain tinnitus in patients without functioning cochleas, or auditory nerves. A second potential problem is the difficulty in relating a high-pitched tinnitus (>4 kHz) to the periodicity principle (frequency coding by means of phase-locking) which is usually limited to periodicities below 4 kHz. However, it is likely that the pitch of tinnitus is not determined by the periodicity information in the correlated activity but rather by which frequency channel(s) are affected by the altered activity.

THE PATHOLOGICAL ENSEMBLE SPONTANEOUS ACTIVITY (ESA) MODEL OF TINNITUS

A useful neurophysiological model of tinnitus has to meet the following criteria (Schreiner and Snyder, 1987):

- electrophysiological correlates of tinnitus should be obtainable from stations of the auditory system;
- the electrophysiological tinnitus correlate should be reliably induced;
- properties of electrophysiologically recordable spontaneous activity must co-vary with psychophysical properties of tinnitus;
- these correlates should reflect the major clinical properties of tinnitus;
- the model should enable a long-term evaluation of the tinnitus correlates.

Fulfillment of these requirements would establish an effective and objective tool in the assessment of properties of tinnitus and serve as a valid correlate to provide objective diagnostic parameters. Consequently, the development of treatments for tinnitus would be enhanced by monitoring the specific therapeutic effects, and in particular, by establishing the pathophysiological mechanisms underlying this symptom. Tinnitus-like effects should become inducible at the level of the cochlea by pharmacological and physical manipulations which are known to cause a tinnitus in humans (e.g., salicylate, noise trauma). Subsequently, the influence of these manipulations on the auditory system has to be investigated by electrophysiological methods. In 1981, Evans and colleagues performed single-fiber recordings of the eighth nerve after the intravenous administration of salicylate and found an increase of the discharge rate. However, the single-unit approach has several limitations that make it less useful for the search for tinnitus correlates. Among the problems are the random and limited sample of fibers/neurons which may grossly underrepresent those frequency ranges that are responsible for the tinnitus generation, and the fact that single unit recordings cannot reveal a temporal correlation between several nerve fibers, a potentially important precondition for the generation of tinnitus.

Other approaches include the registration of neural activity in more central auditory neurons, for example, single unit activity in the inferior colliculus (Jastreboff and Sasaki, 1986) or mass evoked activity in the auditory cortex (Hoke, Feldmann, Pantev, Lütkenhöner, and Lehnertz 1989).

One experimental strategy that we have explored is the recording of the spontaneous ensemble activity (ESA) from the auditory nerve or from other stations along the auditory pathway (Schreiner, Snyder, and Johnstone 1986; Schreiner and Snyder 1987).

In an attempt to verify the usefulness of this approach, Schreiner and Snyder (1987) recorded the ESA with low-impedance electrodes placed near the auditory nerve of the cat. After administration of a potentially tinnitus-inducing drug (sodium salicylate), a characteristic change in the amplitude spectrum of the ESA was often ob-

served. Although subsequent test showed convincingly that the obtained altered ESA did not originate from the auditory nerve itself (Schreiner, Snyder, and Johnstone unpublished observations), the observed phenomena may serve as an example of how the recording of the ESA may contribute to the establishment of a valid electrophysiological model of tinnitus.

Since the ESA is not stimulus-driven and does not contain stimulus-synchronized activity, normal averaging procedures of the time-waveform cannot be applied. Instead, the frequency spectrum of raw traces is obtained and the power spectra of many traces are averaged. The thin line in Figure 10-3A shows such an averaged spectrum of the ESA recorded near the auditory nerve of the anesthetized cat (filter setting 0.1 to 10 kHz, 12 dB/octave). A common feature of ESA spectra is a pronounced spectral peak between 0.8 and 1 to 2 kHz corresponding to the main spectral features of the waveform of action potentials (Dolan, Nuttall, and Avinash 1990). In this animal, administration of sodium salicylate (600 mg/kg IV), a tinnitus-inducing drug, resulted in a pronounced shift in CAP threshold of 30 to 40 dB. In the ESA, two effects were visible. First, the high-frequency peak around 1 kHz diminished (thick line, Figure 10-3A). This reduction in spectral energy could be the result of a decrease of activity in the auditory nerve due to the salicylate, such as a reduction in spontaneous activity and/or a reduction of the transmission of ubiquitous sounds, such as vascular noise, due to the increase in threshold. Second, a pronounced spectral low-frequency peak around 200 Hz became more apparent. Although the cause and site of origin of the 200 Hz peak remains obscure, the spectral maximum clearly reflects a spontaneous process of high temporal coherence and regularity. Event-triggered averaging from prominent peaks of the raw waveform indeed revealed a clear periodicity of 5 msec in the spontaneous activity. It is not clear at this time whether the appearance of the low-frequency peak in the ESA spectrum is due to an "unmasking" of the peak by suppression of the noise background, or

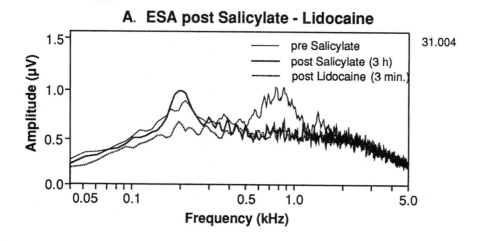

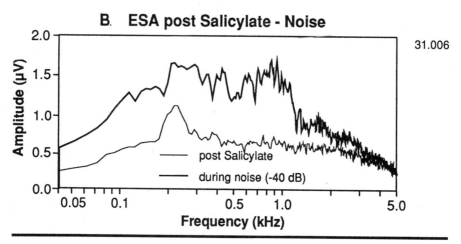

FIGURE 10-3.   ESA. Amplitude power spectrum. (A) The normal spectrum shows a maximum in the high-frequency range around 1 kHz and resembles the spike waveform (plain line). After salicylate i.v. the spectral energy in the high-frequency range dropped and the small peak around 200 Hz showed an increase (bold line). After the injection of lidocaine i.v. the peak can be suppressed transiently (dashed line). (B) The low-frequency peak induced with salicylate i.v. was masked by an increase of the overall spectral energy during the presentation of a white noise stimulus.

whether it reflects a true induction or enhancement of a previously nonexisting or small peak. In any case, this phenomenon can be observed not only after salicylate administration but also after other tinnitus-inducing cochlear lesions.

The intravenous administration of lidocaine (20 mg) always resulted in a pronounced and short lasting (0.5 to 20 min) suppression of the low-frequency peak (dotted line, Figure 10-3A), similar to its effect on tinnitus. This behavior is compatible with the known lidocaine effects, such as lengthening of the refractory period and increase in conduction time, thus resulting in a desynchronization of the apparently more temporally coherent abnormal spontaneous activity. Note that the high-frequency peak around 1 kHz is not restored during the lidocaine effect—the spontaneous activity is not increased or the response thresholds are not normalized.

Masking of tinnitus is a well-investigated phenomenon with far-reaching clinical implications (Vernon 1988). In animals with a residual hearing after salicylate administration, an acoustic stimulation with broadband noise leads to an increase of the overall ESA spectral amplitude across a wide range of frequencies. Under these circumstances, the low-frequency peak at 200 Hz is not a dominant phenomenon any more and may be a reflection of the masking of tinnitus by noise.

The induction of tinnitus with salicylate and its suppression with lidocaine are well-known phenomena (Lenarz 1989) that are seemingly reproduced by the behavior of the low-frequency peak at 200 Hz in the spectrum of the ESA. However, since the mechanisms for the generation and alteration of the low-frequency peak and its site of origin are still uncertain, it is premature to equate this electrophysiological phenomenon with the clinical symptom of tinnitus. Nevertheless, these findings serve as an example of how electrophysiologically verifiable activity patterns in the central auditory system may contribute to our understanding of the origins of tinnitus and eventually, its treatment. It is conceivable that the temporal coherence reflected in the 200 Hz peak may not reflect the property of the altered spontaneous activity entering the central auditory system from the periphery, but rather is the consequence of the altered input on the functional state of central spontaneous activity. In other words, altered peripheral inputs may induce or enhance an oscillatory activity in some frequency channels of central stations, resulting in the percept associated with tinnitus.

DISCUSSION

Different cochlear lesions can cause tinnitus with identical characteristics, for example, loudness, masking characteristics, or pitch. The character is mainly determined by the frequency range, but not by the etiology of the underlying hearing loss. Therefore, it seems useful to postulate and search for a common neurophysiological correlate of tinnitus beyond the cochlea. This neurophysiological correlate should resemble the clinical features of tinnitus and should be recordable from one or several locations within the auditory system. However, up to now such a correlate has not been identified in tinnitus patients due to the lack of knowledge about the pathophysiological mechanisms of tinnitus and the limited access to hidden structures of the auditory pathways. Therefore, it is useful to establish a valid animal model that resembles the present knowledge about the pathophysiology of the auditory system and can explain the clinical features of human tinnitus.

As explained above, tinnitus can be defined as the perceptual correlate of spontaneous neural activity in the auditory system under "no sound conditions". A valid neurophysiological model of tinnitus should meet the following criteria (Schreiner and Snyder, 1987):

1. The electrophysiological tinnitus correlate should be easily and reliably induced by the various mechanisms known to cause tinnitus;
2. The model should cover many, if not all, of the various induction mechanisms of tinnitus and show the common neurophysiological correlate of tinnitus generation and maintenance;
3. Properties of electrophysiologically recordable spontaneous activity have to co-vary with psychophysical tinnitus properties (masking behavior, pitch, residual inhibition);
4. These effects should reflect the major clinical properties of tinnitus (lidocaine effect, glutamate effect, suppression by electrical stimulation, masking phenomenon);
5. The model should enable a long-term evaluation of tinnitus correlates and treatment modalities.

The various models of neural tinnitus mechanisms fulfill these requirements in certain aspects, but most of them show essential limitations that will be briefly discussed below.

As outlined above, one can distinguish between the mechanisms for the *induction* of tinnitus and the mechanisms of *generation and maintenance* of the tinnitus-related percept. The induction mechanisms, in most cases, are located in the cochlea, but they can also be located in the auditory nerve, or even the central auditory pathways. They are the necessary preconditions for the more centrally located tinnitus generators to start producing the abnormal spontaneous activity that seemingly reflects the presence of an acoustic stimulus.

The possible cochlear induction mechanisms are described by the various cochlear-based models (e.g., cochlear motor tinnitus, transduction tinnitus, and signal transfer tinnitus; see Zenner and Ernst, chapter 18) that consider one or several pathophysiological conditions of the cochlea and relate them to tinnitus generation. This approach is not completely satisfactory for several reasons: First, all of these models stand only for one of many possible tinnitus induction mechanisms; second, they all commonly cause a change of the discharge pattern of the attached auditory nerve fibers. Additionally, they cannot explain tinnitus in deaf patients or tinnitus of neural origin. The same reservations apply to the impact of the efferent system, which requires intact or responding outer hair cells. An influence of central auditory structures seems theoretically possible but lacks any evidence by experimental or clinical data.

The same holds true for the gate control theory, which is a mere analogy to a concept of chronic pain (Tonndorf, 1987). There is no experimental or clinical evidence for a dual neural afferent system which gives input to central structures. However, the gate control theory provides a theoretical framework for all neural theories that are based on the mutual relationship of several neural elements.

The neural model of ephaptic transmission seems to be valid in cases of auditory nerve damage (e.g., acoustic neuroma, demyelinating diseases) (Møller 1984; Eggermont 1990). In cases of vascular compression syndrome, the recovery of nerve function in a short time after surgical decompression makes damage of the myelin sheaths less reasonable, but rather argues for a mechanical

neural conduction block. This model can explain the persistence of tinnitus after destructive procedures of the cochlea or auditory nerve sectioning, but does not explain tinnitus in the majority of cases, namely those induced by cochlear lesions.

The concept of correlated neural activity in auditory nerve fibers (Eggermont 1990) attempts to model animal experimental data on basic assumptions drawn from the presently known auditory anatomy and physiology. A merit of this model is that it considers common neurophysiological characteristics of different pathologies that can induce tinnitus in humans. It focuses on the mechanisms of tinnitus generation and maintenance which are similar to the process of encoding and recognition of a real acoustic signal. Corroboration of this model requires the evaluation of the temporal pattern and coherence of at least two otherwise independent afferent auditory nerve fibers, a process that is difficult to accomplish, since the number of fibers that may carry correlated activity may be small compared to the total number of fibers.

One way to establish the existence of a temporal relationship between several neural elements is provided by recording of the ensemble spontaneous activity (ESA). An advantage of this method is that the neural elements that exhibit temporal coherence in their firing pattern do not have to be identified explicitly. On the other hand, if the number of elements that show temporal coherence is small, the resulting signal may be too small to be detectable over the amount of incoherent activity. A main advantage of this approach is that it is not restricted to the auditory nerve, but the ESA can fairly easily be recorded from various locations along the auditory pathways.

The magnitude of potential deviations of a pathological ESA from normal ESA characteristics—for example, the amplitude of a low-frequency peak in the averaged power spectrum—depends on the amount of coherence and the number of elements involved. The observation of a spectrally well-circumscribed maximum in the ESA that can be recorded from different locations in the brain might be explicable by oscillatory or reverberant activity within and between certain structures of the central nervous system (Figure 10-2) (Schreiner et al. unpublished observations). It could be hypothesized that this oscillatory activity is usually not present because of desynchronizing inputs of spontaneous activity to the central stations. Changes in this steady stream of desynchronizing discharges—in particular a decrease, or an increase in coherence, either induced by an acoustic stimulus or by a pathophysiological condition prior to the neuron—may result in the emergence of an oscillatory activity that is interpreted as the presence of an external signal (Møller 1984; Eggermont 1990). Hence, a variety of events at the level of the organ of Corti (e.g., noise trauma with a subsequent destruction of OHCs, potassium intoxication, etc. For review, see Zenner and Ernst, chapter 18) or the auditory nerve (Møller 1984; Eggermont 1990) can possibly contribute to the induction of tinnitus by altering the ability of the spontaneous discharge to desynchronize central oscillations. The altered peripheral activity thus enables the central auditory pathway to generate and maintain a synchronized repetitive activity, resulting in the perception of tinnitus. In this way, the current models of cochlear and neural tinnitus explain the induction mechanisms of tinnitus, based on animal experimental data and the concepts of auditory physiology, but not the mechanisms of tinnitus generation and maintenance.

Current experimental models are only valid to a limited extent in resembling the psychophysical and clinical features of tinnitus. The most important are:

- Tinnitus persists even after destruction of the cochlea or the eighth nerve (Douek, 1987, Wigand et al., 1982);
- Tinnitus can be masked both ipsi- and contralaterally, but its masking behavior differs from an external sound (Feldmann, 1988);
- Tinnitus can show residual inhibition that can exceed the duration of forward masking by orders of magnitude;
- Tinnitus can be transiently suppressed by intra-

venous administration of lidocaine (Lenarz 1986);
- Tinnitus can be transiently suppressed by either DC or AC current (Aran and Cazals, 1981).

For most of the discussed models, these features are not evaluated experimentally, but deduced from theoretical speculations, although some experimental data exist for the single-fiber studies. By contrast, all of these features can be fairly easily evaluated for the ESA, and would reflect specific characteristics of the underlying tinnitus-generating processes.

Tinnitus is a multifactorial symptom in humans. It is therefore important to find a valid experimental approach to simulate its possible sources, and thus to outline means of influencing tinnitus and related phenomena. Among the presented neural models of tinnitus, the pathological ESA provides an opportunity of rationalizing these attempts by serving as a means to describe common neural events as related to the generation of tinnitus. If this experimental approach succeeds, the ESA could be applied to explain the therapeutic efficiency of lidocaine, glutamate, masking, electrical stimulation, and related manipulations in the suppression of tinnitus, and most importantly, could be utilized in the development of new therapeutic strategies.

REFERENCES

Aran, M. and Cazals, Y. 1981. "Electrical Suppression of Tinnitus." In D. Evered and G. Lawrenson, *Tinnitus*, pp. 217–231.

Dolan, D.F., Nuttall, A.L., and Avinash, G. 1990. "Asynchronous Neural Activity Recorded from the Round Window." *Journal of the Acoustical Society of America, 87*, 2621–2627.

Doueck, E. 1987. "Tinnitus following Surgery." In H. Feldmann (Ed.), *Proceedings III International Tinnitus Seminar, Muenster, 1987*, pp. 64–69. Karlsruhe: Harsch Verlag.

Eggermont, J.J. 1990. "On the Pathophysiology of Tinnitus: A Review and Peripheral Model." *Hearing Research, 48*, 111–124.

Evans, E.F., Wilson, J.P., and Borerwe, T.A. 1981. "Animal Modes of Tinnitus." In D. Evered and G. Lawrenson (Eds.), *Tinnitus*, pp. 108–138. *Ciba Foundation 85.* London: Pitman.

Feldmann, H. 1988. "Pathophysiology of Tinnitus." In M. Kitahara (Ed.), *Tinnitus—Pathophysiology and Management*, pp. 7–35. Tokyo/New York: Igaku-Shoin.

Hazell, J.W.P. 1987. "A Cochlear Model for Tinnitus." In H. Feldmann (Ed.), *Proceedings III International Tinnitus Seminar, Muenster, 1987*, pp. 121–128. Karlsruhe: Harsch Verlag.

Hoke, M., Feldmann, H., Pantev, C., Lütkenhöner, B., and Lehnertz, K. 1989. "Objective Evidence of Tinnitus in Auditory Evoked Magnetic Fields." *Hearing Research, 37,* 281–286.

House, J.W. and Brackmann, D.E. 1981. "Tinnitus: Surgical Treatment." In D. Evered and G. Lawrenson (Eds.), *Tinnitus,* pp. 204–212. *Ciba Foundation Symposium 85.* London: Pitman.

Jacobson, G.P., Ahmad, B.K., Moran, J., Newman, C.W., Tepley, N., and Wharton, J. 1991. "Auditory Evoked Magnetic Field (M100-M200) Measurements in Tinnitus and Normal Groups." *Hearing Research, 56,* 44–52.

Jannetta, P.J. 1987. "Microvascular Decompression of the Cochlear Nerve as a Treatment Treatment of Tinnitus." In H. Feldmann (Ed.), *Proceedings III International Tinnitus Seminar, Muenster, 1987*, pp. 348–352. Karlsruhe: Harsch Verlag.

Jastreboff, P.J. and Sasaki, C.T. 1986. "Salicylate-induced Changes in Spontaneous Activity of Single Units in the Inferior Colliculus of the Guinea Pig." *Journal of the Acoustical Society of America, 80,* 1384–1391.

Kiang, N.Y.-S., Moxon, E.C., and Levine, L.A. 1970. "Auditory-nerve Activity in Cats with Normal and Abnormal Cochleas." In G.E.W. Wolstenholme and J. Knight (Eds.), *Sensorineural Hearing Loss,* pp. 241–273. London: Churchill Livingstone.

Lenarz, T. 1986. "Treatment of Tinnitus with Lidocaine and Tocainamide." *Scandinavian Audiology (Supplement), 26,* 49–51.

Lenarz, T. 1989. *Medikamentöse Tinnitustherapie. Klinische und tierexperimentelle Untersuchungen zur Pharmakologie der Hörbahn.* Stuttgart/New York: Thieme.

Lenarz, T. 1992. "Medikamentöse Therapie." In H. Feldmann, T. Lenarz, and H. von Wedel (Eds.), *Tinnitus,* pp. 101–112. Stuttgart/New York: Thieme.

Liberman, M.C. and Kiang, N.Y.-S. 1978. "Acoustic Trauma in Cats. Cochlear Pathology and Auditory Nerve Activity." *Acta Otolaryngologica, Supplement 358,* 1–63.

Lim, D.J. 1986. "Functional Structure of the Organ of Corti." *Hearing Research, 22,* 117–146.

McFadden, D. 1982. *Tinnitus: Facts, Theories, and Treatments.* Washington, DC: National Academic Press.

Melzack, R. and Wall, P.D. 1965. "Pain Mechanisms: A New Theory." *Science, 150,* 971–979.

Møller, A.R. 1984. "Pathophysiology of Tinnitus." *Annals of Otology, Rhinology, and Laryngology, 93,* 39–44.

Møller, M. 1987. "Vascular Compression of the Eighth Nerve as a Cause of Tinnitus." In H. Feldmann (Ed.), *Proceedings III International Tinnitus Seminar, Muenster, 1987*, pp. 340–347. Karlsruhe: Harsch Verlag.

Oliveira, C.A., Schuknecht, H.F., and Glynn, F.J. 1990. "In Search of Cochlear Morphological Correlates for Tinnitus." *Archives of Otolaryngology—Head and Neck Surgery, 116,* 937–939.

Probst, R. 1990. "Otoacoustic Emissions: An Overview." *Advanced Otorhinolaryngology, 44,* 1–91.

Ronis, M.L. 1981. "Panel Discussion." In A. Shulman (Ed.,) *Tinnitus: Proceedings of the First International Tinnitus Seminar. Journal of Laryngology and Otology Supplement 4,* 145–146.

Salvi, R.J. and Ahroon, W.A. 1983. "Tinnitus and Neural Activity." *Journal of Speech and Hearing Research, 26,* 629–632.

Sasaki, C.T., Babitz, L., and Kauer, J.S. 1981. "Tinnitus: Development of a Neurophysiological Correlate." *Laryngoscope, 91,* 2018–2024.

Schacht, J. and Zenner, H.P. 1986. "Evidence That Phosphoinositides Mediate Motility in Cochlear Outer Hair Cells." *Hearing Research, 31,* 155–160.

Schreiner, C.E. 1990. "Oscillatory Activity in the Central Auditory System as a Neurophysiological Correlate of Tinnitus." Personal communication.

Schreiner, C.E. and Snyder, R.L. 1987. "A Physiological Animal Model of Peripheral Tinnitus." In H. Feldmann (Ed.), *Proceedings III International Tinnitus Seminar, Muenster, 1987*, pp. 100–106. Karlsruhe: Harsch Verlag.

Schreiner, C.E., Snyder, R.L., and Johnstone, B.M. 1986. "Effects of Extracochlear Direct Current Stimulation on the Ensemble Nerve Activity of Cats." *Hearing Research, 21,* 213–226.

Siegel, J.H. and Kim, D.O. 1982. "Efferent Neural Control of Cochlear Membranes? Olivocochlear Bundle Stimulation Affects Cochlear Biomechanical Nonlinearity." *Hearing Research, 6,* 171–182.

Tonndorf, J. 1987. "The Origin of Tinnitus: A New Hypothesis in Analogy with Pain." In H. Feldmann (Ed.), *Proceedings III International Tinnitus Seminar, Muenster, 1987,* pp. 70–74. Karlsruhe: Harsch Verlag.

Vernon, J. 1988. "Current Use of Masking for the Relief of Tinnitus." In M. Kitahara (Ed.), *Tinnitus—Pathophysiology and Management,* pp. 96–106. Tokyo/ New York: Igaku-Shoin.

Versnel, H., Prijs, V.F., and Schoonhoven, R. 1992. "Round-window Recorded Potential of Single-fibre Discharge (Unit Response) in Normal and Noise-damaged Cochleas." *Hearing Research, 59,* 157–170.

Wigand, M.E., Hellweg, F.C., and Berg, M. 1982. "Tinnitus nach Eingriffen am achten Hirnnerven." *Laryngology, Rhinology, and Otology, 61,* 132–134.

Zenner, H.P. 1986. "Motile Responses in Outer Hair Cells." *Hearing Research, 22,* 83–90.

Zenner, H.P. and Ernst, A. 1992. "Sound Preprocessing by AC and DC Movements of Cochlear Outer Hair Cells." *Progressive Brain Research,* in press.

Zurek, P.M. 1981. "Spontaneous Narrowband Acoustic Signals Emitted by Human Ears." *Journal of the Acoustical Society of America, 69,* 515–523.

Zwicker, E. 1987. "Objective Otoacoustic Emissions and Their Uncorrelation to Tinnitus." In H. Feldmann (Ed.), *Proceedings III International Tinnitus Seminar, Muenster, 1987,* pp. 75–81. Karlsruhe: Harsch Verlag.

CHAPTER 11

A MODEL FOR COCHLEAR ORIGIN OF SUBJECTIVE TINNITUS

EXCITATORY DRIFT IN THE OPERATING POINT OF INNER HAIR CELLS

ERIC L. LEPAGE
National Acoustic Laboratories, Chatswood, N.S.W., Australia

INTRODUCTION

There are many purported sites for the origin of tinnitus. However, for the most part, the incidence of tinnitus is so strongly connected with the onset of sensorineural hearing loss (whether it be permanent, or temporary due to acoustic overexposure) as to implicate the cochlea as the key site. The objects of this chapter include:

1. to set down an itemized list of salient properties of tinnitus of cochlear origin as reported in the literature;

2. to set down a further itemized characterization of a single relevant case study, like that of Wegel (1931) the only case of which the author has intimate experience;

3. to produce a descriptive treatment of the physiological regulation of tectorial membrane position along the lines suggested by Davis (1954);

4. to show that this model constitutes a testable hypothesis for explaining the origin of the listed items in terms of a *phantom input to the cochlea* (Jastreboff 1990);

5. to observe that the model explains the difficulty of characterizing tinnitus in terms of equivalent external sounds;

6. to observe that the issue of severity is strongly dependent not just on masking influences but also on selective attention—this accounts for the heavy psychological involvement and difficulty of treatment in severe cases; and

7. to observe that much of the difficulty in obtaining a conceptual purchase on the causes of tinnitus stems from the long-held but questionable assumption that hearing sensitivity provides a sensitive measure of the extent of cochlear damage.

PREVIOUSLY REPORTED RELEVANT CHARACTERISTICS

Repeated studies have provided an invaluable characterization of the facets of tinnitus. These relate to basic issues in cochlear physiology and noise-induced hearing loss. A nonexhaustive review of relevant literature provides some key characteristics.

Nature of Sensations

1. The phenomenon can be categorized as *continuous* or *discontinuous* (transient).

2. *Continuous tinnitus* (CT), at least in cases of high frequency hearing loss, or *continuous high-frequency tinnitus* (CHFT), is of a predominantly high-frequency nature (80 percent over 3 kHz, 55 percent over 5 kHz, 42 percent over 7 kHz, Meikle and Taylor-Walsh 1984), but can be of a very low frequency (<100 Hz) (CLFT) (Wilson, 1979).

3. CHFT is heard as narrow bands of noise, likened to the sounds of cicadas; the most debilitating seem to be like externally applied intense sinusoids (Reed, 1960).

4. CT can also be like "water rushing", "sand blasting" (wideband) or in the case of Ménière's syndrome "roaring" and of low frequency (Nodar and Graham, 1965).

5. CT can be uniform or pulsating (Harris, Brismar, and Cronqvist 1979). In cases of otosclerosis, it is frequently dynamic in character, like a bell pealing or hooting noises, causing great difficulty obtaining an auditory assessment.

6. Transient "spontaneous" tinnitus (TST) is invariably unilateral and frequently preceded by a transient nonaudible pressure-like sensation within the affected ear accompanied by dulled hearing acuity (Vernon, Schleuning, Odell, and Hughes 1978).

7. Subjective judgments of tinnitus pitch are highly variable (Harris et al. 1979; Penner, 1983; Burns, 1984).

Loudness and severity

8. The loudness of tinnitus is variable and also depends on ambient noise-level; it becomes louder with decrease in ambient noise-level (Axelsson and Ringdahl 1989).

9. There exists an inherent problem (in common with pain) of assessing severity (Meikle and Taylor-Walsh 1984; Tyler, Aran, and Dauman 1992; Burns, 1984).

10. While on a scale of 1 to 10, most patients rate the severity of their tinnitus between 5 and 8, 76 percent of patients match the loudness of their tinnitus at <6 dB SL (Meikle 1991c).

11. Severe cases require higher masking levels; it often requires sound levels approaching 100 dB to mask the tinnitus (Vernon 1991).

12. Patients "fix" upon their tinnitus (Hazell 1979a); selective attention or focusing is evidently an important component in assessing disability.

Physical/Physiological Attributes

13. The production of beats between an external tone and CT is very rare, even when the tinnitus is tonal (Vernon 1991).

14. Fowler (1944) describes tinnitus as *objective* or *subjective* ("*nonvibratory*").

15. Subjective tinnitus most often has no associated spontaneous otoacoustic emission (Penner, 1992; Shulman, Goldstein, and Bhathal 1992).

16. Ears with tinnitus have much larger cochlear microphonics than unaffected ears (Hazell 1979c)

17. There is a distinction to be made between masking and suppression, which may be electrically induced (Hazell 1979c).

18. Electrical suppression of tinnitus is possible with positive but not negative current-produced auditory sensations (Grapengiesser 1801, see Vernon 1991; Portmann, Cazals, Negrevergne and Aran 1979; Aran 1981).

Possible Causative Factors

19. Purported factors in etiology of tinnitus include: medications including aspirin (Jastreboff, Brennan, Coleman, and Sasaki 1988; Day, Graham, Bieri, Brown, Cairns, Harris, Hounsel, Platt-Hepworth, Reeve, Sambrook, and Smith 1989), oral contraceptives, changes in diet (caffeine and cholesterol), noise exposure (Reed 1960; Man and Naggan 1981; Coles, David, and Haggard 1981; Chung, Gannon, and Mason 1984; Axelsson and Barrenäs 1992), diabetes, and cardiovascular status (Meikle 1991a).

20. Tinnitus may be due to steady mechanical pressure producing a slight but permanent displacement of the tectorial membrane in relation to the hair cells (Davis 1954), and there is a fairly strong connection with this type of origin in Ménière's syndrome (Nodar and Graham 1965), since in Ménière attacks a pressure build-up is histologically well-documented.

21. Barotrauma can produce a change in tinnitus (Farmer 1977; Tonkin and Fagan 1975).

22. Tinnitus can be manipulated by a wide variety of pharmacological agents known to have a direct effect on the cochlea, such as glycerol or ethacrynic acid.

Relation to Incidence of Hearing Loss

23. Like presbyacusis, tinnitus cannot be regarded as an independent disease but a manifestation of accumulative damage or aging, predominantly af-

fecting the 40- to 70-year age group (Meikle, Griest, Press, and Stewart 1991; Coles et al. 1981).
24. Sex distribution for tinnitus reveals (Reed 1960; Bailey 1979); a higher incidence in males (71 percent) than in females (29 percent) (Meikle 1991a).
25. Regarding laterality, it appears more commonly in the left ear (46 percent) than the right (29 percent) (Hazell 1981). "Head" tinnitus apparently constitutes the most severe form.
26. Although continuous high-frequency tinnitus (CHFT) is strongly associated with the onset of hearing loss (Loeb and Smith 1967; Coles et al. 1981), particularly *noise-induced hearing loss* (NIHL), there is a poor correlation with the extent of the hearing loss.

    a. There may be no associated hearing loss; Hazell (1979b) reports a high incidence of tinnitus in people with normal or near normal hearing;

    b. It is frequently associated with mild to moderate hearing losses; and

    c. It can remain following sectioning the auditory nerve to eliminate it, analogous to phantom pain from a severed limb.

27. Continuous tinnitus (CT) seldom impairs hearing threshold by more than 10 dB (Vernon, Johnson, Schleuning, and Mitchell 1980).
28. CT is regarded like a rise in noise level (Tonndorf 1981) by up to 55 dB. Patients frequently complain that tinnitus masks their normal hearing; if they could be rid of the tinnitus they feel they could hear normally (Meikle and Taylor-Walsh 1984; Meikle 1991b; Meikle et al. 1991).

Masking of Tinnitus

29. CT can be masked as can external sounds (Hazell 1979c; Vernon et al. 1978; Vernon et al. 1980).
30. Masking conditions are not predictable; masking is not always possible (*ibid.*);
31. Masking of CHFT is most successful when the hearing loss is minimal (*ibid.*).
32. It is easier to mask a relatively quiet CT (*ibid.*).
33. Tinnitus falls into three categories according to the ease with which it may be masked: 18 per-

cent easy to mask with tones; 52 percent can be masked at low sensation levels but only by tones near in frequency to the tinnitus; 22 percent where excessive levels are needed; plus 8 percent other (*ibid.*).
34. Broadband noise provides effective masking for just under half of those with CHFT (Meikle 1991b).
35. Tinnitus is slightly better masked when in the right ear (Hazell, Williams, and Sheldrake 1979).
36. Masking of tinnitus differs from masking external sounds (Vernon et al. 1980):

    a. An external noise can more easily mask an internal noise-type tinnitus than it can mask another external sound;

    b. The usual upward spread of masking for external sounds below 11 kHz is not the case for tinnitus;

    c. The sensation level of a tone required to mask tinnitus is not necessarily related to the perceived loudness of the tinnitus;

    d. Unlike external sounds that are reinstated once the masking noise is removed, release of the masking sound is often followed by temporary cessation or reduction of the tinnitus (*residual inhibition*, RI).

37. Residual inhibition is more likely to occur with CHFT (Vernon et al. 1978).

SOME NEW OBSERVATIONS— ONE CASE HISTORY

In an area of sensation, like pain, which tends to defy objective quantification, we tend to find patients' descriptions highly non-specific and limited to comparison with everyday sounds, even though the descriptions may change substantially when patients are presented with the actual sounds given as examples. In the author's experience, it is quite rare to find a tinnitus patient who can express the sensory experience of tinnitus in more precise terms by using the languages of science, engineering, or music. To try to bridge this shortfall, the following are a series of personal observations by a single tinnitus sufferer (ELP), a male aged 47, with a background in relevant disciplines such as mathematics, physics, and engineering, plus twenty years researching auditory physiology. More relevant here is his educated ear for analyzing musical sounds, his early training as a concert pianist and organist, and his abiding interest in musical acoustics (which includes thirty-two years' experience tuning pianos). He is experienced at a variety of psychophysical discrimination tasks, such as distinguishing the difference between place pitch and repetition pitch, and esti-

mating relative levels of noise and coherence in various frequency bands. He has contributed to experiments on absolute pitch (Siegel, 1976) that is, he can effortlessly name a note, plus octave, over the musical pitch range without external reference, and hence can determine an equivalent frequency (±0.05 octaves) for external and phantom sounds. Figure 11-1 shows for each ear his puretone airconduction audiograms, plus click-evoked otoacoustic emission spectra obtained using the

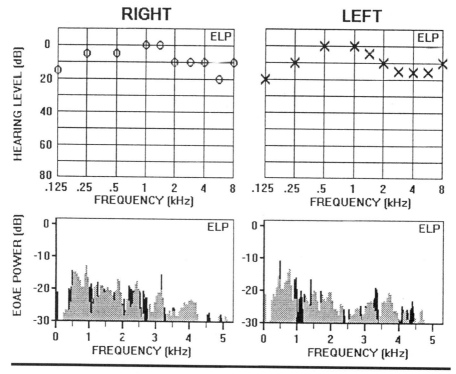

FIGURE 11-1. Audiometric and objective measures of ear function of tinnitus subject ELP. The top two panels show pure-tone audiograms for right and left ears respectively. The lower two panels show the corresponding click-evoked otoacoustic emission spectra obtained using the Otodynamics ILO88 Analyser in standard screening mode (80 μs, 80 dB SPL clicks, average of 260 presentations of the nonlinear click sequence of 4 reversing clicks). The black regions indicate the cross power spectrum for coherent part of the response while the gray regions are for the incoherent part of the response (a measure of external and internal noise sources). The subjective measures indicate mild low- and high-frequency hearing losses, in contrast to the inferred substantial scattered OHC damage indicated by the objective results.

Otodynamics ILO88 Analyser in standard screening mode. The tinnitus of this observer has obviously not been as debilitating as that of some clients, but it can often be very troublesome, either in terms of its loudness at low-level ambient noise conditions, or its interference with perception of low-level sounds. The following list itemizes the prime features of his tinnitus, in order of appearance summarized in Figure 11-2A.

Transient Spontaneous Tinnitus (TST)

38. TST has occurred since early teens; long before any manifestation of continuous tinnitus, it occurred only with a single pitch corresponding to a frequency in the range never below 1 kHz and seldom above 4 kHz.

39. The incidence has been episodic, maybe twenty times per week during periods of frequent music exposure or great tiredness, to less than once per week at other times; total number of occasions estimated to be many thousands.

40. The incidence of TST is estimated to be approximately equally divided between ears, never both ears simultaneously.

41. TST was mostly preceded (and often followed) by feelings of dullness (reduction in auditory sensitivity) and fullness (sensation of pressure) in the same ear. This lasted no more than a few seconds. This sensation is vaguely similar to the change in pressure equalization during ascent or descent of an airplane. It is followed by the TST rising to a peak of around 15 to 20 dB SL, typically in 1 to 2 seconds.

42. The incidence of fluctuant sensations of pressure is far more common than the incidence of TST itself.

43. TST decreased steadily in loudness lasting various lengths of time ranging from 5 seconds for minor disturbances, to 45 seconds for loud cases occurring in very quiet ambient levels, suggesting that the decay of the excitation may be exponential in nature. This possibility is depicted in Figure 11-3A showing sensation level (dB) as a function of time (s). The abscissa is the level above which the disturbance is audible.

44. TST may possess harmonic distortion; the percept is that of an external pure tone with a second harmonic discernible at low background noise levels.

45. Only rarely is TST associated with a specific incidence of overexposure, but high level TST (>80 dB SL) can be evoked by a brief, high-level impulse and is accompanied by an equally strong pressure sensation or even pain.

46. TST is not easily masked by whistling even though a pitch match is readily generated.

Continuous Low-Frequency Tinnitus (CLFT)

47. CLFT first presented after age 40 only in the right ear and is ever-present in conditions of low ambient noise, such as in the quiet of the night.

48. It normally has a sensation level of 5 to 10 dB or even up to 20 dB in an anechoic chamber.

49. The pitch is scarcely discernible; like a broadband rumble centered around 50 Hz. If several pitches are present covering the band, there are no obvious beats. There are no upper harmonics or partials.

50. Masking is readily and rapidly produced, providing the masker has a frequency less than 300 Hz, that is, there is a downward spread of masking for low frequencies. Lower frequencies are more effective maskers, for example, humming. The duration of residual inhibition is a strong function of frequency, extending up to 5 seconds for very low frequencies. A sound of similar sensation level to the tinnitus can readily mask the CLFT. The sensation often has a throbbing quality if the ambient level varies around the masking level, like a car passing down the street outside; even continuous head movement can suppress the CLFT.

51. The period of residual inhibition (RI) depends directly on the strength of the masker in a way which suggests that the perturbation recovery function is exponential. This possibility is depicted in Figure 11-2D showing sensation level (dB) as a function of time (s). Again, the abscissa is the level above which the disturbance is audible, so that the CLFT is always audible except when masked, after which recovery occurs.

52. Experiments have failed to reveal any objective counterpart to the CLFT, that is, a spontaneous emission at very low frequencies which can be masked as above.

53. Sudden counterclockwise rotation of the head accentuates the CLFT; clockwise rotation masks the CLFT very briefly; this phenomenon occurs irrespective the orientation of the head.

Continuous High-Frequency Tinnitus (CHFT)

54. CHFT occurs at frequencies above 8 kHz in both ears simultaneously; there is no musical note value; the pitch is too high; the percept is central. This sounds like a thin tone or set of tones like once was heard emanating from the 10 kHz line-oscillator on a television set. However, unlike external sounds of that frequency that are highly directional, the location of CHFT within the head cannot be controlled or modulated by rotating the head.

55. The sensation level is highly dependent on:
  a. The ambient background noise level, and
  b. The attention paid to it. In low-noise conditions especially, the sensation level can be made to increase substantially over a period of seconds to a minute or more, simply by focusing on the high-frequency "mixture", whereupon a single frequency emerges as dominant. This, however, tends to become more unilateral in origin.

56. Focusing on this single frequency sensation for minutes can cause the sensation level to rise still further with a marked increase in the coherence of the percept.

57. Relief is achieved by diverting attention away from the sensation, more so than by actively trying to ignore it.

Transient High-Frequency Spontaneous Tinnitus (THFST).

58. Most recent in appearance is TST at discrete frequencies above 6 kHz at relatively low sensation levels. No harmonics are discernible at these frequencies.

A PHYSIOLOGICAL MODEL FOR NORMAL OUTER HAIR CELL ACTION

Electromechanical Regulation of Inner Hair Cell Operating Point by the Outer Hair Cells

For many years, theories of cochlear function have been based solely on the finding that a traveling wave, like a water wave, propagates along the basilar membrane, producing vibrational peaks at places corresponding to frequency components in the sound (von Békésy 1960) which are detected as peaks by the hair cells. Since von Békésy's innovative experiments, we have learned that the outer hair cells (OHC) are not just sensory cells; they are also motor cells which presumably were not displaying motor activity during his postmortem experiments. It is now largely accepted that his passive traveling wave picture is incomplete. The OHC activity has fast and slow aspects but the roles of each have yet to be integrated into any comprehensive theory. The fast activity of the OHC (Ashmore 1987; Zenner, Zimmermann, and Gitter 1987; Kachar, Kalinek, Iwasa, Holley, and Lim 1991) is thought to boost the vibration to be large enough to be detectable by the inner hair cells (IHC), even at high frequencies. To model this phenomenon, it was necessary to invoke an amplifier (Neely and Kim, 1983; Davis, 1983) to counteract the viscous effects of the cochlear fluids damping out the sound-produced vibration. Indeed, there are some well-advanced ideas about the origins of tinnitus. Most deal with the assumption that, like spontaneous otoacoustic emissions, tinnitus has its origins in an anomalous boosted mechanical oscillation (e.g. Plinkert, Gitter, and Zenner 1990). However, the incidence of spontaneous emissions is not strongly tied to the incidence of subjective tinnitus (Penner, 1992; Shulman et al. 1992).

What still needs to be considered in depth is the possible role(s) of the slow motility of the OHC—the length changes. These cells have the capacity to change their length by 10 percent (i.e., up to 10 μm) (Zenner, Zimmermann, and Schmitt 1985). The

OHC are like microscopic sausage balloons with a raised internal pressure (Brownell and Shehata 1990). They also have a very specialized cell border which appears to act like a girdle (Brownell and Shehata 1990; Holley and Ashmore 1990). Cell swelling may be due to the cell taking in water and increasing its internal pressure. The girdle appears to have limits to its elasticity and cannot take too much of this. The cell will start to assume a more spherical shape, the swelling starting from its base resulting in shortening of the cell. Eventually the cell can explode and even eject the nucleus (Evans, 1990). When this happens, the cell dies, but in the process of doing so the passive spring in the cell wall returns it toward its original cylindrical shape. Also over a period of time, the cell membrane can degrade, leading to increased compliance (LePage et al. 1992b), suggesting that the cell has become slack.

Isolated outer hair cells display sinusoidal variations in length in response to low-frequency sinusoidal electric stimulation (Brownell, Bader, Bertrand, and deRibaupierre 1985; Zenner et al. 1985). The direction of the length change is a systematic function of frequency and place of origin of the OHC (Canlon, Brundin, and Flock 1988). By contrast, OHC *in vitro*, in an intact explanted segment of the basilar membrane, organ of Corti, and tectorial membrane, display a steady length change superimposed on the oscillating movement (LePage 1993a). This summating behavior ceases when the stimulus is turned off. Direct *in vivo* measurements in the cochleas of guinea pigs have also shown substantial summating displacements of basilar membrane (LePage 1989) and also in the organ of Corti (Brundin, Flock, Khanna, and Ulfendahl 1991). A recent study has failed to replicate these measurements (Cooper and Rhode 1992), highlighting the need for further investigation (LePage 1993). The fact remains that under certain conditions, baseline summating movements of the basilar membrane are observable (LePage 1981; 1987) and mirror the frequency dependence of the summating potential measured simulta-

neously from an electrode on the round window (LePage 1987). Similar results have recently been produced by Brundin, Flock, and Flock 1992. The slow summating movements are prima facie evidence that the OHC regulate the mean position of the basilar membrane, thereby stabilizing the operating point of the inner hair cells (IHC) against global fluctuations in the pressure in the endolymph relative to perilymph pressure.

Figure 11-3A depicts two images of the cross-section of scala media, redrawn from post mortem sections of hydropic cochleas, illustrating that the basilar membrane may undergo substantial baseline variations due to fluctuations in endolymph pressure in the scalar media (SM). In addition, variations in basilar membrane (BM) bias position produced by high-level low-frequency tones have been shown to have a marked influence on cochlear sensitivity (Zwicker 1977; LePage 1981; Patuzzi, Sellick, and Johnstone 1984). Low-level, low-frequency tones have no biasing effect because the baseline regulation process actively compensates for the biasing influence. This same process appears to be intimately linked to the normal mode of stimulation of the IHC. In terms of the model, the position of both BM and TM is either steady or continually moving to some new set point, depending upon the history of the stimulus (LePage 1989; 1992) and descending neural influences via the medial efferent pathway (see Warr 1992 for a recent review). In the presence of a fixed pure tone, the basilar membrane apparently adopts a "biphasic" or "triphasic" pattern of DC displacement that is excitatory at the characteristic frequency (CF) of the place under measurement. Displacements toward ST (strongly suppressive) have been observed for frequencies either side of CF (LePage 1989; 1992).

Assumptions of the Baseline Regulation Model

1. The OHC detect high frequency energy (Brundin, Flock, and Canlon 1989; Iwasa, Minxu,

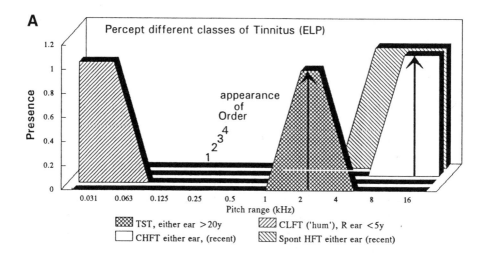

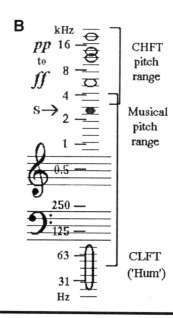

FIGURE 11-2. Relevant features of the subjective tinnitus of ELP. Panels A and B show two diverse representations of the pitch of the continuous high-frequency tinnitus (CHFT), continuous low-frequency tinnitus (CLFT); the mid-range transient spontaneous tinnitus (TST), and the transient spontaneous high-frequency tinnitus (TSHFT). The frequency representation in A shows the order of appearance; the ordinate indicates presence or absence. The TST present since early teens develops at a single frequency mostly in the mid-frequency range, 1 to 4 kHz, and possesses even harmonics. The CLFT developed around age 40 in the right ear only. It has nondiscernible pitch around 50 Hz and has no upper harmonics or timber. The CHFT which has developed since is mostly perceived as tight clusters of pseudo-sinusoids above 8 kHz (as distinct from the percept of broadband noise). The coherence of the combination is strongly dependent on selectively attending to it. A musical representation is

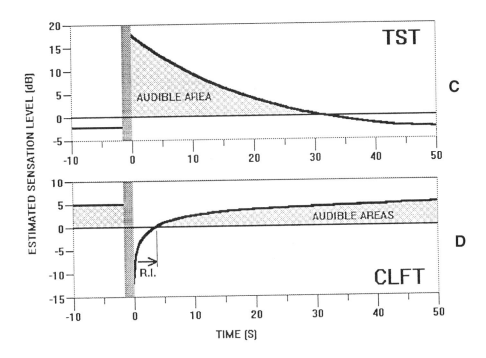

provided in B to illustrate first that *place pitch* may extend to much higher frequencies than does *repetition (musical) pitch*; second, that CHFT may generally be thought of as being above the musical pitch range; and thirdly, that it may be thought of as clusters of pseudo-tones. Once CHFT extends downward into the musical pitch range, as in the case of Smetana's "high E" (2637 Hz, "S" arrow), it may be considerably more debilitating because it is closer to the center of the tonotopy. The indeterminate pitch of the CLFT in the right ear suggests that an apical segment of the cochlear partition has collapsed or sagged, perhaps due to separation of the outer spiral ligament from the bone. The tectorial membrane is now normally set in the position where inner hair cells (IHC) are excited. The central hypothesis is that this is because the normal setpoint for OHC length has permanently drifted (see text). C shows the perceived sensation level of transient spontaneous tinnitus (TST). Prior to some transient disturbance, such as a sudden burst of efferent activity or the death of an OHC, there is no sensation because the IHCs are biased off. In the model, the sudden mismatch of opposing forces holding the tectorial membrane in place leads to a excitatory deflection until the previous equilibrium state can be re-established by the remaining OHC, which now must generate the same net force as before the sick cell stopped contributing its steady tonic force. The presence of second harmonic distortion (Property 44) suggests that TST does involve an oscillation with some mechanical limiting or saturation that may be attributable to the nonlinear electromechanical properties of the OHC. The instability arises when the cochlear partition is displaced from its normal position and because the damping is reduced during such displacement. D shows that CLFT may arise for very similar reasons as TST, despite having very different origins and percepts. The explanation derives from the same baseline regulation model, but now the OHCs are regulating at a different operating point where the tectorial membrane has drifted in the excitatory direction of the IHC. This leads to the percept of a low-frequency hum which can be suppressed if there are sufficient viable surrounding OHCs excited to generate a suppressive displacement. The fact that the sensation has no harmonics suggests the generator is not an oscillation.

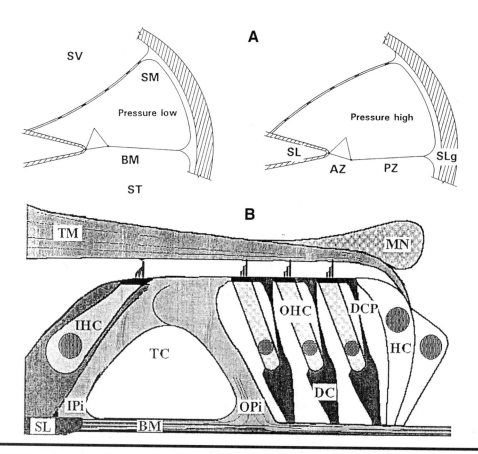

FIGURE 11-3.   Integral action of the basilar membrane, organ of Corti, and tectorial membrane. A contains two views of the cross-section of scala media bordered below by scala tympani (ST) and above by scala vestibuli (SV). The basilar membrane (BM) is divided into two radial segments, the inner arctuate zone (AZ) and the outer pectinate zone (PZ), which is joined to the wall via the spiral ligament (SLg). The PZ is passive in its properties, whereas the AZ embodies the organ of Corti and pillars that make up the arch which is hinged at the spiral lamina (SL). The two images are redrawn from histological sections of the cochlea to illustrate that slow pressure variations in the endolymph relative to pressures in ST and SV cause the basilar membrane and Reissner's membrane to flex inward and outward. Typically the basilar membrane is 150 μm wide in the basal turn, and under experimental conditions may flex up and down by up to 10 μm. Under normal conditions, the OHCs deliver a tonic force to regulate the position of the basilar membrane to compensate for such pressure fluctuations and stabilize hearing sensitivity. B (redrawn from Lim, 1986) shows the key mechanical elements involved in OHC control and IHC stimulation. The OHCs are suspended from the reticular membrane in which are embedded their cuticular plates (black) containing roots of the OHC stereocilia. The reticular membrane itself is supported by the arch made up of the inner and outer pillars (IPi, OPi). The bases of the OHC sit in sockets of the Deiter cells (DC) which are attached to the reticular membrane by the diagonal processes. Attached to the outer rim of the reticular membrane are the Hensen cells (HC). The OHC stereocilia are embedded in the underside of the tectorial membrane (TM), glued by proteoglycand molecules. The IHC stereocilia are not embedded in the TM but brush on its underside. On the upper outer edge of the tectorial membrane is the marginal net (MN).

Li, and Kachard 1991) and *adapt* to it by change in their length (LePage et al. 1993b).

2. The length change of the OHCs is delivered as a change in displacement of the tectorial membrane and to a lesser extent the basilar membrane in opposite phase.

3. The IHCs are simple displacement detectors with stereocilia that brush the underside of the tectorial membrane and are deflected by changes in its position (Figure 11-3B).

4. The IHCs are non-adapting receptors, that is, a constant deflection of the IHC stereocilia (IHCSC) brings about a constant level of depolarization of the IHCs and a constant afferent firing rate (Kiang, Watanabe, Thomas, and Clarke 1965).

5. The IHCs have a sensory bandwidth which does not exceed the bandwidth fixed by maximal firing rates of nerve fibers (speculation).

6. The bandwidth of the primary force generation mechanism by the outer hair cells need not be much greater than that of the IHCs (speculation). Fast length changes have velocities which come within the sensitivity range of sensitive Doppler shift measurement techniques (Sellick, Patuzzi, and Johnstone 1982), which invalidly assume the motion is pure sinusoidal (LePage 1993).

7. In response to a pure tone, the OHCs establish a "triphasic" pattern of baseline shift *in the position of the tectorial membrane* as a function of place, so that the suppression lobes may mechanically bias the IHCs *off* (generate masking) for frequencies either side of CF (speculation).

8. The medial efferent pathway is a negative feedback system which stabilizes the IHC operating point against long-term degradation of the organ of Corti. There are limits to the effectiveness of the stabilization; it requires some OHCs to be present to generate displacements in the suppressive direction (TM moves away from the IHCSC). Total loss of OHCs opens the loop. Partial degradation of the active elements can result in "creep", or drift toward the excitatory direction.

9. Regulation of OHC tonic force must effect regulation of this tension in the radial fibers of the tectorial membrane and basilar membrane through the lever action of the arch (LePage 1990; speculation) which, based on the modified Helmholz model (LePage 1992), will be highest at the base of the cochlea.

In this model, the primary stimulus for high-frequency detection by the IHCs is thus assumed to be OHC length change, modifying the transverse position of the tectorial membrane (Figure 11-3B) by about 10 μm. For sound transduction to occur, the very narrow region of high sensitivity of the IHCs (about 0.1 μm) must be physically aligned with the connection to the OHC. That is, the angle of the tectorial membrane needs to be such that the IHCs are minimally able to respond to deflection of their stereocilia.

Mechanical Action of the Outer Hair Cells

A hypothesis for the manner of action of the OHCs stems from the geometry of the cells that support the OHC, the Deiter cells. These cells have a string-like process which is attached at one end to the cup in which the base of the OHC sits. The other end connects with the reticular membrane one or two cells more apical than their own location (Voldřich and Úlehlová 1987). Rather than being directly supported by the basilar membrane (BM), the base of OHC is thus supported rigidly from the overlying structure in such a manner that elongation of the OHC results in an upwards force upon the reticular membrane in the direction of scalar vestibuli (SV) and a smaller force downwards on the BM in the direction of scalar tympani (ST) (see Figure 11-4A, B, and C). Conversely, a reduction in length of the OHC will cause the tectorial membrane to move towards ST. The OHC elongation is accompanied by a twisting motion longitudinally *along* the reticular membrane, which simultaneously tends to increase the tension, not just in the Deiter processes but in the radial fibers of TM as well. Note that the Deiter cell processes must be diagonal or the OHCs would have no freedom to elongate. Figure 11-4D, E, and F show this process in cross-section so that

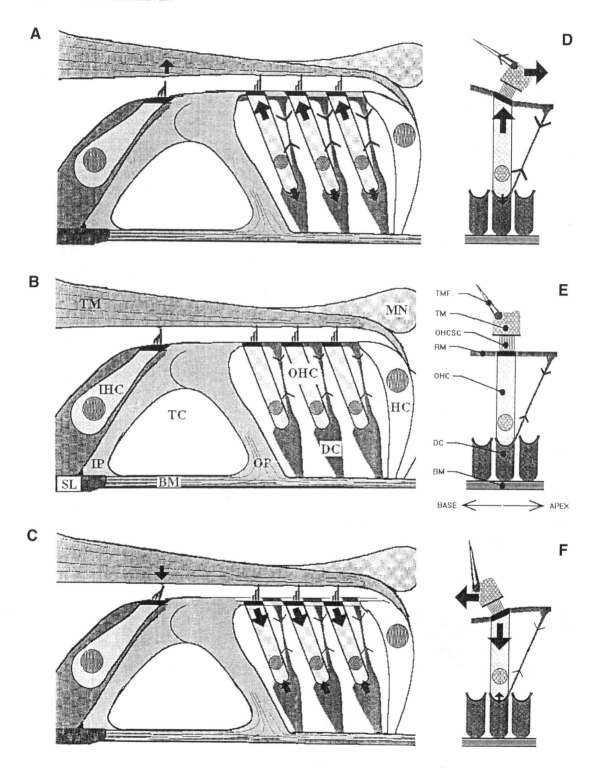

FIGURE 11-4. Regulation of tectorial membrane position. In the traditional view of operation of the organ of Corti, vibratory shear between the reticular membrane (RM) and the tectorial membrane (TM) deflects the OHC stereocilia (OHCSC). In the current picture, the direction of action is reversed. The three pairs of panels (A–D, B–E, C–F) show views of the OHC, RM, and TM seen from a radial cross-sectional view looking from base toward apex (A, B, C; redrawn from Lim, 1986) and the corresponding longitudinal section (D, E, F). Panels A, B, and C show the OHCs at their standard length, which gives rise to the normal operating point of the IHCs (see Figure 11-5). At their standard length, the OHCs exert a tonic longitudinal tensile force upon the diagonal Deiter cell processes (arrows) which are inextensible, like strings. The regulation process requires that there exist a line of static force running radially through the radial fibers of the TM (TMRF), the arch, the BM, and spiral ligament attached to the outer wall of the cochlea, such that the OHCSC act as tiny levers to increase the tension in the TM (see arrow). Preparation artifacts readily show that the TM must be under radial tension, because the TM retracts when separated from the tips of the OHCSC. The torque thus applied across the length of the OHCSC serves to move the arch and the TM up and down, varying the degree of deflection of the IHC stereocilia (IHCSC) in the process. In the panels A and D, elongation of the OHC pushes the reticular membrane upwards, causing flexion in the longitudinal direction. The result is a rotatory movement to the cuticular plates which tends to open the gap and suppress IHC response. The tectorial membrane may be raised well clear of the IHCSC (the separation is limited by string-like trabeculae) removing all excitatory displacement (Figure 11-5, operating position A). Panels B–E and C–F show shortened OHCs, resulting in the generation of shear between the reticular membrane and the tectorial membrane. This shear has both radial and longitudinal components. As shown, clockwise rotation of the arch will close the subtectorial gap, impinging upon the tips of the IHCSC and causing them to slide along the undersurface of the TM known as Hensen's stripe. Any drift in the regulating processes tending to close the subtectorial gap will result in excitation of the IHCs. Various states of IHC excitation are possible (Figure 11-5B, C, and D) resulting from various degrees of rotation of the arch toward ST.

the longitudinal flexing of the reticular membrane can be appreciated. The OHC stereocilia are specialized to withstand this shear force and to maintain tension in the TM and BM (LePage 1990). Each hair cell has three rows of stereocilia. The smaller-length stereocilia are tied together with filaments and butt against the base of the tallest to prevent them deflecting radially toward the modiolus while still allowing them to deflect radially outward freely.

IHC Operating Point in the Normal Cochlea

In normal undamaged cochleas, the OHC *motor unit control system* has ample capacity to control the sensitivity of the IHCs by setting the operating point on the IHC transfer characteristic to some position which the brain normally interprets as no

sound input (Figure 11-5, inset position A). This condition never actually constitutes zero sound input, but rather a sound level currently deemed as background within the frequency band being coded by that IHC. With significant background noise, the IHCs will depolarize to, say, C. In response, the motor unit control system will apply negative feedback to try to reset the operating point back towards the same point A, but the closest position is B. The dynamic range of the primary neuron is thus extended. Only an increase of sound level in that frequency band will be registered, and by definition, will become a signal of interest (see below).

This scheme constitutes a more comprehensive role for the OHCs than pure amplifiers boosting the vibration. It may be a more realistic one because it also provides that the role of the OHCs is

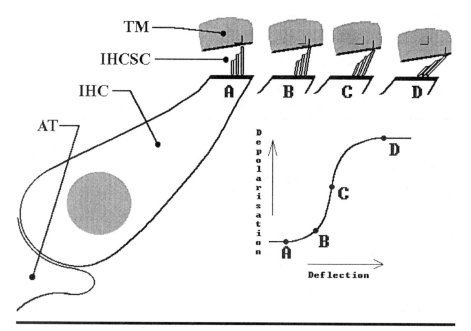

FIGURE 11-5. Shortening of the OHC results in excitation of the IHC. The IHC stereocilia (IHCSC) are deflected by various degrees according to the displacement of the tectorial membrane (TM) under the control of the OHCs. They are believed to slide freely under the TM. In position A, the IHC is maximally polarized. The TM is not touching the IHCSC. Small movements increase the depolarization of the IHC until saturation occurs at D, leading to transmitter release and excitation of the afferent terminal (AT) (see text).

to be the primary detectors of high-frequency energy, delivering their output to the IHCs as a low bandwidth signal containing only the envelope of the sound (LePage 1989). As such it appeals to the principle of Occam's Razor: Why should the IHCs also be envelope detectors, if the OHCs already have an adaptive role, changing their length according to amount of the high-frequency energy reaching them? That is, the baseline regulation function of the OHCs means that the IHCs need not also be specialized for detection of high-frequency vibration. The transition of OHC function from AC amplifiers to AC detectors and integrators occurs over the frequency range 1 to 4 kHz.

In turn, this simple scheme does not specifically require the cochlear amplifier be sharply

tuned with resonant elements in the model proposed by Gold (1948). Frequency selectivity is modeled in the spatial domain as the triphasic pattern of varying OHC length along the cochlear partition (LePage 1987; 1989) depicted in Figure 11-6. Figure 11-6A shows the effect of a variation in the length (greatly exaggerated) of the representative OHC along a 3 mm segment of the cochlear partition in response to a pure tone. Shortening of the OHC results in excitation of the IHC; lengthening results in suppression by virtue of the resulting displacement of the attached tectorial membrane (TM). Figures 11-6B and C assist with visualizing the effect of superimposing a uniform bias component on such a triphasic pattern of excitation. The pattern of Figure 11-6A is inverted so that positive-going (downward) displacements of the TM result in excitation (Figure 11-6B; refer again to Figure 11-5). Such a uniform bias could be established by the medial efferent system as a direct function of sound level, higher sound levels resulting in more positive values of DC bias. In this schematic, the size of the triphasic pattern is fixed for simplicity, and only values of TM displacement resulting in a positive deflection of the IHC stereocilia (IHCSC) (Figure 11-5, point A) are shown. Highly positive peaks (greater than 40 arbitrary units) in the displacement will result in deflections of the IHCSC past setpoint D, resulting in saturation of the IHC electric response as shown. For each level of the stimulus, the IHC frequency-response profiles (Figure 11-6C) are remarkably similar to the iso-SPL frequency response characteristics of single neurons in the squirrel monkey (Geisler, Rhode, and Kennedy 1974, Figure 2), leading to the standard representation of tuning at threshold (dark horizontal line representing the spatial extent of the excitation region).

The property of this model that is highly relevant to tinnitus is that two-tone suppression can occur by virtue of locating the frequency of the suppressing tone so that one or other of the negative phases is spatially aligned with the excitation peak of the primary tone. The central excitation region may be due to a real input, or equally well, a phantom input. In the model, the operating point is controlled very precisely so that any drift in that position will have the effect of varying not only the firing rate of the nerve if the operating point is within the displacement-sensing range of the cell but the number of afferent fibres stimulated—the size of the excitatory region. This scheme provides for suppression of the firing rate by turning off the IHCs with a negative-going displacement of the cochlear partition, produced by efferent control of OHC length. Clearly the size of the excitatory region (mm) depends upon the value of the bias which is under central control.

There is considerable redundancy in the numbers of OHCs. Humans have some 12,000 in each ear at birth (see summary in Kim 1984). Not only

are there three rows, but each *motor unit* will consist of the 20 to 50 OHCs synapsing with a single medial efferent neuron (see Figure 11-7, redrawn from Spoendlin 1970). The scheme allows that different motor units may give rise to differing local values of bias so that the size of the excitatory region for any sound may be varied with respect to any other sound. The neural innervation pattern of these motor units suggests a likely candidate for the improvement in signal-to-noise ratio (SNR). Here the definition of "noise" is any signal in which one has no interest, whether or not it contains information which has meaning if attention were directed at it.

PHANTOM ACOUSTIC INPUT: THE OPERATING POINT DRIFT HYPOTHESIS

Numerous histological studies (e.g., Engstrom, Ades, and Bredberg, 1970; Bohne, Yohman, and Gruner 1987) have shown permanent damage patterns ranging from loss of OHCs, to loss of the supporting cells, to loss of the whole organ of Corti. The lesioned areas may be quite irregular, giving rise to loss of control of the input to the IHC via the tectorial membrane at these locations. The current state of excitation of the IHCs set by the angle of deflection of the IHC stereocilia (IHCSC), is termed its operating (set) point which varies along the transfer curve (refer to Figure 11-5). In the model anything which results in steady deflection of the IHC stereocilia in the excitation direction can be interpreted by the brain as a real acoustic excitation pattern. It is clear that any coding system in which the OHCs are the fundamental detectors, delivering their response to the IHCs as a shift in the baseline position of the tectorial membrane, must incorporate precise regulation of baseline position so that the organ may detect very tiny signals buried in ambient noise. Moreover, the scheme should be able to continue to do so even if the normal range of operation of the mechanism is compromised temporarily or permanently (Property 1). The following speculations stem from the baseline regulation model.

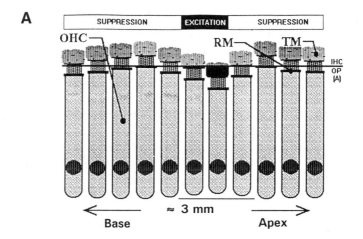

A

SUPPRESSION | EXCITATION | SUPPRESSION

OHC

RM   TM

IHC
OP
(A)

← ≈ 3 mm →

Base   Apex

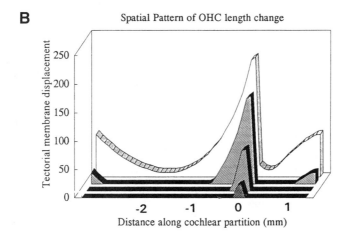

B

Spatial Pattern of OHC length change

Tectorial membrane displacement

250
200
150
100
50
0

-2   -1   0   1

Distance along cochlear partition (mm)

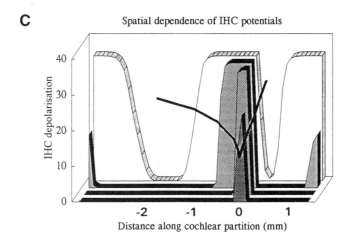

C

Spatial dependence of IHC potentials

IHC depolarisation

40
30
20
10
0

-2   -1   0   1

Distance along cochlear partition (mm)

FIGURE 11-6.   Schematic of the baseline regulation model. A shows a representative sample of outer hair cells (OHC) along a 3 mm *(ca)* length of the cochlear partition under stimulation of a single sinusoidal stimulus. The OHCs sense the mean vibratory stimulus and respond by adjusting their lengths accordingly. This is a dynamic, history-dependent process in which the OHC length varies about some mean length which fixes the transverse position of the tectorial membrane TM. In one of the several possible mechanical schemes, each OHC shortens in order to pull (down) upon the TM, deflecting the IHC stereocilia (IHCSC) and depolarizing the IHCs (as in Figure 11-4). Conversely, the OHCs elongate to lift the TM away from IHCSC to produce suppression. The figure utilizes a "triphasic" (here M-shaped) excitation pattern (the amplitude is exaggerated a hundredfold for display) in which an excitatory region (a downward movement of the TM) is bordered by an inhibitory surround (upward movement of the TM). The relative lengths of the excitatory region versus the inhibitory regions depend strongly on the normal operating point of the OHCs relative to the displacement required to just excite the IHC (OP). Clearly if the OHCs must deliver a power-stroke in the suppressive direction, the level of suppression at any time depends upon the integrity of the force-generation mechanism leading to an elongation of the OHCs. Suppression will be reduced by any agent which tends to disable this force component. Panel C shows how shortening of the OHCs results in a downward movement of the TM and excitation of the IHCs. In panel B, the ordinate represents the deflection of the IHCSC which results from the M-shaped pattern (Panel A), this time inverted to appear W-shaped so that positive indicates cell excitation. Each of the four curves can be thought of as a stimulus-produced pattern upon which is superimposed a different value of DC-bias (the OHC lengths are changing), due, for example, to a broadband stimulus, or a small change in the endocochlear potential—or a global change in OHC turgor pressure. The curve in front represents the value of the bias necessary for the underside of the tectorial membrane to just touch the IHC stereocilia for the excitatory peak at the CF. As the bias is raised, due to a rise in OHC DC-operating point, the frequency band for which the TM is in contact with the IHCSC is increased and the IHC are deflected more at the CF. There are still frequencies removed from CF for which the TM does not contact the IHCSC. As the bias is raised further (OHC length increase) the IHCSC register the whole excitatory peak, but not the suppressive displacements. For the rear curve in the top panel the TM is continuous contact with the IHCSC and so the IHCs are now *excited* by the pattern for all frequencies. It is important to realize that the ability of the OHCs to generate these biases is large (up to *ca.* 10 μm) relative to the stimulus-produced DC-excitation pattern which, at threshold may be of just-detectable amplitude (*ca.* 1 nm), yielding a very different picture of cochlear mechanics from the traditional *traveling wave envelope*. Panel C shows the effect of these displacements on the electrical behavior of the IHCs (refer to Figure 11-5); the ordinate values are arbitrary but may be helpful in thinking in terms of mV depolarization. Assuming that the IHC operating point is at A, the IHC will register the smallest deflection as a tiny depolarization B. Progressively larger deflections will cause more depolarization (C and D), however, because the IHC has a narrow displacement range (*ca.* 0.1μm) the membrane potential will saturate for larger deflections. The resulting pattern of depolarization shows very clearly how the bias plays a very important role in the definition of the tuning curve formed by joining the edges of the excitatory region with straight lines in the horizontal plane. Indeed, the series of profiles mimics strongly the patterns of firing of primary afferent neurons. Note that because of the W-shaped pattern, sinusoidal stimuli at other frequencies will generate a negative bias which will be superimposed on the existing stimulus/bias pattern. This will have the effect of driving the W-shaped excitation pattern downward and the operating point of the IHC back toward A, reducing the level of excitation at the CF and masking the response. As is described in the text, this scheme applies equally well for any pseudo-stimulus excitatory pattern such as seen in Figure 11-8. Provided there are enough OHCs in the neighborhood to generate a negative-going displacement (by elongation, drawing the TM away from the IHCSC), the pseudo stimulus may be masked. The greater the loss of OHCs the smaller the net force they can deliver on elongation and the more difficult it will be to mask.

A

B

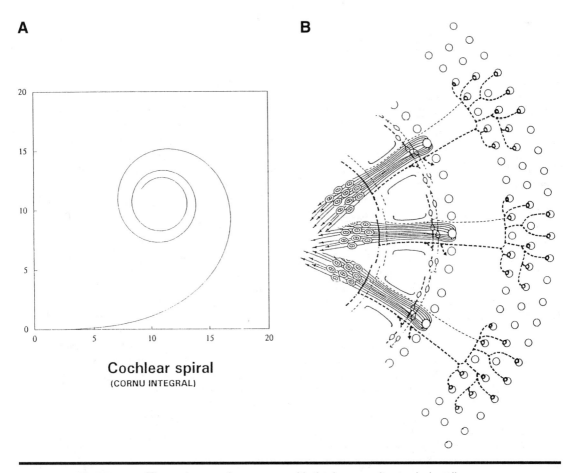

Cochlear spiral
(CORNU INTEGRAL)

FIGURE 11-7. The main neural synapses with the inner and outer hair cells (redrawn from Spoendlin). Panel A shows the form of the cochlear spiral calculated from a Cornu integral. In the Panel B most afferent neurons synapse with the single row of inner hair cells. The dotted lines show the efferent or motor neurons which control patches of outer hair cells or "motor units" (LePage 1989). Three such motor units are shown. The brain would appear to be able to vary the sensitivity of the cochlea for different narrow-frequency bands, independently from those either side. This pattern of innervation offers the possibility for a listener to selectively attend to sounds at specific frequencies (presumably either real or phantom) by setting up a comb-shaped filter (LePage 1989).

Potential Conditions that May Give Rise to Drift in IHC Operating Point

1. IHCs with permanently distorted stereocilia (Saunders, Canton, and Flock 1986; Thorne, Duncan, and Gavin 1986; Canlon, Miller, Flock, and Borg 1987), if still functional, could be interpreted by the brain as a *phantom* or virtual acoustic input.

2. Passive shift of the cochlear partition due to
   a. pressure build-up in scalar media (Figure 11-3A) (see Relevant Characteristics 41 and 42),
   b. changes to the morphology of the TM (Canlon 1987),

c. detachment of the tectorial membrane from the tips of the OHCs (von Békésy 1960),

d. loss of elasticity of the spiral ligament (Voldřich and Úlehlová 1982).

3. Active shift due to a drift in the OHC electromechanical setpoint, for example, due to

a. temporary or permanent change in tonic efferent firing rates (Liberman 1989),

b. loss of regulation in biochemical gradients due to noise (Konishi and Salt 1983), or

c. OHC degeneration, for example, due to

(1) loss of volume and/or length regulation,

(2) loss of force generation per cell, or

(3) decrease in numbers of cells.

The common factor in each of these potential disturbances of regulation is abnormal deflection of the IHC stereocilia in the excitatory direction (Figure 11-5) exciting the afferent terminals. In the first case the permanent deflection is independent of OHC response. In cases 2 and 3, recovery depends on the viability of the remaining OHCs in the neighborhood to perform some regulation.

In cochleas where there is significant permanent OHC loss, the capacity of the remaining OHCs to oppose *drifts* in the setpoint will be reduced, resulting in a reduced range of suppression or excitation. Damaged OHCs may drift in their length, changing the transverse position of the tectorial membrane. The changes in electromechanical setpoint of the OHCs may be expected to be accompanied by changes in the size of the microphonics to external tones (Property 16).

When the OHC drift is sufficient, they may no longer respond to the medial efferent influence and the displacement range over which active baseline restoration can take place will be reduced. Presumably at the limit (complete OHC loss) no suppression can occur since no OHCs exist in the neighborhood to generate a suppressive displacement (cell elongation). Clearly, no permanent loss of OHC function need occur to produce tinnitus. If the mechanical coupling is damaged at any point in the lever system, such as a temporary separation of the tectorial membrane from the tips of the OHC stereocilia, force genera-

tion by the OHCs can no longer maintain that tension and the structure will become slack.

Incessant Character of Continuous Tinnitus

The brain will not be able to distinguish between active deflection by OHC action in response to sound as per the model, mechanical drift due to OHC inactivation, or collapse of the organ of Corti due to acoustic overexposure (Saunders et al. 1986; Harding, Baggot, and Bohne 1992). Constant deflection of the IHC stereocilia produces a constant firing rate, consistent with properties 14, 15, 17–22, 43, 51–53. Therefore, in terms of the model, neither CHFT nor CLFT needs a physical oscillation to generate it, accounting for the lack of perceived beats with an external tone (Properties 13, 49).

Figure 11-8A depicts a localized area of collapse in the structure of the organ of Corti due to loss of OHC turgor, leading to an increased deflection of the stereocilia of the IHCs mimicking a real input (Figure 11-6A). The loudness of the tinnitus will likely depend upon the depth of the deflection. This will be determined by the extent of the OHC lesion and whether all three rows are affected or missing. In turn this will set the number of IHCs being stimulated. If the OHC loss is not extensive but scattered, the condition may constitute a mild wideband tinnitus. The adjacent OHCs can still exert some regulation function; it simply requires a higher level acoustic stimulus to evoke an increase in OHC length which acts to reduce the amount of deflection of IHCs (Figure 11-8C). The sound level required to reduce the depolarization of the IHCs to zero is effectively the masking level (Properties 29–37).

Tinnitus Pitch

If a short length of the cochlear partition were collapsed, or the OHC tonus decreased (Figure 11-8A), the resulting dynamic excitation pattern is similar to the triphasic pattern for a pure tone (Figure 11-6). The model therefore suggests that the percept of this condition will be a place-code input, that is, the percept of a pure sinusoid. To

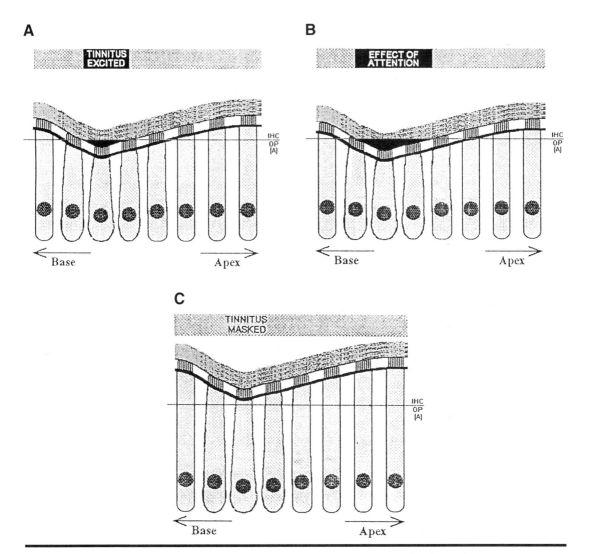

FIGURE 11-8.   Hypothesized origin of subjective tinnitus. Panel A schematizes a short (*ca* 40 µm) segment of degraded OHCs surrounded on either side by healthy OHCs. OHCs tend to shorten with degradation and can no longer extend to deliver tonic force to raise the tectorial membrane. There is consequently a short longitudinal segment of tectorial membrane which is depolarizing IHCs. The black region constitutes the pseudo-input exciting the IHCs (refer again to Figure 11-5). Panel B depicts the hypothesized effect of efferent stimulation of the OHCs resulting in shortening of the OHCs in the region. A longer segment of the tectorial membrane now lies below the threshold stimulus level of the IHCs and so the hypothesized effect of attention is shortening of the OHC leading to a greater number of IHCs and afferent fibers being excited. Elongation of the OHCs (Panel C) due to acoustic or electric stimulation (but not voluntary control via efferent activity) results in suppression of IHC response.

hear harmonics of a fundamental frequency might suggest the existence of a complex waveform propagating along the basilar membrane. Yet for CLFT and CHFT one does not hear anything other than a very "thin" single pitch even when intense (Properties 13,14, 54) without the harmonic richness (repetition pitch) which accompanies a complex time waveform.

The continuous aspects of the tinnitus are also characterized in musical pitch notation in Figure 11-2B. The purpose of this representation was to illustrate just *how high* the pitch of CHFT may be. To the majority of people not generally acquainted with the distinction between *place pitch* and *repetition pitch*, describing a sound as "high-pitched" may tend to convey the impression of the sound of a musical instrument in the high register, such as a trumpet, violin, or piccolo. Indeed, in Smetana's string quartet in E major the composer uses a high E from the first violin apparently to record the sound of his CHFT, yet the note chosen is at 2637 Hz, just 2.6 octaves above A=440 Hz (see "S" arrow, Figure 11-2B). However, the most common and debilitating kind of tinnitus described by clients of the author, particularly those with industrial hearing loss, is between one and two octaves higher again than this—well above the range of periodicity or musical pitch. It seems very few texts on tinnitus have made much distinction between the two types when the pitch of tinnitus is considered. Confusion about the nature of CHFT may exist (Property 7), because place pitch is normally implied in pure-tone pitch-matching experiments. If CLFT ("hum") were due to an oscillation, one might expect to hear upper partials like those for the TST but at least in this case none exist (Property 49).

The audiotape produced by the British Tinnitus Association uses a musical synthesizer to give an "artist's impression" of how different individuals perceive their tinnitus. Interestingly, over half the examples of synthesized tinnitus provided on the tape from the British Tinnitus Association are centered in the low to mid ranges (i.e., <2 kHz). Few kinds of tinnitus have any inherently musical quality about them. They generally appear to fall into broadband noise, multiples of tone-like peaks, or the same amplitude modulated at rates ranging from 0.5 Hz up to 10 Hz (Property 5). Accordingly, one can view broadband noise-induced tinnitus as being due to extensive scattered OHC damage over a length of the cochlear partition, particularly involving the basal end, leading to poor regulation of basilar membrane position. The percept will be like many tones which have no harmonic or phase relationship, depending on the number and location of the lesions.

The hydropic condition is caused by displacement of the basilar membrane position downwards (Figure 11-3A, right side, and Figure 11-5, position D). Ménière's syndrome in particular is marked by large, positive pressure fluctuations that are sensed jointly by the vestibular hair cells as vertigo, and, according to this model, the IHCs as roaring tinnitus. The spectrum of the tinnitus will likely contain a preponderance of low frequencies, because a raised static pressure in the scalar media along the cochlear partition will produce the greatest displacement where the static compliance is greatest (at the apex). Indeed Nodar and Graham (1965) report mostly frequencies below 1 kHz in Ménière syndrome attacks.

Onset of Tinnitus

As the ear ages, the strength of click-evoked otoacoustic emissions decreases, particularly at high frequencies (LePage and Murray 1992), suggesting that either the numbers of OHCs are decreasing or that their functionality decreases. In the regulation model (Property 9), the OHCs at the highest frequency end must sustain the highest static force in the fibers of the TM (Figure 11-4) and the BM (PZ, Figure 11-3) (LePage 1990). The site of greatest tension, and therefore the site most likely to display damage *first*, is the high-frequency region of the cochlea. Tinnitus tends to range from 4 to 12 kHz, judged from pitch-matching experiments in which octave errors frequently occur. Vernon reported one case at 17 kHz which is consistent with our case study here. It is therefore expected that continuous tinnitus will most frequently first present at high frequencies, consistent with Properties 2-4, 23, and 26. However, tinnitus may occur at any pitch, depending on the frequency of acute noise or other trauma and the resulting site(s) of cochlear damage (Property 26).

Many of the synthesized examples produced on the British Tinnitus Association tape contain amplitude modulations, some with a modulation frequency about the heart rate (Property 5). Presumably spurious contractions of the tensor tympani and/or stapedius muscles may also be responsible for pulsations. It follows from the mechanical regulation function of the OHCs that deterioration of that function may lead to sloppy regulation; the system will become slack, and be more subject to perturbing influences, such as minor vascular pulsations or jaw movements (Vernon 1991) which normally do not influence tectorial membrane regulation (Property 42).

This model does not exclude the possibility that physical oscillation may occur simultaneously (LePage 1992) and modulate the percept of setpoint drift (Properties 3, 5). The percept of cicadas and crickets by some sufferers suggests that some physical oscillation may be involved, since the percept of low-frequency amplitude modulation is unlikely to be the result of neural interaction centrally. In this case, the condition may be caused by combination of collapse of the cochlear partition *plus* a spontaneous mechanical oscillation. Certainly, in the case of TST the presence of harmonics (Property 44) suggests that a mechanical oscillation occurs, in which case such unpredictable phenomena should have an objective counterpart.

Exponential-type Behavior: Residual Inhibition

The temporal behavior, particularly the decay of both the TST and CLFT, suggests that the time course of the regulation process is exponential in nature. As is shown in Figures 11-2C and D, this descriptive model has merit because the *same*

baseline-regulation model can apply to *both kinds of tinnitus—the spontaneous and the continuous*—despite their diversity. In the figure, the ordinate corresponds to sensation level for the tinnitus. However, in the case of the CLFT tinnitus, the setpoint for the IHCs has drifted above the audible level where it remains permanently until some transient masking influence occurs. Alternately, in the case of the spontaneous tinnitus, the setpoint is normally just below the sensation level until triggered to go above by some perturbation (Property 45) such as an OHC exploding or a spurious burst of activity in one of the motor units generating a transient bulge in the tectorial membrane. This subsides once the remaining OHCs re-establish their estimate of the "normal" operating point of the IHCs.

The decrease of TST with time (Property 43) suggests that damping of oscillation on the BM is a function of baseline position. Given that a parasitic oscillation has begun, the baseline regulation process will act so as to return the system to a just-stable condition. Indeed, the profile of the OHC length change with place (Figure 11-6) could be tested as controlling damping of the cochlear partition.

In the model, the OHCs normally undergo length changes while a stimulus is maintained, but will return to their prestimulus length when the stimulus is removed. The time it takes for the decay to occur may depend on several factors. There is a strongly nonlinear relationship between OHC potential and the length change (Evans, Hallworth, and Dallos 1991), so it is to be expected that some kind of electrical exponential decay will take place before any mechanical change occurs. Residual inhibition (RI) (Figure 11-2D; Property 36d) could simply be the result of the lag between the electrical driving force and the slow electromechanical response.

Poor Correlation of Tinnitus Incidence with Hearing Loss

Over the history of auditory science, we have become conditioned to think that because the mammalian hearing organ is an exquisitely sensitive mechano-receptor, this is equivalent to the assertion that behavioral thresholds are a sensitive indicator of damage to the organ. An alternative hypothesis is that audiometric thresholds may be a late indicator of damage (LePage 1991), because damage must be extensive before there is a significant change to the audiogram. The field of otoacoustic emissions has resulted in the development of the concept of *cochlear mechanical loss* (Kemp 1989), determined by objective measurement, which is in contrast with the concept of a hearing loss determined psychophysically. Evidence is accumulating that the ear may suffer considerable mechanical damage over a long period of time *before* it is actually manifested as a hearing loss. Click-evoked otoacoustic emissions suggest that loss of motor function (either due to loss of numbers of OHCs or loss of OHC function due for example, to decline in endocochlear potential) may in some cases be determinable many years prior to a loss in hearing sensitivity (Murray and LePage 1990). In this sense the ear "fails gracefully".

By contrast, tinnitus can be manifest at a much earlier stage once there are punctate lesions along the cochlear partition involving only small patches of defunct cells or small regions of mechanical disruption which, due to OHC redundancy, has not yet been revealed as a decline in hearing sensitivity (Properties 26a,b,c). Figure 11-1 illustrates for our case study near-normal thresholds despite the fact that the otoemissions are very low in amplitude, indicating the existence of substantial scattered OHC damage over the length of the cochlea (LePage and Murray 1993).

In the case where substantial high-frequency hearing loss has already occurred, leading to a sloping audiogram, the pitch of the tinnitus is frequently matched with a pure tone of frequency where pure-tone thresholds have risen by 25 to 30 dB (Meikle 1991b) by which stage otoacoustic emissions will have dropped to non-measurable levels (Kemp 1989). This coincidence suggests that there exists a broadband tinnitus at all frequencies, but the tinnitus is identified perceptually

by an edge effect which normally accompanies band-limited noise. One can speculate that this may be due to the presence of a working region of cells bordered on the basal side by a region of substantial damage.

Pure-tone audiometry shows that left ears preferentially have higher permanent losses than right ears. This is registered using otoacoustic emissions as lower emission strengths (LePage and Murray 1993). This suggests that left ears acquire more permanent damage before right ears (Pirilä, Jounio-Ervasti, and Sorri 1991), so it is also not surprising that left ears show a higher percentage of tinnitus (Property 25). If tinnitus is generally less well-developed in the right ear, it follows that with less damage it will be easier to find masking conditions for the right ear than the left ear (Property 35). On the basis of acquired hearing loss, therefore, one might expect to find more tinnitus in males than females (Property 24).

Difficulty of Obtaining Masking Conditions

Not all tinnitus can be easily masked (Properties 30-33). The conditions required for masking seem largely unpredictable, particularly in respect of the frequency of the masker. The variability of masking conditions may be explained in terms of the baseline regulation model. The more extensive the neighborhood of OHC loss, the higher the level of sound required to mask the tinnitus. For scattered OHC loss, a broadband masker will be more effective. Alternately, for a "punctate" lesion, a pure-tone masker may be more effective, its frequency being any frequency over a wide range which will produce a suppressive displacement (refer again to Figure 11-6A and B).

The fact that there is no upward spread of masking for CHFT (Property 36b) stems from the fact that there is no spatial pattern of excitation extending over several millimeters length of the cochlear partition as occurs with an external tone (Figure 11-6). Lesions causing CHFT can be punctate and limited to just a few OHCs extending along the cochlear partition less than 100 μm (Figure 11-8). Indeed, there is no reason to suppose any given relationship between the loudness of tinnitus and that of an external masking tone (Property 36c); the TM displacement patterns due to both pseudo and real tones will depend on the patterns of OHC damage. The ability to mask with an external sound is strongly linked to the ability of the OHCs remaining in the neighborhood to respond to the external sound, to generate a shift of the TM in the suppression or repolarizing direction (returning to point A in Figure 11-5), rather than in the excitatory direction. In Figure 11-8C, the normal cells adjacent to the damaged cells will be able to generate the required extension to suppress IHC response. Eventually they too may fail, resulting in an increase in size of the lesion, leading to a longer excitatory region and a louder percept (Property 11). If the compromised region is small, masking conditions will be easier to obtain (Properties 31-33). As the OHC damage increases, the ability for the fewer remaining OHCs to raise the TM will be less. In the cases where a whole contiguous patch of OHCs is missing, no masking will be possible (Property 30).

Under some circumstances, masking could depend on just a few remaining OHCs. The task is then to set up stimulus conditions to find at what frequency and level they will be caused to extend. This may not be a simple task because the *place* being stimulated by a particular tone apparently does not depend solely on stimulus frequency. At least at higher sound levels, the *place* also normally depends on the level of the stimulus, due to the motor action of the OHCs. Once very high sound levels are necessary for masking (>100 dB SPL), the excitation pattern varies with functional remapping of frequency to place (LePage 1990; 1992) which will tend to move apically depending on the pattern of the loss (Property 30, 32–34).

Location of Tinnitus

Finding an adequate explanation for central tinnitus has perhaps represented one of the most challenging aspects to our understanding and management (Møller 1984). Individuals who have had the eighth nerve sectioned may still experience debilitating tinnitus. While mechanisms proposed for central origin of tinnitus remain equally valid, the baseline regulation model opens the possibility that even central tinnitus stems originally from cochlear dysfunction. The fact that the sensation appears diffusely located within the head may simply reflect that normal binaural processing operations in the brainstem break down when the inputs from both ears cannot be correlated and their relative phases on the basilar membrane be voluntarily manipulated by turning the head. By induction, phantom neural input from just one ear alone following nerve section may be sufficient for maintenance of central tinnitus.

Variability in Severity

Inherent in tinnitus is the fact that there is no adequate measure of its severity (Properties 8-11), which this condition has in common with constant pain. Variation in the apparent loudness of constant level sounds is generally appreciated as a basic property of how we hear, such as what makes a ticking clock basically inaudible during the day yet "loud" in the quiet of the night. It is currently being modelled in terms of an internal *automatic volume control* mechanism (Lyon 1990) such as is commonly used in hearing aids. Although the idea has been intuitively obvious for a long time, it was not until OHC length changes were observed both *in vitro* (Brownell et al. 1985; Zenner, 1986) and *in vivo* (LePage 1981; 1987; 1989) that a physical parameter could be assigned as a likely parameter controlling cochlear sensitivity. This single fact can account for the absence of any absolute sense of loudness in human hearing. Automatic volume control (AVC) systems are adaptive systems which over a time period adapt the detector to registering small signals above background noise level. Typically the adaptation period may be much longer than the repetition rate of information usable by the detector, similar to the visual system, where dark adaptation typically takes a few minutes.

Tinnitus is paradoxically "loudest" in low ambient background levels (Properties 8, 32, 47, 48). Typically a patient complains of trying to get to sleep at night (Axelsson and Ringdahl 1989) when all is quiet and the daily sounds that normally provide masking are absent. The model provides some insight into why this is so. Because of the partial similarity which exists between real acoustic (Figure 11-6) and pseudo inputs (Figure 11-8) (Properties 3-5, 28) we can *re-utilize* the external tone profile in Figure 11-6B to represent a pseudo-tonal input. Broadband noise generates masking, which will generally have the effect of applying a *net* suppressive bias to the TM, because for any frequency component the excitatory region is much shorter than the suppressive region. Suppose that the kind of pathology depicted in Figure 11-8 gives rise to an excitation pattern such as that shown in Figure 11-6B. We can picture the unmasked displacement pattern as the rear profile. The spatial dependence of firing rates of primary fibers (Figure 11-6C) constitutes a significant input to the brainstem. With increasing background noise, we have a situation of increasing broadband suppression, and the displacement profile of the tectorial membrane descends in the hyperpolarizing direction with the consequent disappearance of the profile below the detection range of the IHCs (front profile, Figure 11-6B). It is clear that the excitatory region is now only represented by the tip of the profile, so that under the higher ambient noise conditions only a small number of afferent fibers carry the phantom input, while under broadband masking the pseudo-input is much less significant (Property 34).

Selective Attention and the "Masking" of External Sounds by Tinnitus

There are some aspects where tinnitus behaves like external sounds (Properties 29–35). Conversely there are some aspects where it does not (Properties 36a–d). To approach an understanding of the masking of tinnitus by external sounds and vice versa, it is first necessary to appreciate the general nature of auditory selection or the voluntary control of improvement of signal-to-noise. All active signal processing systems have a "noise floor". Wegel (1931) recognized that all people have tinnitus to the extent that the internal noise of their ears can be appreciated independently when external noise sources are eliminated, or reduced below the internal noise, for example, in an anechoic chamber. Indeed, these are the conditions sought for pure-tone audiometry (Murray and LePage 1991). A pure-tone audiogram is in reality the result of an experiment in selective attention. It is a measure of how well the auditory system can focus on a pure tone when it is being masked by internal noise only. In a normal ear, the internal noise level is low. It is still an open question whether the reason auditory thresholds rise is because there is an effective rise in the internal noise level. However, in terms of the theory, there is no real conceptual need to distinguish between a loss of hearing sensitivity and a rise in internal noise level. This is because the origin of the "pathological noise" need be nothing more than a drift in the setpoint of the IHCs for some length of the cochlear partition, which can no longer be reset by OHC activity of the kind depicted in Figure 11-6. Both result in a decreased ability to select, or identify, the spatial pattern generated on the basilar membrane due to a pure tone—traditionally designated the *traveling wave envelope*—which gives rise to cochlear tuning.

By virtue of being able to consider tinnitus as an internal signal adding to external noise, it is no surprise therefore that there should be a heavy overlay of selective attention-related issues in the perception of tinnitus (Properties 12, 55–57) which constitute a major complication in dealing with the severity of tinnitus. Selective attention has been the subject of considerable research in the areas of neuroscience (see Näätänen 1990 for a recent review) and cognitive psychology (see Johnston and Dark 1986 and Kinchla 1992 for recent reviews). Researchers in both areas have argued for many years about whether there are mechanisms located at the earliest stages of sensory processing that play a role in attention. This has become known as the *peripheral filtering hypothesis* and was first proposed by Hernandez-Peon in 1966. It proposes that exclusion of irrelevant and/or facilitation of relevant information occurs in the sensory pathway, even at the most peripheral levels, by processes under the control of higher brain centers via centrifugal or efferent fibres. It is clear that the OHC motor unit (LePage 1989) with its efferent innervation has the capacity to modify sensory processing in this way. However, data supporting attentional effects at the level of observations of an effect measured at the round window were subsequently criticized for their lack of important controls, but better controlled animal experiments by Oatman and colleagues (Oatman, 1971, 1976; Oatman and Anderson 1977, 1980) demonstrated suppression of irrelevant auditory information at the level of the cochlea. Repeated attempts to find robust evidence of peripheral effects of attention in humans using brainstem auditory evoked responses, however, have been generally unsuccessful (see Hirschhorn and Michie 1991 for a review). This has led some to assert that attention is mediated and implemented by higher-level brain mechanisms. To date, the earliest replicable effect of attention has been observed on cortical evoked potentials with a latency of approximately 50–60 ms and is presumably mediated by cortical mechanisms (Michie, Crawford, Bearpark, and Glue 1990; Näätänen 1990).

Recently, it has been suggested that OHC-motor units may be selectively implicated in attention tasks (LePage 1989). The pattern of efferent innervation (Figure 11-7; see also Warr 1992) strongly suggests that the machinery exists for the central nervous system to influence cochlear sensitivity globally or selectively, depending upon the variation in tonic firing rates of the medial efferent neurons. For example, a comb-shaped filter could be established to match the spectral peaks of any sound signal deemed important to the listener. The effect of such a selection operation is *hypothesized* to increase the excitation of the IHCs through

shortening of the OHCs (Figure 11-8A) so that the size of the excitatory region for a given input is increased still further. Like the brainstem evoked response results, recent experiments show that the effect of attention on otoacoustic emissions, if any, is very small (Puel, Bonfils, and Pujol 1988; Froehlich, Collet, Chanal, and Morgon 1990; Giard, Bouchet, Collet, and Pernier 1992). The outcome of these experiments may be highly paradigm-dependent and also subject-dependent according to the state of cochlear damage in test subjects not revealed by pure-tone audiometry.

The baseline regulation model also suggests that if the postulated motor-controlled selection process is disabled, the sufferer may not be able to ignore either a virtual input (tinnitus), or indeed a real signal input (hyperacusis?). If the process of masking an input depends upon the ability of OHCs to generate a suppressive displacement, decreasing numbers of functional OHCs would mean a reduction in ability to select. Depending upon how auditory selection is governed centrally, an increase in firing rate may accordingly be deemed a "signal of interest" even if it is only caused by a drift in the setpoint, which is outside the control of the efferent feedback loop.

Trying to actively ignore tinnitus by a variety of schemes—for example, biofeedback (House 1978)—may bring variable results *if the efferent system is only programmed to focus* by shortening of selected OHC motor units (Figure 11-8B) (Properties 55–57), that is, if the efferent activity only works in one direction which is not the direction needed to mask the tinnitus (Figure 11-8C). That is, trying to ignore tinnitus, *with effort*, may be rather akin to trying to sleep in a hurry. Mental effort plus an absence of distractions thus serves to focus subject attention on the offending input. One suspects it is not even possible to actively focus attention on something else; because the act of focusing establishes an internal program of arbitrary cycle time of attention-switching between the thing being ignored and its replacement.

Likewise in an experiment to test the relative effectiveness of a broadband masker on tinnitus, or on an external tone, the masker might be predicted to have less effect on the external tone, by virtue that it is possible to focus on the tone (or any coherent input), which is inherently more difficult with a broadband tinnitus (Property 36a).

Relaxation techniques (e.g., Tyler et al. 1992) are therefore more likely to be of benefit clinically, while methods aimed at masking (acoustic or electrical) depend on there remaining sufficient numbers of OHCs in the neighborhood of the lesion capable of raising the TM away from the IHCSC. Pure-tone masking should work well for punctate lesions, while broadband masking will be predictably better for scattered OHC loss.

In the model, if efferent action is unidirectional, a phantom input cannot actually "mask" an external sound, because masking requires generation of a suppressive displacement (TM towards SV) and such masking is not possible at places where OHC loss is complete. In this sense a pseudo-input interferes with external sound reception only in the sense that the internal noise level has risen, requiring external sounds to be higher in level than the maximum voluntary selective improvement normally achievable (*ca.* 10 dB), accounting for the limit to such "pseudo-masking" (Property 27). Since "true" masking is produced only by OHC elongation in response to external tones, masking of external tones is merely a manifestation of a spastic patch of OHCs.

SUMMARY AND CONCLUSIONS

Perhaps the most significant obstacle to progress in tinnitus research has been the lack of a sufficiently tangible and testable model for its origin. The model proposed here for continuous subjective tinnitus is not new, but is an elaboration of a "homeostatic" mechanism for cochlear tinnitus proposed by Stephens and Davis (1938:1983), Davis (1954), and furthered by Tonndorf (1981). Accordingly, this chapter presents the results of an experiment to investigate how many of the salient properties of tinnitus have a potential explanation in the morphology of the organ of Corti, and in

particular, speculations concerning the function of the slow activity of the OHCs. In terms of this theory, phantom acoustic input to the central nervous system is the natural consequence of degradation of OHC activity or an alternate disturbance to a passive mechanical structure such as the spiral ligament. The form of this degradation is essentially loss of OHC control of regulation, resulting in collapse, or static distortion, of the structure, to be contrasted with the more popular notion of a mechanical oscillation. If the resulting position shift is localized it may resemble the triphasic displacement pattern of IHC excitation in response to a pure tone, and thus be regarded by the brain as a real input having the appropriate properties such as no associated spontaneous emissions, no beats with external tones, and no perceived harmonic structure. This hypothesis hinges critically upon the primary afferent synapses at the base of the IHC being essentially non-adapting (Kiang et al. 1965, pp. 73–79.). Apart from refractory effects in neural excitation (Gaumond, Molnar, and Kim 1982), adaptation seen in primary afferent fibers (Kiang et al. 1965) is presumed to be due exclusively to OHC electromechanical adaptation (LePage et al. 1993b).

If, in the vicinity of any damaged region, there are still OHCs with normal functionality, hearing loss may not be manifest at all and masking of the tinnitus will also be possible. This is due to OHC elongation that raises the tectorial membrane and reduces the deflection of the IHC stereocilia. Hence, the model offers the possibility that the incidence of tinnitus and hearing loss not being directly related, while each is directly relatable to the extent of damage to the cochlear partition. When the damage becomes more extensive, it will become increasingly difficult to mask the tinnitus, because there will be fewer OHCs remaining to generate suppressive displacements of the tectorial membrane. Hence, within the framework of OHC motility, it is possible to describe subjective tinnitus of cochlear origin in fairly general terms using a single parameter—steady deflection of the IHC stereocilia—and less generally in terms of tectorial membrane displacement toward scala tympani offering a direct explanation of the roaring tinnitus in Ménière's syndrome. The transient spontaneous tinnitus (TST) described by the author, by virtue of its harmonic content, suggests the existence of a mechanical oscillation that should be detectable as an ear emission if any such event could be captured. More generally, recovery from TST supports the notion that the basilar membrane is maintained in a "conditionally stable" state and that the OHC length is regulated until any parasitic oscillation is just damped out.

Tinnitus can occur at any pitch corresponding to a site of OHC degradation leading to a shift in the direction of IHC excitation. However, when investigators talk of high pitch and low pitch, what they mean and what any sufferer may mean may be quite different because of the different sense in which the term "pitch" is used. The variety of forms of damage range from punctate lesions leading to percepts mimicking pure tones, to damage over a length of the cochlear partition leading to a wideband hiss. In the case of punctate lesions, the "masking" which they perform on real signals will not have any spread. In terms of the model such "pseudo-masking" is not true masking which requires OHC elongation.

Like pain, the severity of tinnitus appears to have a significant attentional component leading to the wide diversity of outcomes of reported investigations. It is observed that the mammalian cochlea receives innervation which theoretically may assist in the selection process at the mechanical level. However, it is known that the process is important in selecting very low level sounds from background noise and that when this selection process becomes disabled, subjects have difficulty in listening as distinct from hearing. Tinnitus may be regarded as an increase in the internal noise of the ear, which, like auditory deficits, becomes clinically significant when the sufferer can no longer select any external signal. This condition is hypothesized to arise when the range of tectorial membrane baseline regulation decreases to the extent that the OHCs cannot generate elongatory

displacements to hyperpolarize the IHCs for frequencies not present in the external signal. On the other hand, by attending to the tinnitus, the brain invokes a motor program which is hypothesized to increase the contrast in the region of the tinnitus relative to the surrounding region. The motor program is hypothesized to work to shorten the OHCs in the region, which has the effect of spreading the excitation region and stimulating a larger number of IHCs. If such a program could be demonstrated in physiological experiment it would go a long way to explaining the "uncertainty principle" which tends to interfere with experiments on tinnitus, and even with individual responses to questionnaires. The act of thinking about the symptoms, for example, How loud is the tinnitus?, modifies the outcome of the experiment.

A model has been presented which establishes a framework for further physiological investigation and at the same time establishes a basis for establishing a stronger understanding of the origins of hearing loss and tinnitus. Many features of tinnitus have a potential explanation in terms of accumulated damage to the motor cells in the cochlea.

The author thanks N. Murray, P.T. Michie, and J. Macrae for helpful comments on the text, particularly to P.T. Michie for contributions to the section on selective attention.

LIST OF ABBREVIATIONS

AVC	Automatic Volume Control
AZ	Arctuate Zone
BM	Basilar Membrane
CF	Characteristic Frequency (for a given location)
CHFT	Continuous High-Frequency Tinnitus
CLFT	Continuous Low-Frequency Tinnitus
CT	Continuous Tinnitus
DC	Deiter Cell
DCP	Deiter Cell (diagonal) Process
HC	Hensen Cells
IHC	Inner Hair Cell

IHCSC   Inner Hair Cell Stereocilia

IPi   Inner Pillar

MN   Marginal Net

MR   Reissner's Membrane

OHC   Outer Hair Cell

OHCSC   Outer Hair Cell Stereocilia

OP   Operating (set) point

OPi   Outer Pillar

PZ   Pectinate Zone

RI   Residual Inhibition

RM   Reticular Membrane

SL   Spiral Lamina

SLg   Spiral Ligament

SM   Scala Media

SNR   Signal-to-Noise Ratio

SPL   Sound Pressure Level

ST   Scala Tympani

SV   Scala Vestibuli

THFST   Transient High-Frequency Spontaneous Tinnitus

TM   Tectorial Membrane

TMF   Tectorial Membrane Fiber

TST   Transient Spontaneous Tinnitus

REFERENCES

Aran, J.-M. 1981. "Electrical Stimulation of the Auditory System and Tinnitus Control." In A. Shulman (chrmn), *Tinnitus. Proceedings of the First International Tinnitus Seminar. Journal of Laryngology and Otology, Supplement 4*, 153–163.

Ashmore J.F. 1987. "A Fast Motile Response in Guinea-Pig Outer Hair Cells: The Cellular Basis of the Cochlear Amplifier." *Journal of Physiology, 388*, 323–347.

Axelsson, A. and Barrenäs, M.-L. 1992. "Tinnitus in Noise-Induced Hearing Loss." In A. Dancer, D. Henderson, R.J. Salvi, and R.P. Hamernik (Eds.), *The Effects of Noise on the Auditory System*, pp. 269–276. Toronto: B.C. Decker.

Axelsson, A. and Ringdahl, A. 1989. "Tinnitus—A Study of its Prevalence and Characteristics." *British Journal of Audiology, 23*, 53–62.

Bailey, Q. 1979. "Audiological Aspects of Tinnitus." *Australian Journal of Audiology, 1*, 19–23.

Békésy, G. von. 1960. *Experiments in Hearing.* New York: McGraw-Hill.

Bohne, B.A., Yohman, L. and Gruner, M.M. 1987. "Cochlear Damage following Interrupted Exposure to High-frequency Noise." *Hearing Research, 29*, 251–264.

British Tinnitus Association, 14-18 West Bar Green, Sheffield S1 2DA, England.

Brownell, W.E., Bader, C.R., Bertrand, D., and de Ribaupierre, Y. 1985. "Evoked Mechanical Responses of Isolated Cochlear Hair Cells." *Science, 227*, 194–195.

Brownell, W.E. and Shehata, W.E. 1990. "The Effect of Cytoplasmic Turgor Pressure on the Static and Dynamic Mechanical Properties of Outer Hair Cells." In P. Dallos, C.D. Geisler, J.W. Matthews, M.A. Ruggero, and C.R. Steele (Eds.), *The mechanics and biophysics of hearing. Lecture notes in biomathematics*, pp. 52–59. New York: Springer-Verlag.

Brundin, L. Flock, Å. and Canlon, B. 1989. "Sound-induced Motility of Isolated Cochlear Outer Cell is Frequency Specific." *Nature, 342*, 814–816.

Brundin, L., Flock, B., and Flock, Å. 1992. "Sound Induced Displacement Response of the Guinea Pig Hearing Organ and Its Relation to the Cochlear Potentials." *Hearing Research, 58*, 175—184.

Brundin, L., Flock, Å., Khanna, S.M., and Ulfendahl, M. 1991. "Frequency-specific Position Shift in the Guinea Pig Organ of Corti." *Neuroscience Letters, 128*, 77–80.

Burns, E.M. 1984. "A Comparison of Variability Among Measurements of Subjective Tinnitus and Objective Stimuli." *Audiology, 23*, 426—440.

Canlon, B. 1987. "Acoustic Overstimulation Alters the Morphology of the Tectorial Membrane." *Hearing Research, 30*, 127–134.

Canlon, B., Brundin L., and Flock, Å. 1988. "Acoustic Stimulation Causes Tonotopic Alterations in the Length of Isolated Outer Hair Cells from the Guinea Pig Hearing Organ." *Proceedings of the National Academy of Science, USA, 85*, 7033–7035.

Canlon, B., Miller, J., Flock, Å., and Borg, E. 1987. "Pure Tone Overstimulation Changes the Micromechanical Properties of the Inner Hair Cell Stereocilia." *Hearing Research. 30*, 65–72.

Chung, D.Y., Gannon, R.P., and Mason, K. 1984. "Factors Affecting the Prevalence of Tinnitus." *Audiology, 23,* 441–452.

Coles, R.R.A., David, A.C. and Haggard, M.P. 1981. "Epidemiology of Tinnitus." *Ciba Foundation Symposium, 85,* 16–34.

Cooper, N.P. and Rhode, W.S. 1992. "Basilar Membrane Mechanics in the Hook Region of Cat and Guinea-Pig Cochleae: Sharp Tuning and Nonlinear in the Absence of Baseline Position Shifts." *Hearing Research, 63,* 163–190.

Crane, H.D. 1982. "IHC-TM Connect-disconnect and Efferent Control." *Journal of the Acoustical Society of America, 72,* 93–101.

Davis, H. 1954. "Tinnitus—Physiological Aspects." *Transcript of the American Academy of Ophthamology and Otology, 58,* 527–528.

Davis, H. 1983. "An Active Process in Cochlear Mechanics." *Hearing Research, 9,* 79–90.

Day, R.O., Graham, G.G., Bieri, D., Brown, M., Cairns D., Harris, G., Hounsell, J., Platt-Hepworth, S., Reeve, R., Sambrook, P.N., and Smith, J. 1989. "Concentration-response Relationships for Salicylate-induced Ototoxicity in Normal Volunteers." *British Journal of Clinical Pharmacology, 28,* 695–702.

Engstrom, H., Ades, H.W., and Bredberg, G. 1970. "Normal Structure of the Organ of Corti and the Effect of Noise-induced Cochlear Damage." In G.E.W. Wolstenhome and J. Knight (Eds.), *Sensorineural hearing loss,* pp. 127–156. Baltimore: Williams and Wilkins.

Evans, B.N. 1990. "Fatal Contractions: Ultrastructural and Electromechanical Changes in Outer Hair Cells following Transmembranous Electrical Stimulation." *Hearing Research, 45,* 265–282.

Evans, B.N., Hallworth, R., and Dallos, P. 1991. "Outer Hair Cell Electromotility: The Sensitivity and Vulnerability of the DC Component." *Hearing Research, 52,* 288–304.

Farmer, J.C. 1977. "Diving Injuries to the Inner Ear." *Annals of Otology, Rhinology, and Laryngology, (Suppl.), 86*(1 Pt.3), 1–20.

Fowler, E.P. 1944. "Head Noises in Normal and Disordered Ears." *Archives of Otolaryngology, 39,* 498–503.

Froehlich, P., Collet, L., Chanal, J.-M., and Morgon, A. 1990. "Variability of the Influence of a Visual Task on the Active Micromechanical Properties of the Cochlea." *Brain Research, 508,* 286–288.

Gaumond, R.P., Molnar, C.E., and Kim, D.O. 1982. "Stimulus and Recovery Dependence of Cat Cochlear Nerve Fiber Spike Discharge Probability." *Journal of Neurophysiology, 48,* 856–873.

Geisler, C.D., Rhode, W.S., and Kennedy, D.T. 1974. "The Responses to Tonal Stimuli of Single Auditory Nerve Fibers and Their Relationships to Basilar Membrane Motion in the Squirrel Monkey." *Journal of Neurophysiology, 37,* 1156–1172.

Giard, M.-H., Bouchet, P., Collet, L., and Pernier, J. 1992. "Auditory Selective Attention at the Cochlear Level." Presented at the 5th International Conference on Cognitive Neurosciences (ICON V), Jerusalem, Israel, June 14–19, 1992.

Gold, T. 1948. "Hearing II. The Physical Basis of the Action of the Cochlea." *Proceedings of the Royal Society of London, B: 135,* 492–498.

Harding, G.W., Baggot, P.J., and Bohne, B.A. 1992. "Height Changes in the Organ of Corti after Noise Exposure." *Hearing Research, 63,* 26–36.

Harris, S., Brismar, J., and Cronqvist, S. 1979. "Pulsatile Tinnitus and Therapeutic Embolization." *Acta Otolaryngologica, 88,* 220–226.

Hazell, J.W.P. 1979a. "Tinnitus." *British Journal of Hospital Medicine, 22,* 468–471.

Hazell, J.W.P. 1979b. "Tinnitus Research. The Current Position." *Hearing, 34*(1), 10–15 (reprinted as RNID pamphlet).

Hazell, J.W.P. 1979c. "A Tinnitus Synthesiser. Physiological Considerations." *Proceedings of the First International Tinnitus Seminar,* New York, 8 June 1979.

Hazell, J.W.P. 1981. "Patterns of Tinnitus: Medical Audiologic Findings." *Journal of Laryngology, Otology, Supplement 4,* 39–47.

Hazell, J.W.P., Williams, G.R., and Sheldrake, J.B. 1979. "Tinnitus Maskers - Success and Failures. A Report on the State of the Art." *Proceedings of the First International Tinnitus Seminar,* New York, 8 June 1979.

Helmholtz. 1875:1954. *On the sensations of tone.* New York: Dover.

Hernandez-Peon, R. 1966. "Physiological mechanisms in attention." In R.W. Russell (Ed.), *Frontiers in Physiological Psychology,* New York: Academic Press.

Hirschhorn, T.N. and Michie, P.T. 1990. "Brainstem Auditory Evoked Potentials (BAEPs) and Selective Attention Revisited." *Psychophysiology, 27,* 495–512.

Holley M.C. and Ashmore, J.F. 1990. "Spectrin, Actin and the Structure of the Cortical Lattice in Mammalian Cochlear Outer Hair Cells." *Journal of Cellular Science, 96,* 283–291.

House, J.W. 1978. "Treatment of Severe Tinnitus with Biofeedback Training." *Laryngoscope, 88,* 406–412.

Iwasa, K.H., Minxu, Li, M.J., and Kachard, B. 1991. "Stretch Sensitivity of the Lateral Wall of the Auditory Outer Hair Cell from the Guinea Pig." *Neuroscience Letters, 133,* 171–174.

Jastreboff, P.J. 1990. "Phantom Auditory Perception (Tinnitus): Mechanisms of Generation and Perception." *Neuroscience Research, 8,* 221–254.

Jastreboff, P.J., Brennan, J.F., Coleman, J.K., and Sasaki, C.T. 1988. "Phantom Auditory Sensation in Rats: An Animal Model for Tinnitus." *Behavioral Neuroscience, 102,* 811–822.

Johnston, W.A. and Dark, V.J. 1986. "Selective Attention." *Annual Review of Psychology, 37,* 43–75.

Kachar, B., Kalinek, F., Iwasa, K., Holley, M., and Lim, D. 1991. "A Novel Membrane-based Mechanism for High Frequency Shape Changes in Outer Hair Cells." Presented at the 28th Workshop on Inner Ear Biology, Tübingen, Sept. 8–11.

Kemp, D.T. 1989. "Otoacoustic Emissions: Basic Facts and Applications." *Audiology in Practice,* 6/3. Amsterdam: Excerpta Medica Medical Communications BV.

Kiang, N.Y.-S., Watanabe, T., Thomas, E.C., and Clarke, L.F. 1965. *Discharge Patterns of Single Fibres in the Cat's Auditory Nerve.* Cambridge, MA: MIT Press.

Kim, D.O. 1984. "Functional Roles of the Inner- and Outer-Hair-Cell Subsystems in the Cochlea and Brainstem." In C.I. Berlin (Ed.), *Hearing Science: Recent Advances,* pp. 241–262. San Diego, CA: College-Hill Press.

Kinchla, R.A. 1992. "Attention." *Annual Review of Psychology, 43,* 711–742.

Konishi, T. and Salt, A.N. 1983. "Electrochemical Profile for Potassium Ions across the Cochlear Hair Cell Membranes of Normal and Noise-exposed Guinea Pigs." *Hearing Research, 11,* 219–234.

LePage, E.L. 1981. *The Role of Nonlinear Mechanical Processes in Mammalian Hearing.* Ph.D. Thesis. The University of Western Australia.

LePage, E.L. 1987. "Frequency-dependent Self-induced Bias of the Basilar Membrane and Its Potential for Controlling Sensitivity and Tuning in the Mammalian Cochlea." *Journal of the Acoustical Society of America, 82,*139–154.

LePage, E.L. 1989. "Functional Role of the Olivocochlear Bundle: A Motor Unit Control System in the Mammalian Cochlea." *Hearing Research, 38,* 177–198.

LePage, E.L. 1990. "Helmholtz Revisited: Direct Mechanical Data Suggest a Physical Model for Dynamic Control of Mapping Frequency to Place along the Cochlear Partition." In P. Dallos, C.D. Geisler, J.W. Matthews, M.A. Ruggero and C.R. Steele (Eds.), *The Mechanics and Biophysics of Hearing,* pp. 278–287. *Lecture Notes in Biomathematics,* New York: Springer-Verlag.

LePage, E.L. 1991. "Hysteresis in Cochlear Mechanics and a Model for Variability in Noise-induced Hearing Loss." In A. Dancer, D. Henderson, R.J. Salvi, and R.P. Hamernik (Eds.), *The Effects of Noise on the Auditory System,* pp. 106–115. Toronto: B.C. Decker.

LePage, E.L. 1992. "Models of Subjective and Objective Tinnitus based on Outer Hair Cell Turgor." In J.-M. Aran and R. Dauman (Eds.), *Proceedings of the Fourth International Tinnitus Seminar,* pp. 73–78. Amsterdam: Kugler Press.

LePage, E.L. 1993. In preparation.

LePage, E.L. and Murray, N.M. 1993. In preparation.

LePage, E.L., Reuter, G., and Zenner, H.P. 1993a. "Summating Baseline Shifts and Mechanical Adaptation in a Guinea Pig Cochlear Explant Shown with Two Displacement Measuring Techniques" (Under revision).

LePage, E.L., Reuter, G. and Zenner, H.P. 1993b. "Threshold for Mechanical Response of Isolated Outer Hair Cells" (Under revision).

Liberman, M.C. 1989. "Rapid Assessment of Sound-evoked Olivocochlear Feedback: Suppression of Compound Action Potentials by Contralateral Sound." *Hearing Research, 38,* 47–56..

Lim, D.J. 1986. "Functional Structure of the Organ of Corti: A Review." *Hearing Research, 22,* 117–146.

Loeb, M. and Smith, R.P. 1967. "Relation of Induced Tinnitus to Physical Characteristics of the Inducing Stimuli." *Journal of the Acoustical Society of America, 42,* 453–455.

Lyon, R.F. 1990. "Automatic Gain Control in Cochlear Mechanics." In *The Mechanics and Biophysics of Hearing,* pp. 395–402. *Lecture notes in biomathematics.* New York: Springer-Verlag.

Man, A. and Naggan, L. 1981. "Characteristics of Tinnitus in Acoustic Trauma." *Audiology, 20,* 72–78.

Meikle, M. 1991a. "The Onset of Tinnitus: Causal and Precipitating Factors." In *Proceedings of the 3rd Bi-Annual Workshop, Tinnitus - Assessment and Re-Habilitation,* pp. 1–3. Melbourne, Australia, 15–17 March 1991.

Meikle, M. 1991b. "How Tinnitus is Related to Hearing Impairment." In *Proceedings of the 3rd Bi-Annual Workshop, Tinnitus - Assessment and Re-Habilitation,* pp. 4–6. Melbourne, Australia, 15–17 March 1991.

Meikle, M. 1991c. "The Issue of Severity: Evaluating the Severity of Tinnitus." In *Proceedings of the 3rd Bi-Annual Workshop, Tinnitus - Assessment and Re-Habilitation,* pp. 7–9. Melbourne, Australia, 15–17 March 1991.

Meikle, M., Griest, S.E., Press, L., and Stewart, B.J. 1991. "Relationships between Tinnitus and Audiometric Variables in a Large Sample of Tinnitus Clinic Patients." In J.-M. Aran and R. Dauman (Eds.), *Proceedings of the Fourth International Tinnitus Seminar,* Amsterdam: Kugler Press.

Meikle, M. and Taylor-Walsh, E. 1984. "Characteristics of Tinnitus and Related Observation in over 1800 Tinnitus Patients." *Journal of Laryngology and Otology, Supplement, 9,* 17–21.

Michie, P.T., Crawford, J.M., Bearpark, H.M., and Glue, L.C. 1990. "The Nature of Selective Attention Effects on Auditory Event-related Potentials." *Biological Psychology, 30,* 219–250.

Møller, A.R. 1984. "Pathophysiology of Tinnitus." *Annals of Otology, Rhinology, and Laryngology, 93,* 39–44.

Murray, N.M. and LePage, E.L. 1990. "Otoacoustic Emissions—Sounds Coming out of the Ear." *Australian Hearing and Deafness Review, 7,* 10–14.

Murray, N.M. and LePage, E.L. 1991. "Estimated Maximum Acceptable Background Noise Levels for Audiometric Testing with Sound-excluding Earphone Enclosures—An Update." *Australian Journal of Audiology, 13,* 47–52.

Näätänen, R. 1990. "The Role of Attention in Auditory Information Processing as Revealed by Event-related Potentials and Other Brain Measures of Cognitive Function." *Behavioral and Brain Sciences, 13,* 201–288.

Neely, S.T. and Kim, D.O. 1983. "An Active Cochlear Model Showing Sharp Tuning and High Sensitivity." *Hearing Research, 9,* 123–130.

Nodar, R.H. and Graham, J.T. 1965. "An Investigation of Frequency Characteristics of Tinnitus Associated with Méniere's Disease." *Archives of Otolaryngology, 82,* 28–31.

Oatman, L.C. 1971. "Role of Visual Attention on Auditory Evoked Potentials in Unanesthetized Cats." *Experimental Neurology, 32,* 341–356.

Oatman, L.C. 1976. "Effects of Visual Attention on the Intensity of Auditory Evoked Potentials." *Experimental Neurology, 51,* 41–53.

Oatman, L.C. and Anderson, B.W. 1977. "Effects of Visual Attention on Tone Burst Evoked Auditory Potentials." *Experimental Neurology, 57,* 200–211.

Oatman, L.C. and Anderson, B.W. 1980. "Suppression of the Auditory Frequency Following Response during Visual Attention." *Electroencephalography and Clinical Neurophysiology, 49,* 314–321.

Patuzzi, R., Sellick, P.M., and Johnstone, B.M. 1984. "The Modulation of the Sensitivity of the Mammalian Cochlea by Low Frequency Tones. I. Primary Afferent Activity." *Hearing Research, 13,* 1–9.

Penner, M.J. 1983. "Variability in Matches to Subjective Tinnitus." *Journal of Speech and Hearing Research, 26,* 263–267.

Penner, M.J. 1992. "Linking Spontaneous Otoacoustic Emissions and Tinnitus." *British Journal of Audiology, 26,* 115–123.

Plinkert, P.K., Gitter, A.H., and Zenner, H.P. 1990. "Tinnitus Associated with Spontaneous Otoacoustic Emissions. Active Outer Hair Cell Movements as Common Origin." *Acta Otolaryngologica (Stockholm), 110,* 342–347.

Pirilä, T., Jounio-Ervasti, K., and Sorri, M. 1991. "Hearing Asymmetry among Left-handed and Right-handed Persons in a Random Population." *Scandinavian Audiology, 20,* 223–226.

Portmann, M., Cazals, Y., Negrevergne, M., and Aran, J.-M., 1979. "Temporary Tinnitus Suppression in Man through Electrical Stimulation of the Cochlea." *Acta Otolaryngologica, 87,* 294–299.

Puel, J.-L., Bonfils, P., and Pujol, R. 1988. "Selective Attention Modifies the Active Micromechanical Properties of the Cochlea." *Brain Research, 447,* 380–383.

Reed, G.F. 1960. "An Audiometric Study of Two Hundred Cases of Subjective Tinnitus." *Archives of Otolaryngology, 71,* 95–104.

Saunders, J.C., Canlon, B., and Flock, Å. 1986. "Changes in Stereocilia Micromechanics Following

Overstimulation in Metabolically Blocked Hair Cells." *Hearing Research, 24,* 217–226.

Sellick, P.M., Patuzzi, R.B., and Johnstone, B.M. 1982. "Measurement of Basilar Membrane Motion in the Guinea Pig Using the Mössbauer Technique." *Journal of the Acoustical Society of America, 72,* 131–141.

Shulman, A., Goldstein, B.A., and Bhathal, B. 1992. "Spontaneous Evoked Otoacoustic Emissions and Tinnitus—Its Correlation/Uncorrelation with Specific Clinical Types of Tinnitus." In J.-M. Aran and R. Dauman (Eds.), *Proceedings of the Fourth International Tinnitus Seminar,* pp. 95–102. Amsterdam: Kugler Press.

Siegel, W. 1976. "The Paradox of Pitch Categories." *Journal of the Acoustical Society of America, 60,* S6.

Spoendlin, H. 1970. "Structural Basis of Peripheral Frequency Analysis." In R. Plomp and G. F. Smoorenburg (Eds.), *Frequency Analysis and Periodicity Detection in Hearing,* pp. 2–40. Leiden: Sijthoff.

Stephens, S.S. and Davis, H. 1938:1983. *Hearing—Its Psychology and Physiology,* pp. 351–352. New York: The American Institute of Physics, Inc.

Thorne, P.R., Duncan, C.E., and Gavin, J.B. 1986. "The Pathogenesis of Stereocilia Abnormalities in Acoustic Trauma." *Hearing Research, 21,* 41–50.

Tonkin, J.P. and Fagan, P. 1975. "Rupture of the Round Window Membrane." *Journal of Laryngology and Otology, 89*(7), 733–756.

Tonndorf, J. 1981. "Stereociliary Dysfunction, a Cause of Sensory Hearing Loss, Recruitment, Poor Speech Discrimination and Tinnitus." *Acta Otolaryngologica, 91,* 469–479.

Tyler, R.S., Aran, J.-M., and Dauman, R. 1992. "Recent Advances in Tinnitus." *American Journal of Audiology, 1/4,* November, 36–44.

Vernon, J. 1991. "Testing and Evaluation of Tinnitus." In *Proceedings of the 3rd Bi-Annual Workshop,*

Tinnitus—Assessment and Re-Habilitation, pp. 10–15. Melbourne, Australia, 15–17 March 1991.

Vernon, J., Johnson, R., Schleuning, A., and Mitchell, C. 1980. "Masking and Tinnitus." *Ear and Hearing, 1,* 5–9.

Vernon, J. and Schleuning, A. 1978. "Tinnitus: A New Management." *Laryngoscope, 88,* 413–419.

Vernon, J., Schleuning, A., Odell, L. and Hughes, F. 1978. "A Tinnitus Clinic." *Ear, Nose and Throat Journal, April,* 58–71.

Voldřich, L. and Úlehlová, L. 1982. "The Role of the Spiral Ligament in Cochlear Mechanics." *Acta Otolaryngologica, 93,* 169–173.

Voldřich, L. and Úlehlová, L. 1987. "Cochlear Micromechanics." *Acta Otolaryngologica, 103,* 661–664.

Warr, W.B. 1992. "Organisation of Olivocochlear Efferent Systems in Mammals." In *Mammalian Auditory Physiology: Neuroanatomy,* pp. 410–448. Springer Handbook of Auditory Research.

Wegel, R.L. 1931. "A study of tinnitus." *Archives of Otolaryngology, 14,* 158–165.

Wilson, S. 1979. "Mystery of People Who Hear the Hum." *New Scientist,* 13th December, 868–870.

Zenner, H.P. 1986. "Motile Responses in Outer Hair Cells." *Hearing Research, 22,* 83–90.

Zenner, H.P., Zimmermann, U., and Schmitt, U. 1985. "Reversible Contraction of Isolated Mammalian Cochlear Hair Cells." *Hearing Research, 18,* 127–133.

Zenner, H.P., Zimmermann U., and Gitter, A.H. 1987. "Fast Motility of Isolated Mammalian Auditory Sensory Cells." *Biochem.Biophys.Res.Comm., 149,* 304–308.

Zwicker, E. 1977. "Masker Period Patterns Produced by Very-low-frequency Maskers and Their Possible Relation to Basilar Membrane Displacement." *Journal of the Acoustical Society of America, 61,* 1031–1040.

A CONVERSATION ABOUT TINNITUS

ROBERT A. LEVINE
Research Associate in Otolaryngology,
Massachusetts Eye and Ear Infirmary

NELSON Y.S. KIANG
Director, Eaton-Peabody Laboratory,
Massachusetts Eye and Ear Infirmary

K: Let us first explain what we will try to do in this conversation. As a practicing otoneurologist, you regularly see tinnitus patients, while as an auditory physiologist, I consider tinnitus to be one of the most challenging intellectual puzzles in understanding hearing. Here we explore our respective ideas on this subject, given the perspectives inherent in our different professional roles, and suggest some approaches for future research.

L: I want to emphasize that we do not do research on tinnitus per se, so aside from some clinical observations and a few odd physiological facts, we can contribute little in the way of new data. We also do not claim that our ideas are necessarily original . . . they do represent our present views.

K: The 1982 National Academy Press volume on *Tinnitus, Facts, Theories and Treatments* put together by Working Group 89 of the Committee on Hearing, Bioacoustics and Biomechanics provides a balanced yet critical assessment of the field which is remarkably current even after more than a decade of increased public awareness (McFadden 1982). The plethora of current ideas on tinnitus is reflected in recent books (e.g., Aran and Dauman 1992; Shulman 1991). There are even some who believe that tinnitus has been "marketed" as a health concern, perhaps more than it should be.

L: For our present purposes we should agree on a definition of tinnitus. Tinnitus is the perception of "primitive" sounds in the absence of external acoustic stimuli. With this definition, we exclude auditory hallucinations such as intelligible voices, but include sounds that could be generated by the body itself, such as sounds relating to blood flow, breathing, middle-ear muscle spasms, opening or closing of the Eustachian tube, and the like. We will concentrate on non-acoustically generated tinnitus, although an exact distinction in some cases could be obscured by a lack of sensitivity in our acoustic detection devices.

K: It should always be emphasized that tinnitus is a symptom, not a disease. There are many ways to produce tinnitus and it is unlikely that a single type of treatment will eradicate all forms of tinnitus. How many tinnitus patients have you seen in the recent past?

L: Perhaps 500 during the past five years. I see anywhere from two to four new patients a week, mostly referred by otolaryngologists.

K: Is tinnitus the presenting symptom for most of these patients?

L: By and large it is their most prominent complaint.

K: What do you generally do with those patients?

L: I take a careful history and perform a physical examination, after which we discuss the etiology and possible attempts at alleviating the symptom. Overall, less than 10 percent have a clear diagnosis (such as Ménière's syndrome, acoustic neuroma, head trauma, medication usage, or acoustic trauma). Because we usually cannot identify an etiology that is treatable, treatment is generally directed toward management of the symptom.

K: Do you do any psychological workup on these patients?

L: In my own evaluation, I try to fathom what major stresses are present in the lives of these patients, assess their anxiety levels, and decide whether they are depressed. Occasionally, I will refer the patient to a consultant for a formal psychiatric evaluation.

K: Is the onset of tinnitus usually difficult to pinpoint in time?

L: Most tend to define the onset within a fairly restricted period of time, such as days or weeks. They begin to notice it at some point, but often can't be specific as to exactly when or where it was first identified. A few can pinpoint the moment because of traumatic exposure to a loud sound such as an explosion.

K: How many of these are acute cases, instead of those who wait for years before they finally decide to come and see you?

L: Most are recent, although many have seen other physicians early on and come to me for another opinion.

K: What do you do for most of these patients? Is response to treatment part of the diagnosis?

L: In general, the patients I see with tinnitus can be distinguished according to their degree of distress related to the tinnitus. At one extreme is the distressed patient for whom the tinnitus is nearly a total preoccupation; at the other end of the spectrum are those who show little distress but are concerned about the significance of this new symptom. My approach is to try to assess whether the patient's response to the tinnitus is at a distressing level. Many patients mainly want to know the significance of the symptom; they often need only to be reassured about the benign nature of the tinnitus. I spend a lot of time going over the fact that my evaluation has revealed no serious medical condition that is causing the tinnitus. Furthermore, I try to put into perspective the fact that tinnitus is a very common symptom that can take different forms. I myself have it, and like most people with this symptom, we acknowledge the presence of the symptom, but otherwise it is of little consequence to our lives and well-being.

For many, the tinnitus is only troublesome during certain situations, such as when they are trying to sleep, or in the evening when they're trying to relax and unwind by reading or watching television. I offer them my own approach to the problem, which usually begins with using simple acoustic maskers (such as a cassette tape of environmental sounds or a noise generator) to suppress the perception of their tinnitus. Masking is harmless and gives patients a feeling that they have some control over their tinnitus.

K: Would you say that there is some sort of residual masking lasting at least a few seconds or so, so that even if the masking sounds are only intermittent, there would be no tinnitus?

L: Clinically, I've never seen anyone who says, "I've put this noise on and then for a several minutes I'm OK." So-called "residual inhibition" does not appear to be important, at least for my patients.

K: How do you decide whether to try medication? Is it after you have tried masking and it doesn't work?

L: No. At the same session when we discuss the coupling between people's level of stress and the distress that they feel from their tinnitus, I usually acknowledge that we are not very good at treating tinnitus per se, but that we have a fair amount of experience in dealing with the stress. Then we talk about different ways of managing stress. This can include social-psychological techniques, such as biofeedback, hypnosis, meditation, cognitive therapy, or various forms of counseling. Any of these techniques can sometimes help to bring the stress level down in a particular individual. I have referred some patients to a psychologist who specializes in biofeedback, but he actually takes a more global view and tries to tailor the psychological approach to what he perceives as the needs of each individual. My overall impression is that he does quite well with many of these people. Medications for anxiety may work well acutely, but in many they do not have any sustained benefit for the long term. If the patient is clearly depressed, I use antidepressant medications (Sullivan, Dobie, Sakai, and Katon 1989). Many of them have a sleep disturbance, as well, and that can be directly addressed. For the sleep disturbance, I usually use tricyclic antidepressants. They are effective and safe medications for sleep, and since sleep disturbance may be a manifestation of depression, at the same time the depression is being treated as well. In any case, I use this as the first stage in treatment of a sleep disorder to break the vicious cycle between the sleeping difficulty and distress of the tinnitus.

K: Do you find when you give antidepressants that the patients adapt to them? Do you have to use increasingly large doses?

L: No. Unlike medications for anxiety, there does not appear to be a tolerance effect for the antidepressants. I usually start on a low dose and then build it up, but once I find the correct dose I usually don't have to adjust it further.

K: In any case, you are managing the patients' response to the tinnitus rather than affecting the tinnitus per se.

L: Yes, that's correct. However, when questioned about the tinnitus, the depressed patient who has responded well to treatment of the depression typically remarks that it is still present but has become just a minor annoyance of little significance. I feel there is a vicious cycle between stress and the distress of tinnitus: the more distressing the tinnitus, the more stress; the more stress, the more distressing the tinnitus.

Changes in the perception of the tinnitus in patients with depression in remission suggests that psychological factors can have a major influence over the perception of tinnitus. Another type of patient I have seen raises a question about whether the basis for tinnitus might have always been present in some of these patients, but only their awareness of the tinnitus changed. This group of patients usually describes a high-pitched tonal tinnitus that is not lateralized to one ear, but is either diffusely located throughout the head or described as being in both ears. In many of these patients the realization of tinnitus begins in association with a highly stressful set of psychosocial circumstances. Their descriptions of tinnitus are essentially identical to the tinnitus of a large proportion of the normal-hearing population who do not complain about their tinnitus. This type of tinnitus can occur in individuals of all age groups, including children.

A second complaint of some of these same distressed patients further suggests that these patients may have had their tinnitus on a long-standing basis, but it never came to their attention, because they were never focused upon their tinnitus before. They also sometimes remark about another type of tinnitus of recent onset that they describe as a crackling sound that occurs when swallowing. Since this second type of tinnitus is the normal experience everyone has due to opening and closing of the Eustachian tube, it was clearly a lifelong experience of these individuals that they now focused upon too, so it became a clinical complaint at about the same time as the more prominent complaint of the tonal tinnitus.

Subjects with spontaneous otoacoustic emissions (SOAEs) are another example. SOAEs can be detected in almost one-third of all normal ears (Schloth 1983). Nearly all of these people are unaware of any tinnitus, but with training they can then hear their SOAEs, so at that point it qualifies to be called tinnitus. Essentially none of the distressed tinnitus patients ever complain of tinnitus corresponding to their SOAEs (Wilson 1986).

K: Would you say that in your own experience there is no drug that will reduce the tinnitus per se?

L: I can't say that categorically. First of all, the literature indicates that tinnitus improves transiently in more than half of patients receiving intravenous lidocaine (Hilders, Hulshof, Vermeij, den Hartigh, and Cohen 1992; Martin and Coleman 1980). However, I have not been using intravenous lidocaine in my patients, because its effect is so transient. I have cared for a few cases when medications appeared to have had a major effect upon the tinnitus. One case was an elderly lady who had an abrupt onset of dizziness, with ataxia and tinnitus. The ataxia and the dizziness gradually resolved but the tinnitus persisted. After a death in the family, she was distraught and given diazepam. She reported that her tinnitus stopped. We picked up on that cue and found that one milligram of diazepam would reliably turn her tinnitus off for twelve hours. This is an extremely small dose (half the smallest routinely available). She seemed to have a very specific response to a very low dose of this medication, but of course this is strictly anecdotal.

K: Did you ever try to use placebos to see whether the tinnitus returns?

L: No, but she had tried other medications that had no effect. Moreover, whenever the diazepam was stopped, she claimed the tinnitus returned within twelve hours. Another patient had had a febrile flu-like illness and had tinnitus ever since, about six months

when I first saw her. I found that doxepin, a tricyclic antidepressant, would apparently stop her tinnitus altogether. We didn't do any placebo trials, but when the antidepressant was discontinued, the tinnitus returned. She's still taking doxepin now after about a year.

K: These particular subjects in whom tinnitus appears to be affected by medications could be studied in better controlled tests. Would you think that there might be a small but significant number of patients whose tinnitus actually goes away with drug treatment?

L: It is quite possible. From a scientific point of view it would be very interesting to study these people, but they are a very small group. There are others who could be studied in whom tinnitus can be reproducibly altered by such manipulations as turning of the eyes in a specific direction or movement of the jaw (Wall, Rosenberg, and Richardson 1987). I have several patients of this type presently.

K: Now and then one hears of drugs such as furosemide that reportedly have some effects on the tinnitus itself (Guth, Risey, Amedee, and Norris 1992). If there are drugs that can affect the peripheral auditory apparatus so as to remove the signals leading to a perception of sound, everyone with tinnitus, including perhaps the distressed patients, might benefit. What is your experience with these drugs?

L: I tried furosemide on half a dozen patients in the more distressed category. None of these patients has had any significant improvement with the use of this medication.

K: A major advance in studying tinnitus would be the availability of an objective measure of tinnitus. As you say, the presence of otoacoustic emissions does not seem to correlate with distress over tinnitus. Evoked cortical magnetic recordings have generated some interest (Hoke, Feldmann, Pantev, Lütkenhöner, and Lehnertz 1989), but more recent reports have not been confirmatory (Jacobson, Ahmad, Moran, Newman, Wharton, and Tepley 1992; Sininger and King 1992). Perhaps "functional imaging" will reveal an objective correlate for certain kinds of tinnitus.

By the way, are the medications that you use for tinnitus patients similar to those used for chronic pain?

L: The main kinds of medications used in chronic pain are antidepressants, major sedatives, and hypnotics. These are the same types of medications I tend to use most frequently for the tinnitus patients. There are many similarities between the problem of chronic pain and tinnitus. Just as in chronic low back pain, the extent of disability is most closely related to psychosocial factors, such as depression, litigation, and job dissatisfaction, it is likely that similar factors are playing a major role in the clinical problem of debilitating tinnitus, as well.

K: If we could find a reliable objective sign for tinnitus, then it might be reasonable to conduct more pharmacological studies on human tinnitus sufferers. Would you say that a decent experimental design should segregate those who are truly distressed by tinnitus and others who have tinnitus but are not particularly disturbed by it?

L: Yes. A measure of the degree of distress being experienced by the patient certainly is one important factor to be incorporated into such a study. At present, one does not know whether the tinnitus of the distressed patients is fundamentally different from the tinnitus of those who are not distressed by it. As I mentioned previously, my experience supports the point of view that the severity of debilitation from tinnitus has to do with the patient's coping mechanisms and not the tinnitus per se (Sullivan, Katon, Dobie, Sakai, Russo, and Harrop-Griffiths 1988).

K: There seem to be perceptually different types of tinnitus. One type has tonal qualities that could be matched to an externally presented tone. Some of these patients have a demonstrable hearing loss, and the tinnitus has a pitch that is related to the boundaries of the presumed lesion. Another type is described as roaring and is frequently reported by patients with Ménière's syndrome. Some types are lateralized, others not. It is my impression that debilitating tinnitus is not associated with any single type of perceptual quality to the tinnitus.

L: That may be correct. The question is whether there are lesions in the auditory system that will cause a debilitating tinnitus in essentially all individuals who are otherwise normal, or is the degree of debilitation associated with tinnitus more related to the intensity of the psychological reaction to the tinnitus? To put it another way, is the problem with debilitating tinnitus chiefly related to the auditory system in a narrow sense, or to problems with levels of the nervous system that are less modality specific?

K: From subjects with spontaneous acoustic emissions we can conclude that the continuous presence of a sound in the ear is not of itself sufficient to develop distressing tinnitus. There must be other factors. If for a great many people there is some internally generated sound that is ordinarily masked by background noise, it is still only in a few individuals where special conditions create the impression of phantom sounds strong enough to be bothersome. Even for these people it is possible to cope with the situation most, if not all, of the time. Another way of posing the question is "Are there physiological conditions in which the perception of phantom sounds (tinnitus) is so overwhelming that no amount of forbearance or distraction can long withstand the intrusion?"

In this context, there are a few suggestions from auditory physiology that perceptual mechanisms are far more complex than was classically realized. The ubiquitous presence of feedback control pathways at almost all levels of the system provides a great many potential ways for the system to malfunction so as to produce phantom perceptions. There appear to be many possible reasons for having such feedback loops. Some parts enable a peripheral sensing device with limited dynamic range to be used over a much broader dynamic range. Others serve to highlight properties of the stimulus needed for specific auditory functions. Some must enable the coding of stimulus properties into perceptually meaningful constructs, such as a moving sound source in space. The fact that problems of tinnitus concern perceptions of "primitive" sounds suggests perhaps relatively peripheral mechanisms.

L: In practice, we don't encounter even simple hallucinations, such as a moving sound source, although some use very descriptive terms to characterize the percept.

K: Do many profoundly deaf patients come to consult you about tinnitus?

L: Very few. Two come to mind. One was profoundly deaf, complained of hyperacusis, and was depressed. She responded nicely to an antidepressant and was able to return to work. The antidepressant dose had to be continually readjusted to minimize side effects. She is presently considering a cochlear implant. The other patient was totally deaf from birth, so I am puzzled to know what he really meant by tinnitus, considering that he has never experienced any kind of sound. Most cochlear implant patients are virtually completely deaf and many have tinnitus. A large proportion report that their tinnitus goes away at least temporarily immediately after the implants.

K: One way to think about tinnitus in deaf patients is that somewhere in the brain there is a feedback control system. Normally this system utilizes an automatic gain control (AGC) for auditory inputs from the auditory nerve. When there is no afferent activity to the AGC from the auditory nerve (as probably occurs from a

deaf ear), the gain of this system would increase. Consequently, any spontaneous activity into the AGC from other parts of the auditory system would be interpreted as a loud sound.[1] This is analogous to the automatic volume control in a radio. When a radio station is broadcasting (whether transmitting sounds or silence), there is no static, because the carrier signal is always present. However, when the radio station goes off the air, the amplification of internal background noise goes up and we hear static. Any external afferent input to the brain would reduce the gain to a tolerable level. Such a mechanism could be the basis for suppression of tinnitus with noise masking in hearing patients. It may also account for observations that electrical stimulation applied transcutaneously, transtympanically, or through a cochlear implant may improve tinnitus (Berliner and Cunningham 1987).

L: My impression is that the results for electrical stimulation are very variable, yet virtually all the studies report some subjects whose tinnitus symptoms are alleviated with electrical stimulation (Lyttkens, Lindberg, Scott, and Melin 1986).

K: One question is whether there is something similar about the tinnitus of the subjects who appear to respond to a particular treatment mode. Is the nature of the tinnitus the same in all such subjects? If, as seems certain to be the case, there are many forms of tinnitus, controlled studies are needed where people with the same type of tinnitus are grouped together. Unfortunately, we do not know whether the groupings should be based on etiology, psychophysical attributes, or duration of severity of response. Common sense suggests we use many points of similarity.

L: I agree. If the effect of diazepam on tinnitus

[1]In barbiturate anesthetized cats, destroying the cochlea acutely eliminates (at least initially) spontaneous activity in ventral cochlear nucleus neurons in acute experiments, but not some dorsal cochlear nucleus neurons (Koerber, Pfeiffer, Warr, and Kiang 1966) Increased activity was not observed. However, the sampling of units was small and we do not know what the chronic effects are. In any case, the residual intrinsic activity could be thought of as internal noise which could be amplified by some AGC mechanism.

were to be studied in a group of 1000 subjects, my one patient who seems to respond would have been lost. One would conclude that diazepam has no demonstrable value.

K: Let's examine some specific mechanisms which we suggested previously for the type of tinnitus that results from acoustic trauma or ototoxic drugs, where there is a demonstrable inner ear lesion and the pitch of the tinnitus is often matched to the pitch of a tone that would be represented by a place in the cochlea close to the lesion (Kiang, Moxon, and Levine 1970). Based on our finding that the auditory nerve fibers from the damaged regions of the cochlea not only were unresponsive to sounds but generally had no spontaneous activity, we developed the idea that certain patterns of activity in the ensemble of auditory nerve fibers could give rise to a phantom perception of sound because the patterns resemble those generated by certain sound stimuli (Kiang 1988). Another mechanism is based on many studies of otoacoustic emissions and distortion products in which attempts are made to localize the site of inner ear damage and correlate it with the perceived pitch of the patient's tinnitus. Presumably in these instances, the altered patterns of activity in the nerve are produced by the presence of sound generated in the inner ear.

There is also a concept that some kinds of tinnitus are like hemifacial spasm or tic douloureux in being caused by tortuous blood vessels (vascular loops) overlying the relevant cranial nerve (Jannetta 1980; Møller 1992). Perhaps in these cases abnormal patterns of activity are generated in the auditory nerve by such a strategically placed vascular loop. In animals one can examine auditory nerve activity directly (although usually in anesthetized preparations), so there are animal models for conditions that would be normally accompanied by tinnitus in humans. The ototoxic and acoustic trauma lesions are such examples (Kiang et al. 1970). Another is salycilate-induced tinnitus. This model is based on finding increased activity of single units recorded from the auditory nerve (Evans and Borerwe 1982) or inferior colliculus (Jastreboff and Sasaki 1986). Also, there are behavioral studies of rats suggesting that rats develop tinnitus with high doses of salycilates (Jastreboff, Brennan, and Sasaki 1988). The idea of using calcium channel blockers as treatment for tinnitus is in part based on this model. Presumably everyone can get tinnitus from raised salicylate level. That's how the medication is often monitored for patients with arthritis who require high doses of salicylates. The dose of the salicylate is raised until tinnitus starts, at which point the dose is lowered to the point where the tinnitus disappears.

L: Acoustic neuroma patients are interesting because they nearly all have tinnitus. The usual estimate is over 80 percent. Another fascinating aspect to the phenomenon of tinnitus is that for over half of these patients their tinnitus will be unimproved even after surgery when the eighth nerve has been sectioned (House and Brackmann 1981). Some surgeons have cut the auditory or vestibular nerves to relieve tinnitus in some desperate patients (Fisch 1970). As with acoustic neuroma patients, the result is unpredictable (Jackson 1985). Clearly the persistence of tinnitus following transection of the auditory nerve suggests that even though, initially, the genesis of the tinnitus might be at the cochlear or auditory nerve level, once the tinnitus is chronic, mechanisms develop in the central nervous system that, by themselves, are sufficient to perpetuate the tinnitus.

K: Acoutic neuromas are space-occupying lesions that presumably compress neurons and blood vessels. As far as I know, acute compression doesn't result in increased neuronal activity, although chronic compression could conceivably do so. The dogma is that compression blocks or decreases the conduction velocity of axonal spike discharges. It is also possible that there are chemical factors associated with such tumors, which would result in increased neural discharges but there are no relevant data to support such an idea. One usually finds that on the tumor side there is an increased latency in brainstem auditory evoked potentials, which is consistent with slowing of conduction velocity. So what would be the basis for tinnitus with this condition? Perhaps it is the blocked activity in some but not all auditory nerve fibers as a result of compression, which could produce patterns of auditory nerve fiber activity that is similar to those produced by some sounds, so that a central processor (e.g., cochlear nucleus) interprets the pattern of activity across this family of auditory nerve fibers as a (phantom) sound. Møller (1987) has suggested that tinnitus might result from ephaptic coupling from damaged axons in the auditory nerves of acoustic tumor patients. He suggests that synchronization of discharges from this coupling could be interpreted as tinnitus by higher levels of the auditory nervous system, again because the ensemble activity resembles the activity produced by sounds.

Have you ever had an acoustic tumor patient who was of the severely distressed type?

L: No. In general I have not observed severe depression in acoustic neuroma patients and certainly not because of the tinnitus. They have other concerns.

K: And when these patients have tinnitus, do they always localize it to the affected ear?

L: Always, without exception.

K: And that is always the case with Ménière's syndrome, as well. Don't they usually localize it to the ear in which hearing loss is demonstrable?

L: Yes, that has always been my experience.

K: Ordinarily a perceived sound is lateralized to the side of greater stimulation. In this view, the tinnitus should be referred to the normal ear, because that's the side that generates more neural activity. For the two really good examples that we have of a peripheral origin, acoustic tumors and Ménière's syndrome, it

would be critical to establish whether the afflicted side contributes more instead of less auditory nerve activity than the normal side.

L: Yes, but in practice that could be difficult to establish in human subjects.

K: Lateralization of tinnitus in unilateral acoustic neuroma cases is actually of considerable interest to auditory physiologists, because from our discussion, it is possible that it is the ear delivering less overall input to the brain that is associated with the tinnitus. One of the most interesting problems with tinnitus is how diminished activity can lead to the perception of phantom sounds. Perhaps the idea about altered distribution of activity amongst the many auditory nerve fibers could apply here as well.

Let us examine some of the implications of this idea about lateralization. An argument can be made for an AGC that must precede the mechanism for lateralization of sounds. Assume for the moment that there is a neural mechanism for lateralizing sounds based on comparing the level of input neural activity from the two sides in comparable frequency channels, and that the perceptual lateralization machinery involves the superior olivary complex. If the auditory nerve input to the cochlear nucleus on the afflicted side has reduced activity, producing a lateralized tinnitus, then the hypothetical AGC mechanism might well involve the cochlear nucleus.

This is an interesting line of argument that could be explored more vigorously. What about patients with one dead ear? If they subsequently develop a tumor on the previously good side, what is the tinnitus like?

L: I don't know, but it is worth examining.

K: Because there is normally always spontaneous activity in the normal auditory nerve, the central processor receives activity from both sides, even in the absence of sound. We know that when hair cells are gone, there is no spontaneous activity in the auditory nerve fibers that innervated these hair cells. This activity would not normally be temporally correlated across neurons even from one ear much less binaurally (Kiang 1990). If there is reduced input from one side with an acoustic tumor, the perceptual machinery can apparently interpret this as a sound coming from the afflicted side. This cannot be the normal condition in which one tends to localize a sound source to the side with a preponderance of activity. Presumably timing cues are not relevant in tumor cases, but perhaps they might be, if abnormally bursty activity is present. If, however, before the lateralization machinery there is an AGC which actually increases the gain on the side with less input activity, then one could lateralize a perceived sound to the affected side.

We need not assume that the conscious perception of laterality necessarily builds on the brainstem lateralization machinery located at the superior olivary complex level (although fine timing cues seem likely to be processed there). It is conceivable, even likely, that direct comparison of inputs from both sides occurs at many levels of the system. There are plenty of projections that bypass the superior olivary complex to reach the nuclei of the lateral lemnisci or inferior colliculi. Moreover, the idea of gain controls need not imply only a single level of control. There may be gain control mechanisms that precede the lateralization machinery and others that follow it. Perhaps the wide range of effects encompassed by a single term "tinnitus" contributes to confusion in the sense that any specific hypothesis that would explain one type of tinnitus could fail when applied to other types.

One consistently reported finding about tinnitus is that its loudness is usually matched to externally presented sounds of only a few decibels above threshold (Reed 1960). This suggests that there may be an inappropriate assignment of loudness to the tinnitus. Some patients with tinnitus also complain of hyperacusis, the perception of sounds as being unusually loud. Let us suppose that in the normal system, individual peripheral elements have a

restricted dynamic range, much smaller than the overall dynamic range covered by the whole organism. Evolutionarily it became possible to extend the dynamic range by using feedback gain controls. The incoming signals are subject to adjustable gains that are controlled by a feedback loop so that higher level stimuli automatically turn down the gain. However, the feedback signal is also sent to the perceptual mechanism so that the true level can be appreciated psychophysically. Such a mechanism could exist at many different levels of the system, but the medial olivocochlear efferent neurons are interesting in this regard (Kiang, Guinan, Liberman, Brown, and Eddington 1987). These neurons have cell bodies in the lower brainstem, and axons that send one branch to the outer hair cells and another to the cochlear nucleus. The branch to the cochlea is thought to activate outer hair cells (OHC) so as to attenuate the responses of inner hair cells (IHC) to sound stimuli. This arc could act as an automatic gain control device (AGC) to keep the responses of auditory nerve fibers below saturation level. The branch to the cochlear nucleus could serve as a weighting factor that tells some components in the nucleus where the gain of the OHCs is set. It is also possible (but not essential) that the small afferent unmyelinated neurons innervating OHCs, the type II efferents (Brown 1993) can signal to the central nervous system the status of the OHC part of the loop.

Now picture what could happen if the OHCs, but not the IHCs, are damaged so that the mechanical or mechanico-electrical gain control for IHCs is inactivated and the system operates in an open-loop condition. The medial olivocochlear efferents will be activated as usual by sound stimuli, but the cochlear effect on OHCs is inoperative. However, the cochlear nucleus branch would still signal that the peripheral gain is turned down even when it was not effective. Thus, any level of auditory nerve activity would be perceived as represent-

↓ b. "informant" is MOCB branch
to CN

ing a higher stimulus level than would have been the case if the OHCs were intact. A very low sound signal generated perhaps by an abnormal cochlear machinery might then be interpreted as a very loud sound. This hypothesis might be tested in patients with vestibular neuronectomies as the medial olivocochlear efferents run in the inferior vestibular branch and are severed when the vestibular nerve is cut for intractable vertigo. In this type of surgery, the auditory nerve is intended to be spared. Unfortunately, the situation is complicated by the fact that most of these patients have tinnitus or hearing loss even before the surgery.

L: Are there different types of injuries to the inner ear that would involve the feedback system to different degrees?

K: Probably. There are different types of peripheral injuries, but how they relate to presence of tinnitus or degree of disability is speculative. For instance, disabling only the inner hair cells might not affect this gain control mechanism selectively. It would simply reduce afferent input to the cochlear nucleus, and have no effect on the activity of the medial olivocochlear efferents. So one prediction could be that the exclusive loss of inner hair cells might not lead to tinnitus unless higher level feedback loops are involved.

L: The medial olivocochlear efferent system is bilateral and consensual. What are the consequences for tinnitus?

K: One can ask what happens to tinnitus of unilateral origin when the other ear is stimulated. If the efferent circuits to one ear with tinnitus are eliminated, stimulating the other ear should have interesting effects on the tinnitus, depending on whether the branch to the cochlear nucleus is also gone. Unfortunately, we do not know whether loss of OHCs or cutting the branch of the medial olivocochlear efferents to the OHCs results in retrograde degeneration of the medial olivocochlear ef-

ferent cell body, or if the cochlear nucleus branch is a sustaining collateral. One way to ask the question is why certain people do not have tinnitus. Perhaps whether the medial olivocochlear efferent dies back completely or only up to the branch going to the cochlear nucleus is the determining factor for whether such a lesion results in tinnitus or not.

L: Can you give more detail about how the type II afferents that apparently are excited by OHCs could play a role in tinnitus?

K: We don't know the circuitry for type II afferents well enough yet, but the input to the central gain control center(s) might not be the information coming in from type I cells, but could be the information provided by type II neurons, or some combination of these two types of cochlear afferents. The type II system would be frequency specific. Increased activity in the type II afferents could reduce the gain of some of the CNS AGCs. If the OHCs or type II nerve fibers were disabled, then there would be no type II activity coming in, so the gain might always be set at some high level, and tinnitus could result.

If an ear lacks the type II fibers but has normal type I inputs, it might still continue to process the meaningful information carried by sound, but the gain control for loudness would be compromised. Then it might be possible to have tinnitus even with normal thresholds. Again this mechanism might also account for the hyperacusis associated with some tinnitus.

L: I want to introduce one other observation. Some event on one side of the face can be associated with a tinnitus on the same side. One of my patients, an audiologist, had a tooth abscess, and developed a tinnitus localized to the same side as the tooth. When the abscess resolved, the tinnitus stopped. Another patient developed facial pain on his right side apparently due to overactivity of his facial muscles, and shortly thereafter tinnitus began on the same side. Another patient had tinnitus and neck pain of a musculo-skeletal nature. She could put her head in a certain position, such that the pain would stop and her tinnitus would stop. I currently have four patients who can turn on or off their tinnitus at will by various manipulations, such as pushing the jaw or temple. There is literature, too, that relates the TMJ syndrome to tinnitus. I find it hard to conceptualize what's going on, but I can testify to the clinical facts.

K: It sounds as if it is possible to have cross-coupling of activity across modalities. There are inputs to the cochlear nucleus from the somatosensory and vestibular systems (Young, Nelken, and Conley 1993; McCue and Guinan 1993). There are also central inputs to the cochlear nucleus. This would be another interesting issue to explore with functional magnetic resonance imaging.

L: What about central lesions? Are there theoretical candidates for critical places where lesions could lead to tinnitus?

K: You have studied auditory responses of multiple sclerosis (MS) patients. Do they ever have tinnitus that correlates in any way with their lesions? If there are some who complained about tinnitus, do their lesions involve specific regions of the brain? MS lesions probably do not generate increased activity, although increased activity could result from blocking central inhibitory mechanisms. It doesn't seem to be the case that widespread MS lesions throughout the brain lead to tinnitus or heightened sensory awareness of any sensory modality. Is that right?

L: I believe that is right. However, MS patients commonly complain of paresthesias and can have paroxysmal symptoms, including pain and itching. About 1 percent have trigeminal neuralgia (Rushton and Olafsonn 1965), brief episodes of excruciating unilateral facial pain. In these cases, usually a lesion is present at the root entry zone of the trigeminal nerve on the same side as the pain.

K: It would be very helpful to explore with functional imaging the brains of some of these patients.

L: What about sensory systems other than audition or pain? Are there phantom perceptions? In neurology we hear about patients with persistent odors or taste but not visual phantoms.

K: Perhaps the purported lack of centrifugal (efferent) inputs to the retina is significant. It may be that a broader look at sensory disorders might give us valuable clues to tinnitus, but at the moment, there is no obvious new insight that I gain by so doing.

L: Perhaps we should sum up our conclusions from this conversation.

K: There are many ways to generate a perception of sound when there is no externally presented acoustic stimulus. Our speculations suggest that decreased activity in the auditory nerve could result in increased activity in the cochlear nucleus in some cases with well-lateralized tinnitus. We've examined various ideas that feedback mechanisms and AGCs involving the cochlea and the CNS might interact and play a role in tinnitus. Finally, we have discussed how altered patterns of activity in the auditory nerve could give rise to a phantom perception of sound.

While these mechanisms are all very interesting and instructive to auditory scientists, the clinically important cases of tinnitus appear to involve breakdowns in coping mechanisms more than auditory sensations per se. The central and still unanswered question is, Is disabling tinnitus the elevation of a relatively innocuous everyday experience into a malignant obsession, or is it a symptom that arises when the perceptual machinery signals overload when there is no overload at the sensory input end? These issues will be decided by data and not speculation.

This work was supported in part by NIH grant P01 DC 00119.

REFERENCES

Aran, J.-M. and Dauman, R. 1992. *Tinnitus 91. Proceedings of the Fourth International Tinnitus Seminar.* Amsterdam: Kugler.

Berliner, K.I. and Cunningham, J.K. 1987. "Tinnitus Suppression in Cochlear Implantation." In J.W.P. Hazell (Ed.), *Tinnitus,* pp. 118–130. Edinburgh: Churchill Livingstone.

Brown, M.C. 1993. "Anatomical and Physiological Studies of Type I and Type II Spiral Ganglion Neurons." In *The Mammalian Cochlear Nuclei: Organization and Function* Plenum.

Evans, E.F. and Borerwe, T.A. 1982. "Ototoxic Effects of Sodium Salicylate on the Responses of Single Cochlear Nerve Fibers and Their Spontaneous Activity." *British Journal of Audiology, 16,* 101–108.

Feldmann, H. 1971. "Homolateral and Contralateral Masking of Tinnitus by Noise-bands and Pure Tones." *Audiology, 10,* 138–144.

Fisch, U. 1970. "Transtemporal Surgery of the Internal Auditory Canal." *Advanced Otology, Rhinology, and Laryngology, 17,* 203–240.

Guth, P.S., Risey, J., Amedee, R., and Norris, C.H. 1992. "A Pharmacological Approach to the Treatment of Tinnitus." In J.-M. Aran and R. Dauman (Eds.), *Tinnitus 91. Proceedings of the Fourth International Tinnitus Seminar, Bordeaux, France, August 27–30, 1991,* pp. 115–118. Amsterdam: Kugler.

Hilders, C.G.J.M., Hulshof, J.H., Vermeij, P., den Hartigh, J., and Cohen, A.F. 1992. "Further Investigations into the Effect of Lidocaine in the Treatment of Tinnitus." In J.-M. Aran and R. Dauman (Eds.), *Tinnitus 91. Proceedings of the Fourth International Tinnitus Seminar, Bordeaux, France, August 27–30, 1991.* Amsterdam: Kugler.

Hoke, M., Feldmann, H., Pantev, C., Lütkenhöner, B., and Lehnertz, K. 1989. "Objective Evidence of Tinnitus in Auditory Evoked Magnetic Fields." *Hearing Research, 37,* 281–286.

House, J.W. and Brackmann, D.E. 1981. "Tinnitus: Surgical Treatment." In D. Evered and G. Lawrenson (Eds.), *Tinnitus, Ciba Foundation Symposium 85,* pp. 204–216. London: Pitman.

Jackson, P. 1985. "A Comparison of the Effects of Eighth Nerve Section with Lidocaine on Tinnitus." *Journal of Laryngology, 99,* 663–666.

Jacobson, G.P., Ahmad, B.K., Moran, J., Newman, C.W., Wharton, J., and Tepley, N. 1992. "Auditory Evoked Field (M100-M200) Measurements in Tinnitus and Normal Groups." In J.-M. Aran and R. Dauman (Eds.), *Tinnitus 91. Proceedings of the Fourth International Tinnitus Seminar, Bordeaux, France, August 27–30, 1991,* pp. 317–322. Amsterdam: Kugler.

Jannetta, P.J. 1980. "Neurovascular Compression in Cranial Nerve and Systemic Disease." *Annals of Surgery, 192,* 518–524.

Jastreboff, P.J., Brennan, J.F., and Sasaki, C.T. 1988. "Phantom Auditory Sensation in Rats: An Animal Model for Tinnitus." *Behavioral Neuroscience, 102,* 811–822.

Jastreboff, P.J. and Sasaki, C.T. 1986. "Salicylate-induced Changes in Spontaneous Activity of Single Units in the Inferior Colliculus of the Guinea Pig." *Journal of the Acoustic Society of America, 80,* 1384–1391.

Kiang, N.Y.S. 1988. "An Auditory Physiologist's View of Ménière's Syndrome." In J.B. Nadol (Ed.), *Second International Symposium on Ménière's Disease,* pp. 13–24. Amsterdam: Kugler & Ghedini.

Kiang, N.Y.S. 1990. "Curious Oddments of Auditory-nerve Studies." *Hearing Research, 49,* 1–16.

Kiang, N.Y.S., Guinan, J.J., Jr., Liberman, M.C., Brown, M.C., and Eddington, D.K. 1987. "Feedback Control Mechanisms of the Auditory Periphery: Implications for Cochlear Implants." In P. Banfai (Ed.), *Cochlear Implant: Current Situation,* pp. 131–151. Duren: International Cochlear Implant Symposium.

Kiang, N.Y.S., Moxon, E.C., and Levine, R.A. 1970. "Auditory-nerve Activity in Cats with Normal and Abnormal Cochleas." In G.E.W. Wolstenholme and J. Knight (Eds.), *Sensorineural Hearing Loss,* pp. 241–273. London: J. & A. Churchill.

Koerber, K.C., Pfeiffer, R.R., Warr, W.B., and Kiang, N.Y.S. 1966. "Spontaneous Spike Discharges from Single Units in the Cochlear Nucleus after Destruction of the Cochlea." *Experimental Neurology, 16*(2), 119–130.

Lyttkens, L., Lindberg, P., Scott, B., and Melin, L. 1986. "Treatment of Tinnitus by External Electrical Stimulation." *Scandinavian Audiology, 15,* 157–164.

Martin, F.W. and Coleman, B.H. 1980. "Tinnitus: A Double-blind Crossover Controlled Trial to Evaluate the Use of Lignocaine." *Clinical Otolaryngology, 5,* 3–11.

McCue, M.P. and Guinan, J.J. Jr. 1993. "Acoustic Responses from Primary Afferent Neurons of the Mammalian Sacculus." *Association for Research in Otolaryngology, Abstracts of the Sixteenth Midwinter Research Meeting, 33.*

McFadden, D. 1982. *Tinnitus: Facts, Theories, and Treatments.* Washington, DC: National Academy Press.

Møller, A.R. 1987. "Can Injury to the Auditory Nerve Cause Tinnitus." In H. Feldmann (Ed.), *Proceedings III International Tinnitus Seminar,* pp. 58–63. Karlsruhe: Harsch Verlag.

Møller, A.R. 1992. "Central Neurophysiological Processes in Tinnitus." In J.-M. Aran and R. Dauman (Eds.), *Tinnitus 91. Proceedings of the Fourth International Tinnitus Seminar, Bordeaux, France, August 27–30, 1991.* Amsterdam: Kugler.

Reed, G.F. 1960. "An Audiometric Study of Two Hundred Cases of Subjective Tinnitus." *Archives of Otolaryngology, 71,* 94–104.

Rushton, J.G. and Olafsonn, R.A. 1965. "Trigeminal Neuralgia Associated with Multiple Sclerosis." *Archives of Neurology, 13,* 383–386.

Schloth, E. 1983. "Relation between Spectral Composition of Spontaneous Oto-acoustic Emissions and Fine Structure of Threshold in Quiet." *Acustica, 53,* 250–256.

Shulman, A. 1991. *Tinnitus: Diagnosis/Treatment.* Philadelphia: Lea & Febiger.

Sininger, Y. and King, A. 1992. "Dipole Source Analysis of Cortical Auditory Evoked Potentials in Tinnitus." *ARO Midwinter Research Meeting, 111.*

Sullivan, M.D., Dobie, R.A., Sakai, C.S., and Katon, W.J. 1989. "Treatment of Depressed Tinnitus Patients with Nortriptyline." *Annals of Otology, Rhinology, and Laryngology, 98,* 867–872.

Sullivan, M.D., Katon, W.J., Dobie, R.A., Sakai, C.S., Russo, J., and Harrop-Griffiths, J. 1988. "Disabling Tinnitus: Association with Affective Disorder." *General Hospital Psychiatry, 10,* 285–291.

Wall, M., Rosenberg, M., and Richardson, D. 1987. "Gaze-evoked Tinnitus." *Neurology, 37,* 1034–1036.

Wilson, J.P. 1986. "Otoacoustic Emissions and Tinnitus." *Scandinavian Audiology, Supplement, 25,* 109–119.

Young, E.D., Nelken, I., and Conley, R.A. 1993. "Cochlear Nucleus Responses Evoked from the Dorsal Column (Somatosensory) Nuclei." *ARO Midwinter Research Meeting, 16,* 124.

CHAPTER 13

SPECTRAL ANALYSIS OF BRAIN ACTIVITY IN THE STUDY OF TINNITUS

WILLIAM HAL MARTIN
Temple University Medical School

THE PROBLEM

A few years ago the Garfield Auditory Research Laboratory was encouraged to evaluate the effectiveness of a bioflavinoid, Ginkgo biloba, in the treatment of tinnitus. We had reviewed the predominately European literature on extract of Ginkgo biloba and were encouraged by the results (Chesseboeuf, Herard, and Trevin 1979; Claussen and Claussen 1981; Meyer 1986; Natali, Rachinel, and Pouyat 1979). A six-month double-blind treatment and placebo-controlled study was designed using 40 volunteers with chronic tinnitus of various and often unknown etiology. Pitch and loudness matching and minimum masking measurements were made monthly during the study. We were disappointed to find that the loudness and minimum masking measures varied by over 300 percent in both the treatment and *placebo* groups. This magnitude of variability precludes statistical analysis for subtle changes. The sources of the variability could include physiologic or emotional/psychoperceptual factors. It is apparent to clinicians who work with tinnitus sufferers that a person's general well-being affects the perceived loudness and annoyance of the tinnitus. Stress and exhaustion are factors which have been commonly reported to aggravate the disorder. As important as perception is to the management of tinnitus, it may work against studies aimed at understanding physiologic mechanisms. Without a lucid understanding of the various processes

which result in tinnitus, developing effective treatments is left to lucky guesses and chance.

As a result of this experience, our laboratory has abandoned treatment studies in order to pursue the development of an objective quantitative measurement technique which reflects the physiologic activity underlying the perceptual phenomenon we call tinnitus.

BACKGROUND

Objective evidence of tinnitus has been difficult to demonstrate. The most promising and exciting work came in 1989 from a group in Germany that reported significant differences in the auditory evoked magnetic fields recorded from tinnitus and non-tinnitus groups (Hoke, Feldmann, Pantev, Lütkenhöner, and Lehnertz 1989; Pantev, Hoke, Lütkenhöner, Lehnertz, and Kumph 1989). Unfortunately, extensive attempts to replicate these findings have been unsuccessful (Jacobson, Ahmad, Moran, Newman, Tepley, and Wharton 1991; Colding-Jørgensen, Lauritzen, Johnsen, Mikkelsen, and Salvmark 1992; Jacobson, Ahmad, Moran, Newman, Wharton, and Tepley 1992).

Another interesting study demonstrating what may be the effects of tinnitus was presented by Jastreboff, Ikner, and Hassen (1992). Auditory brainstem responses (ABRs) were recorded from age, gender, and hearing matched groups of seven individuals that either did or did not have tinnitus.

The tinnitus and non-tinnitus groups were differentiated from each other using a modified analysis of variance for partially correlated data method. The tinnitus and non-tinnitus ABRs were compared in the frequency and time domains. The groups were significantly different in their spectral content at 100 and 600 Hz, and there was increased energy in the tinnitus group at 200 Hz compared to the non-tinnitus controls. The ABRs differed in the time domain as well. There were significant differences in the ABRs during the negativity following wave V and during wave VI. The working hypothesis was not that the ABR actually records the tinnitus activity, but that it may reflect changes in the auditory pathway function resulting from chronic peripheral activity, or changes in the evoked potentials due to the presence of increased or modified physiologic noise. The physiologic activity underlying tinnitus would presumably be a continuous signal and would be, by design, eliminated from the ABR by the averaging process. So this technique does not measure tinnitus, but its "shadow" on the normal processing performed by the auditory pathway.

High doses of salicylate have long been known to cause tinnitus in humans. Jastreboff and colleagues (Jastreboff, Brennan, Coleman, and Sasaki 1988a; Jastreboff, Brennan, and Sasaki 1988b; Jastreboff 1990) have demonstrated that salicylate treatment can cause auditory sensations in rats. This suggests that similar mechanisms are responsible for salicylate-induced tinnitus in humans and other animals. Evans and colleagues (Evans, Wilson, and Borerwe 1981) studied the single-unit firing rates of cochlear fibers in cats before and after salicylate infusion. They noted that the firing rates and patterns were significantly affected by the salicylate treatment. Jastreboff and Sasaki (1986) treated guinea pigs with salicylates and were able to induce changes in the firing rates of single units in the inferior colliculus. Salicylate was also used by Schreiner and Snyder (1987) to modify the activity of the auditory nerve in the cat. Bipolar electrodes were placed upon the exposed auditory nerve and the ensemble spontaneous activity was recorded.

The spectral characteristics of the activity were affected by salicylate treatment. Specifically, there was an increase in activity near 200 Hz that occurred after treatment with salicylates. They suggested that the spectral change may have reflected the presence of tinnitus. This study introduced the possibility of using spectral averaging to identify changes in spontaneous neural activity. Spectral averaging was performed by Dolan and colleagues (Dolan, Nuttall, and Avinash 1990) on recordings of spontaneous activity from the round window of guinea pigs (without salicylate treatment). This demonstrated that such recordings could be made relatively noninvasively.

SPECTRAL AVERAGING

Spectral averaging (technically, incoherent spectral averaging) is a process which allows the identification and quantification of continuous signals that have consistent frequency characteristics. During incoherent spectral averaging, frequency and amplitude are measured, but phase measures are not considered. In contrast, coherent spectral averaging incorporates phase information but requires the sweep to be time-locked to the signal (Figure 13-1). Incoherent spectral averaging does not increase the signal-to-noise ratio as does time domain averaging and coherent spectral averaging. Instead, it allows the identification of consistent features in the average power spectrum. Therefore, spectral averaging lends itself to the measurement of signals which are continuous and unable to be time-locked to a stimulus (as in the case of evoked potentials).

Spectral averaging can be performed by automated systems which have predetermined response characteristics and capabilities. It can also be performed by modifying systems which have been designed to do averaging in the time domain (like evoked potential systems).

During time domain averaging for evoked potentials, electrical activity from the scalp is continuously amplified and filtered by a preamplifier. During a specific period of time, usually linked to

Spectral averaging: Coherent vs. Incoherent

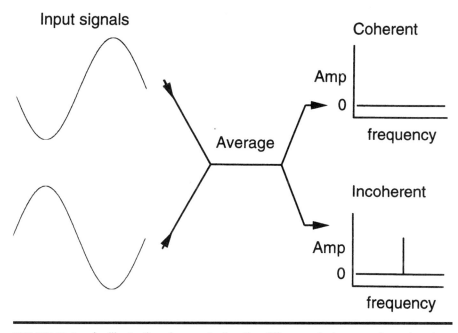

FIGURE 13-1. An illustration demonstrating the difference between coherent and incoherent spectral averaging. Phase is utilized during *coherent* averaging and results in the cancellation of signals which are 180° out of phase and result in no spectral activity (upper right). Phase is disregarded during *incoherent* spectral averaging, and energy at the frequency of the signal is represented in the spectral average regardless of the phase of the signal (lower right). (This figure was conceived and suggested by Dr. David Stapells.)

the occurrence of a stimulus, a single sweep of that activity is recorded by the analog-to-digital converter of the system. This process divides the time period during the sweep into a sequence of data points or samples, each of which is stored in the computer's memory with an associated voltage value. The voltage values from many sweeps are averaged continuously. This increases the ability to identify signals time-locked to the stimulus or the trigger of the sweep in the averaged response. Averaging will serve to reduce the amount of noise in the averaged response, since the noise should not be time-locked to the sweep. Averag-

ing is less effective at reducing noise whenever the frequency of the noise is a multiple of the rate at which the sweeps are being acquired.

Frequency domain averaging (i.e., spectral averaging) is similar to time-domain averaging during the initial stages. The electrical activity is amplified, filtered, and digitized. However, each digitized time domain sweep undergoes a Fourier transform to convert the response from the time to frequency domain. Finally, the spectrum of each sweep is averaged and stored. Averaging is required to reduce the frequency-to-frequency variability. The final spectrum represents the average energy at each represented frequency over the time period during which the sweeps were recorded. If there is stable activity at a particular frequency, it will be represented as a peak in the averaged spectrum.

Factors which affect the range and resolution of the frequencies represented include the duration of the time-domain recording sweep, the number of data points sampled during that sweep, the characteristics of the Fourier-transform window, and the filter characteristics (cut-off and slope) of the preamplifier in the recording system. Long sweep durations and low high-pass filtering are required to sample low frequencies and to increase the frequency resolution of the average. High sampling rates and high low-pass filtering are required to sample high frequencies. The Fourier-transform window determines the "leakage" of energy to side lobes of the primary frequency (this is the same principal as acoustic splatter).

If we hypothesize that there is some relatively stable and continuous electrical activity generated within the auditory system which is perceived as tinnitus, then it may be possible to use spectral averaging to quantify this activity. This hypothesis is the basis for the following studies in cats and man.

ANALYSIS OF AUDITORY NERVE ACTIVITY IN THE CAT

The results of a study of the spectral analysis of cat auditory nerve activity (Martin, Schwegler, Scheibelhoffer, and Ronis 1993) are summarized below.

The work of Schreiner and Snyder (1987) indicated that spectral changes in bipolar recordings of auditory nerve activity could be induced by treating cats with salicylates. Dolan and colleagues (1990) demonstrated that the spectrum of activity of the auditory nerve could be recorded from the round window in guinea pigs. The purpose of our study in the cat was to 1) confirm the results of Schreiner and Snyder, using bipolar electrodes to perform spectral analysis of auditory nerve activity before and after salicylate treatment; 2) attempt other recording methods for spectral averaging, including monopolar auditory nerve and round window recordings; and 3) evaluate the effects of lidocaine on the spectrum of spontaneous auditory nerve activity. The lidocaine test was performed because lidocaine injection has been demonstrated to cause temporary relief of tinnitus in humans (Martin and Coleman 1980; Melding, Goodey, and Thorne 1978; Shea and Harell 1978).

Methods

Twelve adult cats were anesthetized and prepared for surgery. All recordings were made in an acoustically and electrically shielded booth, and no acoustic stimuli were presented during spectral averaging. The auditory nerve and round window were exposed, and platinum-iridium electrodes were placed and fixed in place. Bipolar and monopolar auditory nerve and round window spectral averaging was performed. The activity was amplified over a bandwidth of 10 Hz to 5 kHz (6 dB/oct) and digitized at a sampling rate of 16 kHz/channel using an 8-bit analog-to-digital converter. Each sweep of 4096 points was multiplied by a Hanning window followed by a fast Fourier transform (FFT) to determine the power spectrum. The spectra of up to 4096 sweeps were averaged to calculate the average power spectrum. These parameters permitted analysis of a spectral range from 0 Hz to 8 kHz (limited to 50 Hz to 2 kHz by the preamplifier bandwidth) with a frequency resolution of 4 Hz/point.

Auditory brainstem responses (ABRs) to click stimuli were monitored to evaluate changes in peripheral auditory function and the integrity of the auditory pathway during the surgical procedure and treatment with salicylate.

Sodium salicylate (150 mg/kg, intravenous) was injected slowly into 10 of the cats following baseline spectral averaging and ABR recordings. The other 2 cats were injected with saline volumes equivalent to the salicylate injections. All animals were then monitored and spectral averaging was performed for 3 to 4 hours. At this time, the salicy-late-treated animals were injected with lidocaine (6 mg/kg, intravenous) and an additional 30 minutes of spectral averaging was performed. All of the animals remained anesthetized throughout the procedure and were euthanized at the end of the study.

Results

It should be noted that salicylates create profound physiologic stress on cats. Respiration rates and temperatures fluctuated during the initial 2 hours after salicylate injection. The ABRs often revealed elevated peripheral hearing thresholds. Surgical exposure often resulted in increases of

the I-IV interpeak interval. In addition, lidocaine injection was fatal in 3 of the 10 cats.

Spectral analysis of the auditory nerve activity revealed marked changes in the pre- and post-salicylate conditions using the bipolar (Figures 13-2, 13-3, 13-4), monopolar (Figures 13-4, 13-6, 13-7) and round window (Figure 13-5) recording conditions. A peak of energy, typically centered near 200 Hz, and a second higher frequency broad peak (Figure 13-2) were identified in all of the cats treated with salicylate by 3 hours after injection. The 200 Hz peak was very consistently recorded where the later, broad peak was highly variably across animals. Neither of the peaks were identified in the pre-salicylate baseline recordings or in

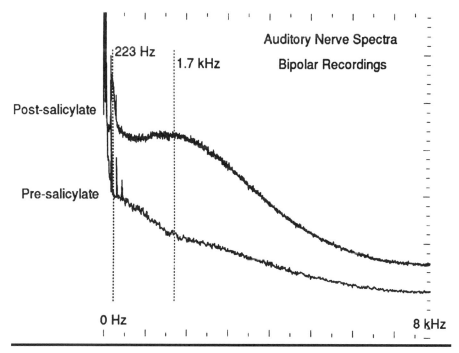

FIGURE 13-2. Power spectra of the spontaneous auditory nerve activity recorded from an anesthetized cat using bipolar recording electrodes. The lower curve was recorded prior to salicylate treatment and was typical of baseline recordings in all of the cats. The upper curve was recorded 3 hours after an intravenous injection of sodium salicylate. Two peaks are identified by the vertical cursors; one at 223 Hz and the other at 1.7 kHz. The sharp spikes are harmonics of 60 Hz noise. (From Martin et al. 1993)

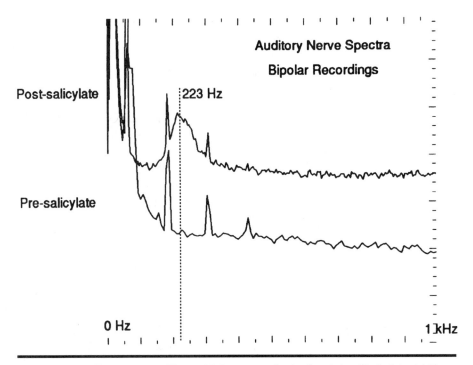

FIGURE 13-3.   The same as Figure 13-2, except the horizontal scale is 0 to 1 kHz instead of 0 to 8 kHz. (From Martin et al. 1993)

the 2 control animals treated with saline instead of salicylate (Figure 13-7). The 200 Hz peak was temporarily eliminated or reduced in amplitude when the animals were treated with lidocaine (Figures 13-4 and 13-6). The peak was also abolished by the death of the animal. In one animal, a series of spectral averages revealed that the center frequency of the salicylate induced peak changed over time (Figure 13-6). The peak was initially observed at 156 Hz and increased to 172 Hz over a 1.5 hour period. Treatment with lidocaine resulted in an immediate decrease in amplitude and center frequency to 160 Hz.

Discussion

Spectral analysis revealed changes in the cat auditory nerve firing patterns resulting from treatment with sodium salicylate. These changes in activity

were most clearly visible in monopolar recordings from the auditory nerve, but were identified using bipolar (as in Schreiner and Snyder) and round window recording conditions as well. The round window recordings were comparatively noninvasive and suggested that this technique may be the basis for future evaluations of auditory nerve function in both animals and man.

Several factors link the changes in auditory nerve function with tinnitus:

1. The 200 Hz peak is a consequence of salicylate treatment at levels which would result in tinnitus in humans and which have induced phantom auditory behavior in rats (Jastreboff, Hansen, Sasaki, and Sasaki 1988c).

2. The changes in the auditory nerve activity resulting from salicylates were reduced or eliminated by intravenous lidocaine for 10 to 20

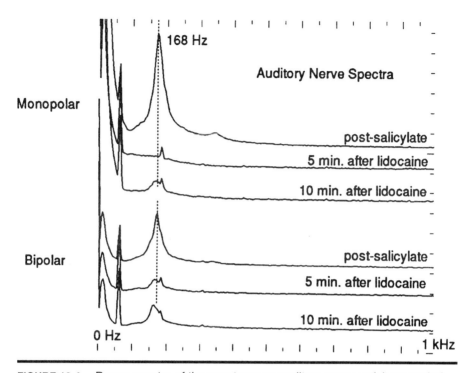

FIGURE 13-4. Power spectra of the spontaneous auditory nerve activity recorded from a cat demonstrating the difference between monopolar (upper 3 records) and bipolar (lower 3 records) electrode montages, and showing the effects of lidocaine. All records were recorded from the same animal (however, a different animal than used for the records in Figure 13-2). The post-salicylate records were recorded 2 hours after salicylate treatment. The other recordings were made either 5 or 10 minutes after intravenous lidocaine treatment. Note that the monopolar peak in the post-salicylate treatment recordings was over twice the amplitude of the bipolar counterpart. This could have been due to a reduction in common mode rejection of the auditory nerve activity which would be greater in bipolar recordings than monopolar. Also note that the 168 Hz peak was temporarily reduced or eliminated by the lidocaine. (From Martin et al. 1993)

minutes. Lidocaine has been reported to temporarily eliminate or reduce tinnitus in humans, provided it is introduced systemically, and not topically, to the tympanic membrane (Martin and Coleman 1980; Melding et al. 1978; Shea and Harell 1978).

3. The center frequency of the activity resulting from salicylate treatment varied over time. Many tinnitus sufferers report that their tinnitus may

change in pitch. This perceptual change may have a physiologic correlate.

4. This peak is absent when treatments which do not induce tinnitus (saline control injections) are performed. The peak could not be electrical artifact because it was abolished by death.

Unfortunately, none of the cats was able to tell us that it was hearing tinnitus after being treated

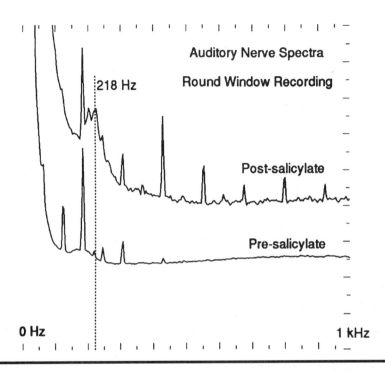

FIGURE 13-5. Spectral analysis of cat spontaneous auditory nerve activity recorded from the round window in the pre-salicylate (lower) and 2 hours after salicylate treatment (upper). As in Figure 13-2, the sharp spikes represent harmonics of 60 Hz noise. Note that the peak at 218 Hz was recorded from the round window. This is significant in that it suggests that this activity may be recorded in a relatively non-invasive approach. (From Martin et al. 1993)

with salicylates. Neither could the cats describe to us changes in pitch over time, or a decrease in the loudness of the tinnitus following lidocaine treatments. Nonetheless, we were encouraged by these results and decided to perform similar recordings on humans.

ANALYSIS OF AUDITORY NERVE ACTIVITY IN HUMANS

Intraoperative monitoring of auditory pathway function during neurologic and otologic surgeries is one of the clinical responsibilities we have that affords us the unique opportunity of performing recordings directly from the exposed human brain. While providing protective information to the surgical team, we may also acquire data that can be used to help understand the workings and failings of neural processing.

Having our initial hypothesis still in mind—that physiologic events related to tinnitus may be able to be recorded from the auditory nervous system—we have performed spectral averaging on the activity recorded from the auditory nerves of several humans. We have not attempted to induce tinnitus in these subjects as was done in the animal experiments. Instead, subjects were classified by whether or not they had tinnitus before or after their surgeries.

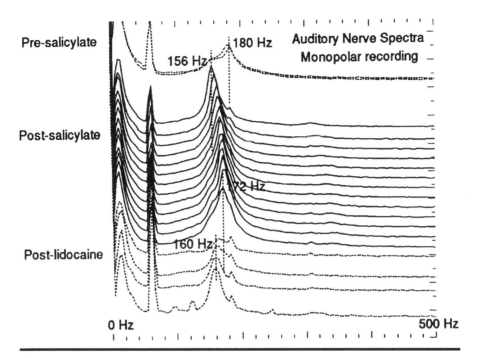

FIGURE 13-6. A chronological sequence (top to bottom) of spectra from recordings of spontaneous auditory nerve activity from a cat. The uppermost recordings (dotted lines) show two superimposed spectra recorded after placement of the monopolar electrode on the auditory nerve and prior to salicylate injection. A small shoulder of activity at 156 Hz rides on the shoulder of a noise harmonic of 180 Hz. The middle group (solid lines) were recorded sequentially (top to bottom) over a 1.5 hour period beginning 2 hours after salicylate injection. The peak of activity changed from 156 Hz to 172 Hz during that time, while remaining stable in amplitude. The lower (dotted) records were obtained over a 20-minute period after injection with lidocaine. The peak temporarily decreased in amplitude and decreased in center frequency from 172 Hz to 160 Hz. (From Martin et al. 1993)

Methods

The subjects were 14 adults undergoing neurosurgical procedures in the cerebellopontine angle in which intraoperative monitoring was required for protection of "at-risk" neural tissue. The various etiologies of these patients are presented in Table 13-1. They were not classified by hearing loss, age, or gender. All of the subjects who complained of tinnitus had the type which could be described as continuous (ringing, hissing, buzzing) rather than linked to mechanical disorders (pulsatile). No formal tinnitus matching or masking procedures were performed on these subjects. The subjects were asked if they had any long term (over 6 months) history of tinnitus, if they had tinnitus on the morning of the surgery, and if they had immediate post-operative tinnitus. These classifications are also presented in Table 13-1.

All recordings were made in an unshielded op-

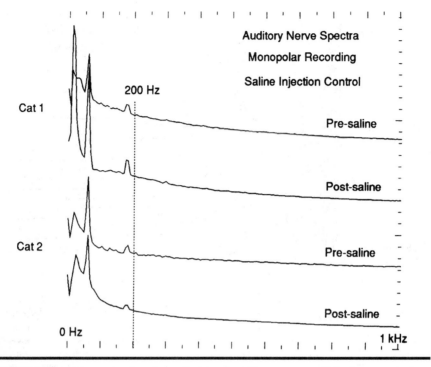

FIGURE 13-7. Power spectra of spontaneous auditory nerve activity from control cats treated with saline instead of sodium salicylate. No spectral changes were noted that would have resulted from the surgical procedure, the injection or any other aspect of the experimental procedure. A cursor was placed at 200 Hz as a reference point. This supported the conclusion that the spectral changes observed in the other 10 cats were induced by the salicylate. (From Martin et al. 1993)

erating room, however, no acoustic stimuli were presented during spectral averaging. The auditory nerve was exposed and a wick electrode was located on the proximal section of the nerve, near the brainstem. The wick electrode (made of cottonoid sutured to insulated silver wire) was connected to the noninverting input of the preamplifier. The inverting input was located on either the contralateral mastoid, the ipsilateral mastoid, or the ipsilateral muscle flap of the surgical opening. The latter location resulted in recordings with the lowest amount of 60 Hz noise and harmonics. Auditory nerve spectral averaging was performed

during breaks which occurred at unscheduled times during the procedure (e.g., obtaining special instrumentation or adjusting the microscope). The activity was amplified over a bandwidth of 100 Hz to 2 kHz (6 dB/oct) and digitized at a sampling rate of 12.5 kHz/channel using an 12-bit analog-to-digital converter. Each sweep of 8192 points was multiplied by a Hanning window followed by a fast Fourier transform (FFT) to determine the power spectrum. The spectra of 100 to 500 sweeps were averaged to calculate the average power spectrum. Spectral analysis was possible from 0 Hz to 6.25 kHz (limited to 100 Hz to 2 kHz by the

TABLE 13-1. Surgical Procedures and Results

SUBJECT	PROCEDURE	HISTORY/ PRE/POST	AN PEAK	POST-OP HEARING
1.	Vestibular n. section	+ / + / +	yes	yes
2.	Vestibular n. section	+ / + / -	yes	yes
3.	Vestibular schwannoma resection	+ / + / +	yes	no
4.	Trigeminal n. section	+ / + / +	yes	yes
5.	Cerebellar hemangioma	- / - / -	no	yes
6.	Vestibular schwannoma resection	+ / + / +	yes	no
7.	Vestibular n. section	+ / - / -	yes	yes
8.	Vestibular n. section	+ / + / +	yes	yes
9.	Vestibular n. section	+ / + / +	yes	yes
10.	CPA tumor	+ / + / +	yes	no
11.	ICA aneurysm clip	- / - / +	yes	yes
12.	Trigeminal n. decompression	+ / + / -	yes	yes
13.	Facial n. decompression	- / - / -	yes	no
14.	Vestibular schwannoma resection	- / - / -	no	no

preamplifier bandwidth) with a frequency resolution of 1.5 Hz/point.

Results

A prominent peak in the spectral average near 200 Hz was present in 12 of the 14 subjects (Figure 13-8, Table 13-1). Eleven of the 12 patients with a spectral peak near 200 Hz also had a pre- or postoperative history of tinnitus. The remaining subject of the 12 having the 200 Hz peak had no pre- or postoperative history of tinnitus. However, that subject also lost all hearing function during the procedure.

No spectral peak at or near 200 Hz could be identified in 2 of the subjects. Neither of these subjects had a history of pre- or postoperative tinnitus (Figures 13-9, 13-10; Table 13-1). One had normal postoperative hearing, and one lost hearing completely during the procedure.

Additional recordings were made in some subjects from nonauditory structures. In one patient, the 200 Hz peak was present when recording from the auditory nerve, but not when recording from the brainstem surface (Figure 13-11). In another patient, the 200 Hz peak was present in auditory nerve recordings, but not in recordings from the pons (Figure 13-12). In a third example, no peak was identified from the auditory nerve, the cerebellum or the retracted muscle flap (Figure 13-10).

Discussion

The acquisition and analysis of data from human subjects is still in progress. One limitation of this study is the selection of subjects. Only those patients who are undergoing a neurosurgical procedure requiring intraoperative evoked potential monitoring are available. This has limited the number of "control" subjects.

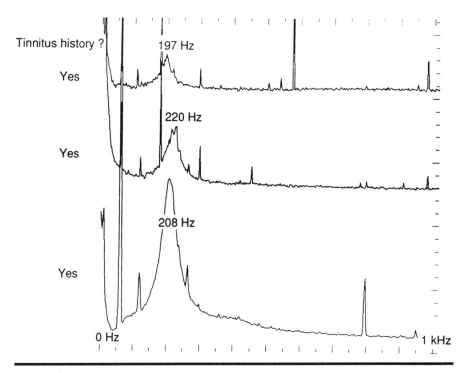

FIGURE 13-8. Examples of power spectra of spontaneous auditory nerve activity recorded from human subjects having a history of tinnitus. Recordings were made during neurosurgical procedures while a wick electrode was placed on the proximal auditory nerve. These are representative of the result identified in 12 of the 14 subjects listed in Table 13-1.

It is remarkable that a spectral peak of 200 Hz was identified in the subjects which had pre- or postoperative tinnitus, and not in those without tinnitus. The one exceptional case was that of a subject who had the peak at the time of the recording, yet had no tinnitus experience. It is significant that this subject lost all hearing during the surgery. The initial procedure was a facial nerve decompression. During the procedure, it was found that she had an arteriovenous malformation (AVM) at the base of the auditory nerve as well. Her hearing loss was secondary to removal of the AVM. It is impossible to rule out that during the procedure a traumatic event occurred which may have affected the auditory nerve in such a manner as to have caused tinnitus. Møller, Møller, Jannetta, and Jho (1992a) have described tinnitus resulting from vascular compression of the auditory nerve. It may be that tinnitus was present during the spectral averaging, but that all auditory function was lost during removal of the AVM. This might account for the absence of pre- or postoperative tinnitus experience.

SUMMARY

The human and animal works suggest that there is a relationship between the 200 Hz peak and tinnitus. This is surprising in multiple ways and brings up the following questions:

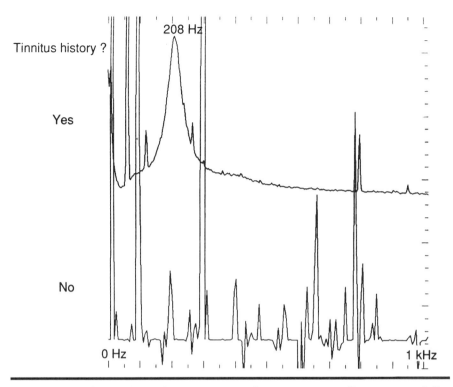

FIGURE 13-9. Comparison of power spectra of spontaneous auditory nerve activity recorded from one human subject with preoperative tinnitus (upper) and one no pre- or postoperative tinnitus history whatsoever (lower). It should be noted that the sharp spikes in both traces are the result of 60 Hz noise and its harmonics.

Is the 200 Hz peak in cats and humans an artifact? One factor likely to cause consistent activity across experiments would be the presence of some external artifact. Acoustic signals were reduced in the cat experiments by using an acoustically shielded booth. This luxury could not be afforded in the operating room. However, in both recording conditions, recordings were made in which the 200 Hz peak was not obtained. In the animal experiments, the peak was not present in the pre-salicylate conditions, the saline control studies, the lidocaine injections, and in expired animals. In the human studies, the response was not recorded from the brainstem, pons, cerebellum, or muscle flap, or in 2 of the subjects, from the auditory nerve.

These results strongly argue against the peak as being an a electric or acoustic artifact.

Why is the change in spectra resulting from salicylate treatment in cats nearly identical to spectra identified in humans having varied etiologies? If the 200 Hz peak is related to tinnitus, it suggests a common pathway or physiologic basis for the phenomenon in multiple etiologies. Based upon the proposed mechanisms for tinnitus (Jastreboff 1990; Hazell and Jastreboff 1990), this seems unlikely. Cochlear mechanisms which may result in tinnitus include mechanical uncoupling of the outer hair cell (OHC) stereocilia from the basilar membrane (Tonndorf 1980) and the "edge effect"

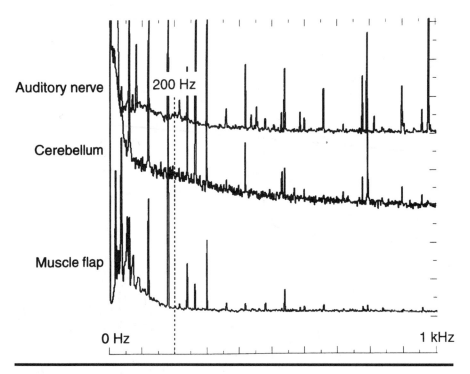

FIGURE 13-10. Power spectra recorded from the auditory nerve (upper), cerebellum (middle), and muscle flap (lower) of a patient with no preoperative history of tinnitus. A vertical cursor (dotted line) was placed at 200 Hz as a reference point.

(Kiang, Moxon, and Levine 1970; Jastreboff 1990). Free moving stereocilia could produce an increase in the physiologic noise, but it would not necessarily be near 200 Hz in all cases. The "edge effect" proposes that the OHCs immediately adjacent to a region of basilar membrane damage would be hyperactive. This is supported in that tinnitus is often tonal or narrowband in quality, implying a limited region of cochlear generation. Tinnitus is often markedly lateralized implying peripheral origin. This type of tinnitus is often associated with sensory neural hearing loss (i.e., cochlear damage). Often the frequency (or more correctly, the perceived pitch) of the tinnitus is near to the frequency of the hearing loss. This mechanism is also an unlikely candidate as a

source of consistent 200 Hz activity in the auditory nerve.

Møller (1984) suggested that in pathologies of the auditory nerve which result in demyelinization, there could be crosstalk between individual fibers, which would result in a synchronized signal being transmitted to the brain. Normally, the random firing of the auditory nerve fibers in the absence of a stimulus would produce a "white noise"-like signal which would be interpreted by the brain as silence. The pathologic synchronization due to crosstalk between fibers would be interpreted as sound by the brain. This helps explain the basis for tinnitus in the absence of cochlear function. However, this mechanism would not account for the 200 Hz peak resulting from salicylate treatments, or the human

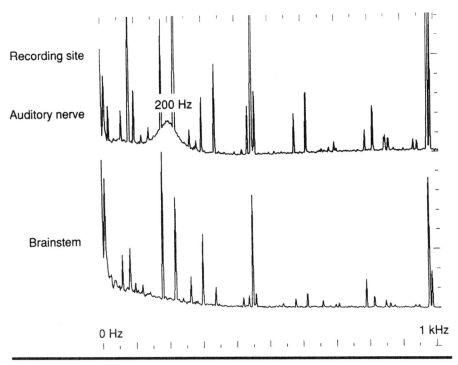

FIGURE 13-11.   Power spectra recorded from the auditory nerve (upper) and brainstem (lower) from a human subject with a history of preoperative tinnitus.

cases in which the auditory nerve had not been compromised.

Efferent fibers from the olivocochlear bundle to the cochlea have been repeatedly demonstrated to innervate the OHCs and to be regulatory (primarily inhibitory) in function. It is postulated that a region of OHC dysfunction could result in a decrease of afferent activity for that given frequency of information (Hazell 1987). To improve sound detection, the efferents which form the OCB might *reduce* their normal regulatory inhibition resulting in hyperactivity of the adjacent "healthy" OHCs. The normal ambient noise within the cochlea would be released and result in aberrant signals at frequencies near that of the damage (hearing loss). A problem with this model is that it requires ambient acoustic signals to produce tinnitus. Most sufferers report an increase

(not decrease) in their tinnitus awareness in quiet. There are, however, some examples of tinnitus exacerbation in quiet settings.

The extralemniscal pathways have been demonstrated to be in contact with the auditory pathway and have indirect effects on some types of tinnitus (Møller, Møller, and Yokota 1992b), yet there is no evidence that this activity would produce an abnormal *auditory nerve* activity as observed in these studies.

It is possible that the 200 Hz activity is related to abnormal efferent pathway activity. This would account for the ability to identify the 200 Hz peak in salicylate induced and other types of tinnitus. Collet (1993) and Veuillet and associates (Veuillet, Collet, Disant, and Morgon 1992) have linked abnormal efferent pathway activity to tinnitus by demonstrating that TEOAE could be suppressed by

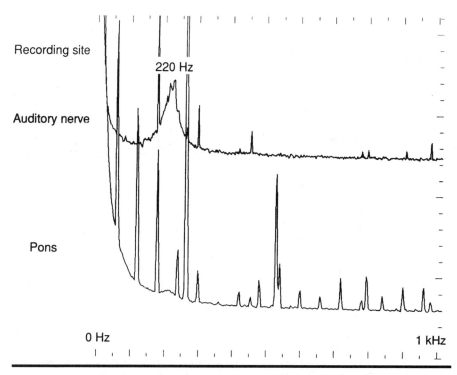

FIGURE 13-12.   Power spectra recorded from the auditory nerve (upper) and pons (lower) from a human subject with a history of preoperative tinnitus.

presenting contralateral white noise of 30 dB SL or higher in normal subjects. In over 300 tinnitus subjects, the TEOAE on the tinnitus side tended not to be suppressed by the contralateral masking (Collet 1993). This suggests the possible involvement of the medial olivocochlear bundle efferents in tinnitus and could represent the increase in spontaneous activity near 200 Hz.

Why 200 Hz?   At first glance, activity at 200 Hz matches nicely with the increase energy in the ABR spectra of tinnitus sufferers compared to non-tinnitus controls noted by Jastreboff, Ikner, and Hassen (1992; mentioned in the Background section of this chapter). This would be convenient; however, the activity noted by Jastreboff is an increase in the 200 Hz component of the stimulus

locked evoked potential, and not representative of a continuous signal. The 200 Hz peak identified by spectral averaging would be averaged out in the normal process of acquiring the ABR. Therefore, the similarity ends at the numeric value. It is difficult to postulate why there might be an increase in activity at 200 Hz or why the activity above and below 200 Hz may selectively decrease. This will have to be determined by extensive studies employing single-unit recordings in parallel with recording from the auditory nerve as a whole.

Is the 200 Hz peak related to tinnitus?   The animal and human evidence, thus far, indicate a link between the spectral peak and tinnitus. Unfortunately, one cannot rule out that the peak is merely an indicator of a peripheral auditory disorder resulting in aberrant auditory neural activity. Studies must be performed in subjects who have tinnitus and no peripheral auditory dysfunction.

CONCLUSIONS

Spectral analysis of neural activity opens new doors to the study of tinnitus. It provides a means to study continuous low amplitude normal and abnormal auditory activity in animals and humans. It opens the door to noninvasive work in multiple species and provides a quantitative tool for evaluating what looks and acts like tinnitus. As of today, the most likely candidate for the spectral peak near 200 Hz is activity from the efferent auditory system. As in all aspects of tinnitus, much work remains to be done, especially employing subjects having tinnitus in the absence of peripheral hearing disorders.

None of the spectral analysis studies performed by our laboratory could have been performed without the expertise and assistance of John Schwegler, M.A., our resident physicist, mathematician, and systems specialist. Hillel Pratt, Ph.D. assisted in the acquisition of the human data. The surgeons who were instrumental in providing patients as subjects for this study include Drs. William Buchheit, Eugene Flamm, Max Ronis, Seth Rosenberg, and Robert Rosenwasser. Insightful review and critique were provided by David Stapells, Ph.D.

The original work presented in this chapter was supported by the Garifeld Foundation, the Bernard Fishman Foundation, and Biomedical Research Support Grant SO7 RR05417 from the National Institutes of Health.

REFERENCES

Chesseboeuf, L., Herard, J., and Trevin, J. 1979. "Comparative Study of Two Vasoregulators in Syndromes of Deafness and Vertigo." *Medecine du Nord et de l'Est, 5,* 534.

Claussen, E. and Claussen, C-F. 1981. "Comparative Study on the Treatment of Dizziness and Tinnitus with Rokan." *Proceedings dem Geselschaft Fur Neurootologie und Aequilibriometrie, 7,* 471–485.

Colding-Jørgensen, E., Lauritzen, M., Johnsen, N.J., Mikkelsen, K.B. and Salvmark, K. 1991. "On the Auditory Evoked Magnetic P200 Peak as an Objective Measure of Tinnitus." In J.-M. Aran and R. Dauman (Eds.), *Proceedings of the Fourth International Tinnitus Seminar, Bordeaux, France,* pp. 321–326, Amsterdam/New York: Kugler Publications.

Collet, L. 1993. "Using Otoacoustic Emissions to Explore the Medial Olivocochlear System: Clinical Application." *Proceedings and Abstracts of the Thirteenth Congress of the International Electric Response Audiometry Study Group,* Abstract B4, p. 26, Park City, September, 1993.

Dolan, D.F., Nutall, A.L., and Avinash, G. 1990. "Asynchronous Neural Activity Recorded from the Round Window." *Journal of the Acoustical Society of America, 87,* 2621–2627.

Evans, E.F., Wilson, J.P., and Borerwe, T.A. 1981. "Animal Models of Tinnitus." In *Tinnitus, Ciba Foundation Symposium, 85,* pp. 108–138. London: Pitman.

Hazell, J.W.P. 1987. "A Cochlear Model for Tinnitus." In H. Feldmann (Ed.), *Proceedings III International Tinnitus Seminar, Munster, 1987,* pp. 121–128. Karlsruhe: Harsch Verlag.

Hazell, J.W.P. and Jastreboff, P.J. 1990. "Tinnitus I: Auditory Mechanisms: a Model for Tinnitus and Hearing Impairment." *Journal of Otolaryngology, 19,* 1–5.

Hoke, M., Feldmann, H., Pantev, C., Lütkenhöner, B., and Lehnertz, K. 1989. "Objective Evidence of Tinnitus in Auditory Evoked Magnetic Fields." *Hearing Research, 37,* 281–286.

Jacobson, G.P., Ahmad, B.K., Moran, J., Newman, C.W., Tepley, N., and Wharton, J. 1991. "Auditory Evoked Cortical Magnetic Field (M100-M200) Measurements in Tinnitus and Normal Groups." *Hearing Research, 56*(1–2), 44–52.

Jacobson, G.P., Ahmad, B.K., Moran, J., Newman, C.W., Wharton, J., and Tepley, N. 1992. "Auditory Evoked Cortical Magnetic Field (M100-M200) Measurements in Tinnitus and Normal Groups." In J.-M. Aran and R. Dauman (Eds.), *Tinnitus '91,* pp. 317–322. Amsterdam/New York: Kugler Publications.

Jastreboff, P.J. 1990. "Phantom Auditory Perception (Tinnitus); Mechanisms of Generation and Perception." *Neuroscience Research, 8,* 221–254.

Jastreboff, P.J., Brennan, J.F., Coleman, J.K., and Sasaki, C.T. 1988a. "Phantom Auditory Sensation in Rats: An Animal Model for Tinnitus." *Behavioral Neuroscience, 102,* 811–822.

Jastreboff, P.J., Brennan, J.F., and Sasaki, C.T. 1988b.

"An Animal Model for Tinnitus." *Laryngoscope, 98,* 280–286.

Jastreboff, P.J., Hansen, R., Sasaki, P.G., and Sasaki, C.T. 1988c. "Differential Uptake of Salicylate in Serum, Cerebrospinal Fluid, and Perilymph." *Archives of Otolaryngology—Head and Neck Surgery, 112,* 1050–1053.

Jastreboff, P.J., Ikner, C.L., and Hassen, A. 1992. "An Approach to the Objective Evaluation of Tinnitus in Humans." In J.-M. Aran and R. Dauman (Eds.), *Tinnitus '91,* pp. 331–339. Amsterdam/New York: Kugler Publications.

Jastreboff, P.J. and Sasaki, C.T. 1986. "Salicylate-induced Changes in Spontaneous Activity of Single Units in the Inferior Colliculus of the Guinea Pig." *Journal of the Acoustical Society of America, 80,* 1384–1391.

Kiang, N.Y.S., Moxon, E.C., and Levine, R.A. 1970. "Auditory-nerve Activity in Cats with Normal and Abnormal Cochleas." In D.E.W. Wolstenholme and J. Knignt (Eds.), *Ciba Foundation Symposium on Sensorineural Hearing Loss,* pp. 241–273. London: Churchill.

Martin, F.W. and Coleman, B.H. 1980. "Tinnitus: A Double Blind Crossover Controlled Trial to Evaluate the Use of Lignocaine." *Clinical Otolaryngology (Oxford), 5,* 3–11.

Martin, W.H., Schwegler, J.W., Scheibelhoffer, J., and Ronis, M.L. 1993. "Salicylate-induced Changes in Cat Auditory Nerve Activity." *The Laryngoscope, 103,* 600–604.

Melding, P.S., Goodey, R.J., and Thorne, P.R. 1978. "The Use of Intravenous Lidocaine in the Diagnosis and Treatment of Tinnitus." *Journal of Laryngology and Otology, 92,* 115–121.

Meyer, B. 1986. "A Multicenter Randomized Double-blind Study of Ginkgo biloba versus Placebo in the Treatment of Tinnitus." *Presse Medicale, 15,* 1562–1564.

Møller, A.R. 1984. "Pathophysiology of Tinnitus." *Annals of Otology, Rhinology, and Laryngology, 93,* 39–44.

Møller, A. R., Møller, M.B., Jannetta, P.J., and Jho, H.D. 1992a. "Compound Action Potentials Recorded from the Exposed Eighth Nerve in Patients with Intractable Tinnitus." *Laryngoscope, 102,* 187–197.

Møller, A. R., Møller, M.B., and Yokota, M. 1992b. "Some Forms of Tinnitus May Involve the Extra-lemniscal Auditory Pathway." *Laryngoscope, 102,* 1165–1171.

Natali, R., Rachinel, J., and Pouyat, P.M. 1979. "Comparative Crossover Trial of Two Vasoactive Drugs in E.N.T. Practice." *Cahiers d'Otorhinolaryngologie, 2,* 185–190.

Pantev, C., Hoke, M., Lütkenhöner, B., Lehnertz, K., and Kumph, W. 1989. "Tinnitus Remission Objectified by Neuromagnetic Measurements." *Hearing Research, 40,* 261–264.

Schreiner, C.E. and Snyder, R.L. 1987. "A Physiological Animal Model of Peripheral Tinnitus." In H. Feldmann (Ed.), *Proceedings III International Tinnitus Seminar, Munster, 1987,* pp. 100–106. Karlsruhe: Harsch Verlag.

Shea, J.J. and Harell, M. 1978. "Management of Tinnitus Aurium with Lidocaine and Carbamazepine." *Laryngoscope, 88,* 1477–1484.

Tonndorf, J. 1981. "Tinnitus and Physiological Correlates of the Cochlea-vestibular System: Peripheral; Central." *Journal of Laryngology, Suppl. 4,* 18–20.

Veuillet, E. Collet, L., Disant, F., and Morgon, A. 1992. "Tinnitus and Medial Cochlear Efferent System." In J.-M. Aran and R. Dauman (Eds.), *Tinnitus '91,* pp. 205–209. Amsterdam/New York: Kugler Publications.

CHAPTER 14

THE INTERACTION OF CENTRAL AND PERIPHERAL MECHANISMS IN TINNITUS

MARY B. MEIKLE
Oregon Health Sciences University

Speculation concerning the mechanisms responsible for subjective tinnitus has ranged from mechanical processes in the cochlea (Evans, Wilson, and Borerwe 1982; Kemp 1981, 1982; Tonndorf 1980; Wilson and Sutton 1981) to abnormal activity of cochlear nerve fibers (Burns 1968; Eggermont 1984, 1990; Feldmann 1971; Goodhill 1954; Jastreboff and Sasaki 1986; Møller 1984; Penner 1980; Salvi and Ahroon 1983; Stevens and Davis 1938), possibly resulting from loss of efferent control mechanisms (Donaldson 1978; Hazell 1987), to central nervous system mechanisms called into play by deafferentation (Atkinson 1944; Kiang, Moxon, and Levine 1970; Sasaki, Kauer, and Babitz 1980; Tonndorf 1987; Vernon and Meikle 1985), abnormal patterning of neural inputs from the periphery (Jastreboff 1990), or epileptiform types of activity inherent to the brain (Emmett and Shea 1980; Melding, Goodey, and Thorne 1978). Such theorizing takes as its starting point the existing anatomical and physiological knowledge concerning damage or disease processes. That approach has generated a number of potentially valuable insights, and is justified by the well-known fact that tinnitus accompanies many different forms of auditory pathology (Fowler 1944); (also see General Discussion in Evered and Lawrenson 1981, pp. 232–237).

A somewhat different approach forms the starting point for the present discussion. In 1981 we established the Tinnitus Data Registry, a computerized database containing medical, audiological, and tinnitus-related information obtained from patients attending the Tinnitus Clinic of the Oregon Health Sciences University. A wealth of information from over 1600 patients is now available, including quantitative and qualitative measures of the attributes of tinnitus and their relation to hearing loss (Meikle and Griest 1989, 1991, 1992; Meikle, Griest, Press, and Stewart 1992). That phenomenological information can shed new light on neural mechanisms that might underlie tinnitus.

In the section entitled Audiological Correlates of Tinnitus, audiological and other data are presented which provide strong evidence that central as well as peripheral mechanisms appear to be involved in generating the various tinnitus localizations and pitch matches observed in the Tinnitus Clinic. The data imply that the localization and pitch of tinnitus may, initially at least, reflect the anatomical locus of peripheral auditory damage in a relatively straightforward manner. However, the evidence also suggests the existence of neural mechanisms that appear capable of modifying the initial auditory processes. These mechanisms, which are in all likelihood central, appear to be capable of transforming the initially perceived localization and pitch into resultant perceptions that are less clearly related to the anatomic locus of peripheral damage. The available evidence strongly supports the concept that there are dynamic processes which tend in many cases to alter the perceived tinnitus over time.

The section on Physiological Mechanisms introduces several physiological mechanisms that could (1) generate tinnitus-related neural activity from damaged zones at the auditory periphery, and (2) transform its central representation in ways that are consistent with the tinnitus characteristics observed in Tinnitus Clinic patients. These suggestions are based in large part on physiological work in the somatosensory system, because of the well-known analogies between the cutaneous and auditory senses. In an earlier discussion we emphasized the many similarities between tinnitus and pain (Vernon and Meikle 1985). Since that time, physiological evidence concerning central auditory-system plasticity has shown that central auditory structures can exhibit changes that are very similar to those observed in central somatosensory regions following peripheral damage. The present discussion extends the analogy between tinnitus and pain by relating recent physiological findings in both the auditory and cutaneous modalities to possible tinnitus mechanisms.

Whether or not the mechanisms suggested here do in fact account for the many varieties of tinnitus that have been observed, they do, nevertheless, serve to focus the discussion in regard to a specific conceptual framework. In this conceptualization, the most common location for initiation of tinnitus is the auditory end-organ, although abnormal functioning at higher auditory structures could equally well serve to initiate a phantom auditory perception. Regardless of where in the auditory system the aberrant activity originates, cochleotopic representation and the tendency for sensory percepts to be referred to the corresponding peripheral locus probably come into play. However, normal auditory processing has difficulty accounting for the observed pitch, loudness, and localization in many cases of tinnitus. Instead, it appears that deviations from a simple tonotopic mapping of abnormal auditory neural activity act so as to modify the resulting tinnitus percept. That is, abnormal central neural

mechanisms appear to extend, shift, or otherwise distort the neural map that gives rise to the perception of tinnitus pitch. Such deviations would also be expected to influence loudness perceptions, in a manner to be described below in the section on Relevance of the Model to the Perceived Loudness of Tinnitus. Further, deviations from the normal balance between binaural neural representations of sound localization would be expected to affect the neural map of auditory space within which tinnitus sensations are localized (Relevance of the Model to the Perceived Localization of Tinnitus, below). Thus, the physiological mechanisms suggested below may help to explain the range of tinnitus percepts typically encountered in the Tinnitus Clinic population.

AUDIOLOGICAL CORRELATES OF TINNITUS: EVIDENCE FOR BOTH PERIPHERAL AND CENTRAL DETERMINANTS

It should be emphasized that the data in the Tinnitus Data Registry are derived from patients with clinically significant tinnitus—that is, individuals whose tinnitus is sufficiently noticeable and/or disabling that it is their primary complaint in seeking professional help. Tinnitus in such individuals is likely to be more severe than in patients for whom the tinnitus is not the primary complaint. Tinnitus Clinic patients probably also display more severe levels of tinnitus than are typical for the general population of individuals in the U.S. with tinnitus—for example, the tinnitus severity ratings selected by Tinnitus Clinic patients tend to be higher than those selected by the general membership of the American Tinnitus Association (1986).

Unpublished observations that we have obtained in individuals with mild or weak tinnitus indicate that such tinnitus is often difficult to match to external sounds as the tinnitus tends to disappear when testing is initiated. Such lability of tinnitus perceptions is *not* typical of Tinnitus Clinic patients, in the majority of whom the tinnitus has stabilized, making it possible to obtain reliable measures of both qualitative and quantitative aspects of tinnitus (Graham and Newby 1962; Hazell, Wood, Cooper, Stephens, Corcoran, Coles, Baskill, and Sheldrake 1985; Meikle and Griest 1987, 1991; Meikle, Schuff, and Griest 1987; Nodar 1978; Vernon 1988; Vernon and Meikle 1981, 1988).

Tinnitus Pitch

Assuming that the pitch-matching procedures are performed with care to avoid loudness differences, residual inhibition, and octave confusions (Vernon 1987; Vernon and Meikle 1981, 1988), most Tinnitus Clinic patients are easily capable of matching the pitch of their tinnitus to external tones. The range of pitch matches for our present sample of 1033 tinnitus patients extends from 80 Hz to 16,000 Hz. Figure 14-1 summarizes the prevalence of the various pitch matches by grouping them in five successive frequency intervals.

An interesting result becomes evident from these Tinnitus Clinic data if we compute the mean audiograms for the five different pitch groups. As Figure 14-2 shows, the group with lowest pitch (<1500 Hz) has the greatest amount of hearing loss, and conversely the group with highest pitch (> 8500 Hz) has the least hearing loss. In between those two extremes, the hearing levels (HLs) for the three intermediate-pitch groups maintain an orderly progression, with the amount of hearing loss inversely related to the pitch of tinnitus. Statistical analysis of the audiometric data for the five groups indicates a highly significant association (p<.0001) between the pitch of tinnitus and the amount of hearing loss. Thus, to the extent that pure tone thresholds are primarily indicative of peripheral types of hearing impairment (Berlin and Lowe 1972; Davis and Silverman 1970), it is

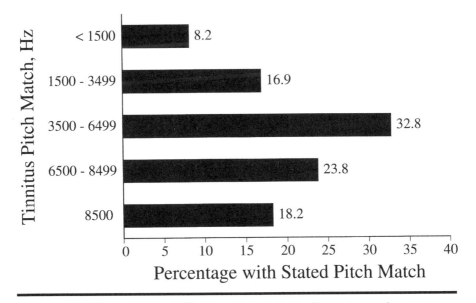

FIGURE 14-1. Pitch matches in Tinnitus Clinic patients. Percentages shown are based on a total of 946 patients who matched the pitch of their predominant tinnitus sound. (87 patients out of the total sample of 1033 were unable to perform the necessary pitch match, because of hearing difficulties or because their tinnitus was too complex or variable to match to a single value.)

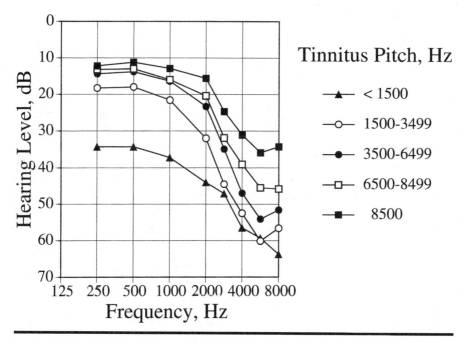

FIGURE 14-2.   Relation between tinnitus pitch and the audiogram. Mean thresholds are plotted for the right ear for each of the 5 pitch groups summarized in Figure 14-1. Repeated-measures ANOVA (5 pitch groups x 8 audiogram frequencies) demonstrated a highly significant relationship between tinnitus pitch and hearing thresholds ($p < .0001$).

clear that peripheral hearing losses exert a strong effect on the perceived pitch of tinnitus.

On the other hand, if we consider the audiograms within a group of individuals selected so as to have identical pitch matches, there are large individual differences in regard to the audiometric configurations observed. Figure 14-3 gives some idea of the wide variation of audiograms in a subset of patients with unilateral tinnitus who matched their tinnitus pitch to 3 kHz. That frequency was chosen quite arbitrarily, because it is a pitch match identified by a relatively large number of patients. For this analysis, the selection was also restricted to patients with tinnitus consisting of only one sound; there was a total of 16 patients meeting these selection criteria. The six cases shown in Figure 14-3 are not excep-

tional, but were chosen because they are representative of the various types of audiograms within the group.

It is clear from Figure 14-3 that the pitch of unilateral 3 kHz tinnitus need not correspond to any consistent audiometric configuration. It thus seems unlikely that the hearing impairment by itself constitutes the sole determinant of the pitch of tinnitus. Rather, one or more additional factors must be operating to generate similar pitch matches in such widely divergent audiometric configurations. A tenable hypothesis is that these other factor(s) are operating in the central nervous system. The net conclusion from the data displayed in Figures 14-2 and 14-3 is that the pitch of tinnitus is likely to be under the control of both peripheral and central mechanisms.

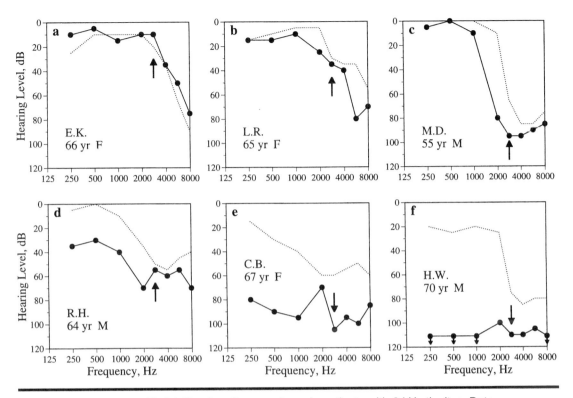

FIGURE 14-3.   Variability of audiogram shape in patients with 3 kHz tinnitus. Data are shown for 6 representative patients selected to illustrate the range of audiometric variations in the group with unilateral 3 kHz tinnitus. Thresholds for the tinnitus ear are plotted using filled circles and heavy lines; dotted lines show thresholds for the contralateral ear. Arrows indicate tinnitus pitch matches at 3 kHz. Tinnitus precipitating circumstances identified by patients were: (a) head cold; (b) unknown (no noise exposure); (c) military helicopters, 9 years; (d) World War II combat noise; (e) radical mastoid surgery; (f) sudden hearing loss, with prior exposure to damaging occupational noise.

Tinnitus Localization

In previous work we have discussed the relationship between audiometric configurations and the perceived localization of tinnitus (Meikle and Griest 1987). More recently we made use of the method of Principal Components Analysis to analyze the audiometric data for the same 1033 Tinnitus Clinic patients described in the preceding section (Meikle et al. 1992). We showed that fac-

tor analysis techniques succeeded in identifying an "Asymmetry Factor"—that is, a factor was extracted from the audiometric data which effectively quantified the individual variations within the Clinic population in regard to interaural acuity differences. We then found that this Asymmetry Factor was strongly related to the localization of tinnitus, as shown in Figure 14-4.

It is clear that patients with non-lateralized tinnitus (those reporting tinnitus that is perceived

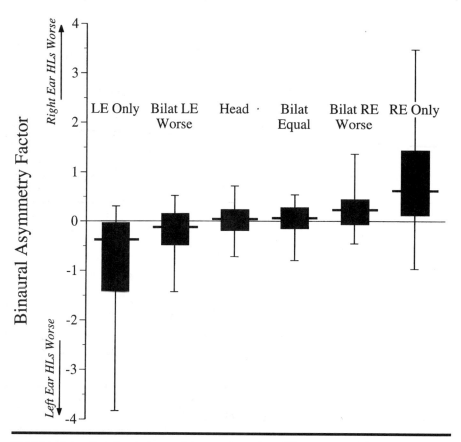

FIGURE 14-4.   Relation between interaural hearing differences and the perceived localization of tinnitus. Box-and-whisker plots (Tukey, 1977) of the distributions of patients' factor scores on the Binaural Asymmetry Factor. The Tinnitus Clinic patients were divided into 6 groups based on their tinnitus localization, as shown. Positive values of the Factor indicate right-ear HLs are worse; negative values indicate left-ear HLs worse. Each black box encloses the range from the 25th to the 75th percentile for that group (median factor scores for each group are indicated by short horizontal line transecting each box); vertical lines or "whiskers" connect the 5th and 95th percentiles. One-way ANOVA showed the relation between hearing asymmetry and tinnitus localization to be highly significant (p<.0001).

"in the head" or in "both ears equally") tend to have audiometric configurations that are bilaterally symmetrical. By contrast, patients reporting unilateral tinnitus tend to have highly asymmetrical audiograms, with the greater hearing loss on the side where the tinnitus is localized. Intermedi-

ate levels of audiometric asymmetry are displayed by patients with bilateral tinnitus that is louder on one side than on the other. Statistical analysis of the data illustrated in Figure 14-4 indicates that there is a strong association (p<.0001) between the localization of tinnitus and the extent and direction of audiometric asymmetry, as quantified by the Asymmetry Factor. The relative magnitude and location of the hearing loss thus appears to play an important role in establishing the perceived localization of tinnitus. To the extent that the audiogram measures peripheral hearing loss, peripheral mechanisms would appear to exert considerable control over tinnitus localizations.

Despite that generalization, there are patients in whom the tinnitus localization is *not* concordant with the degree of hearing asymmetry. This can be demonstrated especially clearly in individuals who exhibit marked differences between the acuity of the two ears. Within that group there is a small percentage who localize their tinnitus to the better-hearing side (Meikle and Griest 1987). Figure 14-5 shows representative examples of such individuals. From these and a number of similar cases it is clear that the extent and nature of peripheral hearing loss cannot be the only determinants of tinnitus localization. Despite the strong association between the hearing loss and the localization of tinnitus as revealed above in Figure 14-4, it is clear that other factors must also be contributing to the perceived localization of tinnitus in cases such as those displayed in Figure 14-5. Again, a plausible inference is that these other factors involve central neural mechanisms.

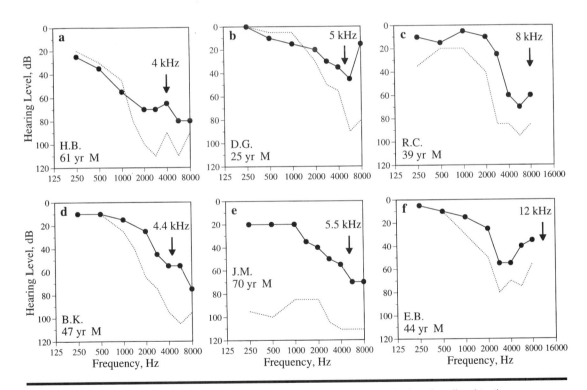

FIGURE 14-5. Representative audiograms for patients with tinnitus localized to the better-hearing ear. Thresholds for the tinnitus ear are shown by filled circles and heavy lines; dotted lines show thresholds for the contralateral ear. Arrows indicate the frequencies matching the tinnitus pitch in each case.

Additional Evidence for Concurrent Involvement of Central and Peripheral Tinnitus Mechanisms

The preceding discussions made use of group comparisons, and did not address the question whether tinnitus within a single individual might involve both peripheral and central mechanisms. Conceivably, the localization and pitch of tinnitus could be dictated solely by peripheral factors in certain individuals (those with tinnitus resulting solely from peripheral auditory disorders), while central factors might be operative in other patients whose tinnitus developed as the result of central pathology (e.g., brain trauma or disease, or systemic conditions that can affect the central nervous system such as hypertension, atherosclerosis, metabolic dysfunction, and so forth). However, there is evidence of multiple causality in many tinnitus cases, and it seems very likely that both central and peripheral tinnitus mechanisms are operating together in many tinnitus patients. Moreover, it is probable that central mechanisms can come into play in individuals who have only experienced peripheral types of hearing damage. Support for that assertion comes from several lines of clinical evidence.

First, there is an interesting group of patients whose tinnitus started in one ear and over time gradually became bilateral—*with the identical sound perceived on both sides*. Of the 1033 patients currently available for analysis in the Tinnitus Data Registry, 140, or nearly 14 percent reported that this type of change occurred (in 8 percent the tinnitus started on the left, while in 6 percent the tinnitus was noted first on the right). Within this group, 66 patients reported either centrally acting etiological circumstances (such as head injury) acting alone, or else reported a combination of peripheral and centrally acting causal factors. In the remaining 74 patients the precipitating factors, when any could be identified, were exclusively peripheral (most commonly, exposure to excessive noise).

The striking fact here is that when these patients later detected tinnitus in a second location,

that tinnitus appeared to be identical in pitch and sound quality to the tinnitus still being perceived in the first location; as far as the patients were concerned, it was "the same sound". Such unanimity is hard to explain if strictly peripheral processes account for the tinnitus perceptions, for it seems highly improbable that noise-induced damage or other peripheral insults would produce precisely the same anatomical pattern of dysfunction on each side, even in the unlikely event that the two ears of an individual are exposed to exactly equivalent events. The more typical situation is for the two ears in any given individual to express different degrees of peripheral pathology, as indicated by dissimilarities between the audiograms in the two ears of most individuals (Phillips, Trune, and Mitchell 1990).

The conclusion that seems unavoidable in these cases of bilateral, identical tinnitus is that mechanism(s) must exist within the central nervous system that are capable of causing peripherally induced tinnitus to be perceived bilaterally once it has become established as a unilateral perception. That is, there appears to be some type of CNS plasticity that accounts for the transition from unilateral to bilateral tinnitus having the same characteristics on both sides. This phenomenon, which has also been noted in previous observations from a very different clinical population (Atkinson 1944), is reminiscent of the "mirror image" duplication of central pain sensations that appear to spread from one side of the body to the other (Livingston 1943).

A second line of evidence implicating the participation of central factors in peripherally induced tinnitus involves the tendency of tinnitus sensations to persist despite section or destruction of the auditory nerve on the side where the tinnitus is perceived (Dandy 1941; House and Brackmann 1981). The fact that the tinnitus persisting after nerve section continues to exhibit clearly definable pitch and other specific spectral characteristics, typically reported in terms normally used to describe external sounds, suggests that there is some central neural process that is capable of mimicking the sensory characteristics of normal auditory stimuli that formerly elicited hearing sensations from the operated ear.

A related situation is that of near-total hearing loss accompanied by tinnitus. Although we can never know how many or which neural units may remain in an ear with "no usable hearing", (e.g., HLs > 90 dB at all frequencies), we can infer that the active neuronal population is probably very sparse, and may be functioning abnormally. The fact that individuals who report hearing tinnitus in the "dead" ear are able to provide reliable matches for the pitch when appropriate stimuli are presented to the other ear (e.g., Figure 14-3f), indicates that the spectral characteristics of their tinnitus are relatively independent of the precise location and extent of cochlear damage in the affected ear.

PHYSIOLOGICAL MECHANISMS FOR THE PERCEIVED ATTRIBUTES OF TINNITUS

In the normal individual it appears that auditory percepts such as the pitch, loudness, and localization of sounds are the combined result of peripheral encoding processes acted upon by central neural mechanisms. The normal central mechanisms undoubtedly exert various types of transformations upon the afferent neural activity that encodes stimulus dimensions such as sound frequency, intensity, and location in space. It is clear that abnormalities of functioning could be interposed at any stage in this complex sequence of events, starting at the auditory periphery and continuing into the CNS where the final level of conscious perception is attained. For example, the normal mechanisms for preserving tonotopic organization or for processing binaural inputs might be missing or functioning abnormally. Therefore, in the abnormal perceptual states accompanying hearing loss, neural transformations that are as yet unknown may well be operating on the neural activity within the auditory system, whether or not that activity is elicited by sound. Keeping in mind that conscious perceptions are likely to be dependent on activity at relatively higher levels within the auditory CNS (Jenkins and

Merzenich 1987), we must next consider what is known about CNS transformations imposed upon afferent neural activity in damaged or dysfunctional sensory systems.

The Pitch of Tinnitus: Evidence of "Tonotopic Remodelling"?

If most individuals' hearing losses affected only a single frequency or a narrow band of frequencies, we could understand why their tinnitus so often sounds like ringing or has a definite tonal character (Graham and Newby 1962; Meikle and Griest 1991; Meikle and Walsh 1984). The difficulty, however, is that almost all tinnitus patients exhibit hearing losses over a broad range of frequencies (Meikle and Griest 1989; Meikle et al. 1992). The problem for the physiologist then is to account for the narrowband nature of tinnitus when the underlying pathological processes affect hearing over a broad range of frequencies.

As was previously discussed, there is a clear and systematic association between the pitch of tinnitus and the audiogram, while at the same time there are substantial audiometric differences between many of the individuals who perceive the same tinnitus pitch. Evidently, some neural mechanism is operating that imposes a general tendency toward roughly similar pitch matches in the majority of individuals with a given pattern of peripheral auditory damage, while at the same time permitting substantial and apparently idiosyncratic departures from that pitch in a portion of the group.

A candidate for this neural mechanism is supplied by evidence from electrophysiological studies in animals. The phenomenon was first discovered in the somatosensory system, and consists in the demonstration that deafferentation can markedly alter somatotopic representation—that is, the mapping of peripheral stimulation onto the sensory cortex and other central nervous sites (Devor 1988; Kaas, Merzenich, and Killackey 1983; McMahon and Wall 1983). This type of CNS plasticity has been called "somatopic remodelling" (Devor

1988), and it results in a distorted sensory map within the CNS structures in question. So far, the most detailed information comes from investigations carried out in somatosensory cortex of cats, primates, and bats (Kaas 1991; Kaas et al. 1983). However, many studies have now shown that somatosensory neurons at various levels of the CNS develop expanded or shifted receptive fields after trauma to the peripheral neurons from which they receive input (Cook, Woolf, Wall, and McMahon 1987; Devor 1988; McMahon and Wall 1983, 1984; Mendell 1984; Wall and Egger 1971).

As a result of such injury-induced plasticity in the somatosensory system, there is substantial capacity for central neural structures (including the spinal cord, the dorsal column nuclei, specific sensory nuclei in the thalamus, and the primary sensory cortex) to alter their somatotopic mapping of cutaneous stimuli following deafferentation (Devor and Wall 1978; McMahon and Wall 1983, 1984; Merzenich and Jenkins 1983; Millar, Basbaum, and Wall 1976; Wall and Cusick 1984). These alterations can occur within minutes (Carrasco, Prazma, Faber, Triana, and Pillsbury 1990; Devor and Wall 1978; Dostrovsky, Millar, and Wall 1976; Merzenich, Kaas, Wall, Sur, Nelson, and Felleman 1983), and can persist for years (Pons, Garraghty, Ommaya, Kaas, Taub, and Mishkin 1991). Although the most typical change is for a CNS neuron to enlarge its receptive field by spreading out to include peripheral stimulation sites immediately adjacent to those that were initially effective (Merzenich, Nelson, Stryker, Cynder, Shoppmann, and Zook 1984) the alteration can involve much larger changes in the relationship between the body site that is stimulated and the resulting CNS location that responds to that stimulation (Kaas 1991). Large changes in the somatosensory cortex (e.g., expansion of the responsive cortical region by as much as 14 mm) appear however to be attainable only after long periods such as several years following deafferentation (Pons et al. 1991).

In the auditory system the analog for the cutaneous receptive field is the "frequency response area" (Harrison, Nagasawa, Smith, Stanton, and Mount 1991), in which neuronal responses are plotted as a function of sound frequency and intensity. Peripheral damage to the auditory system has been shown to produce enlargement of the frequency response areas of neurons in the inferior colliculus (Salvi, Powers, and Saunders 1992a, Salvi, Powers, Saunders, Boettcher, and Clock 1992b). Abnormally large response areas have also been reported in the auditory cortex of the cat (Harrison et al. 1991), in which "W-shaped" response areas for cortical neurons have been described following sound-induced damage to the cochlea. The expansion of response areas in cortical neurons might of course reflect response alterations at various subcortical levels.

Even more impressive are the damage-induced alterations in the mapping of acoustical stimuli onto the corresponding cortical response areas that have recently been demonstrated (Harrison et al. 1991; Rajan, Irvine, Calford, and Wise 1992; Robertson and Irvine 1989). For example, in one cat treated previously with the ototoxic drug amikacin to produce marked high-frequency hearing loss starting at about 4 kHz, the cortical representation for the highest frequencies was lost, and the cortical region devoted to frequencies in the 6 to 7 kHz band expanded until it occupied 74 percent of the total primary auditory area (Harrison et al. 1991). In effect, the frequencies corresponding to the low-frequency border of the cochlear damage preempted the cortical areas that originally had responded to higher frequencies.

Such results, which have been obtained in both guinea pigs and cats, suggest that it may be a common occurrence following peripheral damage for acoustical stimulation to shift its excitation pattern in the CNS. Following injury to the cochlear end organ, cortical regions that formerly responded primarily to inputs from the damaged cochlear regions do not become "silent". Instead, they alter their behavior by responding to stimuli that excite undamaged regions of the cochlea, usually regions that are adjacent to the damaged portion. What is most surprising is the magnitude of this "tonotopic remodelling"—in some cases, a very large region of auditory cortex comes to respond to a single, narrowly restricted range of tones (Harrison et al. 1991; Robertson and Irvine 1989).

Work in a number of different neural systems indicates that the reorganization of sensory maps in the CNS is a commonly occurring, perhaps universal, result of peripheral nerve damage. In addition to the somatosensory and auditory research cited above, such changes have been observed in motor cortex and in motor regions of the spinal cord following injury to the corresponding peripheral tissues (Jacobs and Donoghue 1991; Woolf 1983); and in visual portions of the CNS following interruption of visual afferent input (Eysel 1982; Kaas, Krubitzer, Chino, Langston, Polley, and Blair 1990). Thus the conclusion seems justified that response plasticity in the CNS is a widespread phenomenon following peripheral damage or other peripheral events that alter the usual pattern of afferent sensory input.

At the cellular level, it is not yet clear what mechanisms are responsible for the remodelling of sensory maps in the various CNS structures where these changes have been observed. Although there is at present considerably more data for the somatosensory system than for the auditory system, this topic remains controversial. According to recent discussions, there seems to be little evidence for neuronal sprouting in somatosensory regions of the brain, although axonal sprouting has been reported in the spinal cord (Devor 1988). Another likely candidate, strengthening of previously existing "weak" synaptic connections (e.g., by removing surrounding inhibitory influences), depends on the existence of terminal arborizations of afferent neurons having the appropriate anatomical relationships to the deafferented regions of the brain (Eysel 1982; Jacobs and Donoghue 1991; Merzenich and Jenkins 1983). Such terminations have been shown to be capable of accounting for at most 1 to 2 mm of displacement of the

responsive area in the cortex. The expansion of cortical somatotopic representations by 10 to 14 mm (as in the case of the macaques with forelimbs deafferented 12 years previous to recording) (Pons et al. 1991), probably can best be accounted for by proposing somatotopic remodelling at subcortical levels where the dimensions of the somatotopic maps are smaller than in the cortex. Because of the divergence of centripetal neural connections, a 1 to 2 mm alteration in one or more subcortical locations might be expected to result in much larger areal spread of the remodelled zone at the cortical level (Devor 1988).

In the auditory domain, the extent of areal dislocation of receptive fields for particular sound frequencies was found to be on the order of 5 mm approximately one year following peripheral auditory damage, an amount which also exceeds the limits of normal dendritic arborizations in the auditory cortex of the cat (Harrison et al. 1991). Therefore, Harrison agrees with Kaas and colleagues (1991) in suggesting that the cochleotopic remapping probably represents both cortical changes and the cumulative effects of a "series of smaller reorganizations at lower levels in the system" (Harrison et al. 1991).

The evidence cited above suggests that many of the Tinnitus Clinic patients are likely to be affected by distortions of tonotopic representation, and that in such patients, auditory stimulation that excites cochlear elements located at or near the border of damage would activate CNS regions that are larger than normal. That suggestion may prove to be testable in humans if CNS imaging and spatial analysis techniques continue to improve in sensitivity and resolution (Belliveau, Kennedy, McKinstry, Buchbinder, Weisskoff, Cohen, Vevea, Brady, and Rosen 1991; Cheyne, Kristeva, and Deecke 1991; Fox, Raichle, Mintun, and Dence 1988; Pantev, Hoke, Lütkenhöner, and Lehnertz 1989). The next question is therefore, what mechanisms exist that could lead to sustained activation of the cochlea or the CNS in the absence of discernible external sound?

The Chronic Nature of Tinnitus: What Sustains It?

Much has been written about the capacity of the somatosensory CNS to sustain pain sensations after the initial peripheral damage has healed (reviewed in Fields 1990, Waxman 1988). This very large body of work contains many suggestions concerning neural mechanisms subserving chronic pain, including such topics as "central pain" (Fields, Dubner, and Cervero 1985), "deafferentation pain" (Fields 1990) "phantom pain" (Wall and Devor 1982), and so on. From this literature we know that the somatosensory system is easily capable of sustaining pain sensations indefinitely. One of the most interesting points of similarity between the somatic and the auditory sensory systems is that tinnitus can resemble chronic pain in many regards, including the frequent persistence of both tinnitus and pain despite attempts to cut or block the relevant afferent pathways (Atkinson 1944; Tonndorf 1987; Vernon and Meikle 1985).

Continued, long-term perception of pain referred to the periphery, despite the absence of detectable somatic stimulation, presents the same problem for somatosensory physiologists as that encountered by auditory physiologists in attempting to explain the persistence of tinnitus. That is, what maintains the neural activity that is perceived as pain by the somatosensory system or as tinnitus by the auditory system? Which are the neural elements that are likely to be maintaining continued activity despite the absence of corresponding external stimuli?

CNS Sensitization in the Somatosensory System.

Recent research into the physiological mechanisms responsible for abnormal, chronic pain has resulted in the demonstration that certain types of spinal cord neurons can become hyperexcitable when exposed to noxious stimulation (Devor 1988; Hoheisel and Mense 1989; Roberts 1986). The process begins when there is intense or traumatizing stimulation of peripheral tissue, following which there is a dramatic alteration of the responses of spinal neurons that receive input from the traumatized region (Roberts 1986). Prior to trauma, so-called "wide-dynamic-range neurons" respond vigorously to inputs from pain receptors (projecting centrally via small-diameter unmyelinated fibers), but respond only weakly to stimulation of low-threshold mechanoreceptors (projecting centrally via larger-diameter myelinated fibers) (Maixner, Dubner, Bushnell, Kenshalo, and Oliveras 1986; Roberts 1986). After traumatic or noxious stimulation of the skin (e.g., pinching, crushing, cutting, burning, etc.) the spinal neurons become more responsive to all types of input (Cook et al. 1987; Hoheisel and Mense 1989; Kramis, Gillette, and Roberts 1991; Roberts 1986; Roberts and Kramis 1990). In particular, the sensitization causes them to respond strongly to gentle mechanical stimulation of the skin that formerly caused only a minimal response or was even subthreshold. In effect, the sensitized neurons now exhibit increased gain for all sensory inputs that succeed in activating them. According to one hypothesis concerning the mechanisms responsible for chronic pain, sensitization or hyperexcitability of the wide-dynamic-range neurons represents the first step in the process of setting up sustained neural activity responsible for chronic pain (Roberts 1986; Roberts and Kramis 1990).

Sensitized Responding by CNS Neurons to Normally Ineffective Sympathetic Activity.

The second step in setting up persistent pain, as proposed by Roberts and his associates, involves tonic activation of peripheral mechanoreceptors by sympathetic efferents that terminate in their vicinity (Roberts 1986; Roberts and Kramis 1990). Normally, this tonic sympathetic activity passes unnoticed; however, after peripheral trauma has sensitized the CNS, they propose that the tonic activity of sympathetic efferents, and the resulting activation of low-threshold mechanoreceptors, becomes an adequate stimulus for provoking vigorous, continual activation of wide-dynamic-range neurons in the spinal cord—the same neurons which formerly responded primarily to pain inputs. The sympathetic activation of peripheral mechanoreceptors could occur either synaptically or through localized release of neurotransmitters, but in either case the sympathetic activity would produce continuously maintained activation of wide-dynamic-range neurons, and therefore continuously maintained pain sensations. It is important to note that not all peripheral trauma results in persistent pain, and that individuals differ widely not only in regard to the type and extent of permanent damage they sustain, but also in regard to the presence or absence of chronic pain states. Consistent with that observation, not all peripheral somatic trauma causes spinal cord sensitization. That fact will become relevant to the discussion below, when it is considered that not all hearing-impaired individuals develop tinnitus.

Sensitization and Sympathetic Activation in the Auditory System. Because of the many similarities already noted between tinnitus and pain (Aran and Cazals 1981; Tonndorf 1987; Vernon and Meikle 1985), it appears reasonable to suggest that somewhat similar mechanisms might be at work in producing abnormal responses following peripheral auditory damage. Noxious stimulation of the auditory periphery appears capable both of damaging the cochlear end-organ and sensitizing the CNS neurons onto which the affected VIII nerve fibers synapse. Sensitization as indicated by decreased thresholds to electrical stimulation has been demonstrated in the cochlear nucleus and inferior colliculus following damaging exposures to intense sound (Gerken 1979; Gerken, Saunders, and Paul 1984; Gerken, Simhadri-Sumithra, and Bhat 1986). When testing of evoked responses is done using acoustical stimuli, decreased thresholds and/or increased response amplitudes have been reported following acoustic overstimulation (Lonsbury-Martin and Martin 1981; Salvi et al. 1992a, 1992b; Salvi, Saunders, Gratton, Arehole, and Powers 1990). There is also preliminary evidence for increases in the background or resting activity in some higher auditory centers when animals are exposed to tinnitus-inducing agents such as salicylates (Jastreboff and Sasaki 1987) or dam-

aging levels of noise (Lonsbury-Martin and Martin 1981; Salvi 1976). Thus, the auditory system appears to resemble the somatosensory system in that noxious peripheral stimulation can increase the excitability of neural elements in the CNS.

In a sensitized condition, the central auditory neurons would be expected to respond unusually vigorously to inputs that were formerly inadequate for eliciting central neural responses. Thus, it seems reasonable to suggest that tinnitus may be the perceptual outcome when certain auditory CNS neurons, in a manner analogous to the spinal cord wide-dynamic-range neurons, respond to peripheral damage or debility by becoming sensitized to previously ineffective and innocuous stimuli.

The scheme proposed by Roberts and his colleagues (1986, 1990) is suggestive regarding possible sympathetic actions in generating tinnitus. Although the anatomical details are not yet complete, there is considerable work which indicates a significant sympathetic innervation of the cochlea. One portion of the sympathetic innervation to the cochlea is associated with blood vessels, while a separate portion appears to be unrelated to any vascular function (Brechtelsbauer, Prazma, Garrett, Carrasco, and Pillsbury 1990; Densert and Flock 1974; Ross 1973; Spoendlin 1988; Spoendlin and Lichtensteiger 1966). The terminal portions of the nonvascular sympathetic efferents appear to be closely intermingled with cochlear nerve afferents just medial to the habenula perforata. Physiological investigation has shown that surgical excision of the superior cervical ganglion decreases the amplitude of suprathreshold auditory nerve responses (Hultcrantz, Nuttall, Brown, and Lawrence 1982). Further, electrical stimulation of the ganglion increases the amplitude of auditory nerve responses (Pickles 1979). If activity in the sympathetic fibers can excite cochlear nerve fibers in humans, tonic sympathetic activity might well be capable of eliciting or modulating ongoing cochlear nerve activity in such a way as to evoke sensations of sound in the absence of acoustic stimulation. The suggestion that tinnitus might be dependent on sympathetic activation also fits well with the fact that a substantial percentage of Tinnitus Clinic patients report that stress, fatigue, and anxiety make their tinnitus worse (Meikle et al. 1987) (also see Evered and Lawrenson 1981, pp. 232–238). These observations suggest that alterations of sympathetic tone may exert measurable physiological effects at some level of the auditory system.

There is also evidence of sympathetic effects on cochlear blood flow (Beausaing-Linder and Hultcrantz 1980; Dengerink and Wright 1988; Miller, Ren, Laurikainen, Quirk, and Nuttall 1992), possibly mediated by the perivascular sympathetic efferents (Carrasco et al. 1990). Sympathetic modulation of cochlear blood flow might thus contribute to sensations of pulsating tinnitus, a type of tinnitus that is reported by some patients (Hazell 1981). In our experience, tinnitus that has a pulsating quality is most often described as an intermittent accompaniment superimposed on otherwise constant ringing, hissing, or other types of sounds (Meikle and Whitney 1984). The inconsistent nature of the pulsations in many patients might indicate that such pulsations are dependent on dynamically changing states such as local or systemic levels of sympathetic activity.

The hypothesis that the sympathetic system may be involved in generating tinnitus is an old one, dating back to the work of Lempert, Atkinson, and others who attempted to relieve tinnitus by sympathetic ganglion block or extirpation (Atkinson 1944; Lempert 1946; Passe 1953). It might be objected that the earlier work did not bolster the argument in favor of sympathetic involvement in tinnitus, as surgical interference with sympathetic effects on the ear apparently did not achieve widespread or lasting success. However, the methods used for evaluating tinnitus were then crude, and little evidence was offered to substantiate the reported tinnitus relief apart from anecdotal or testimonial types of information. Furthermore, the surgical approach was quite invasive and likely to generate unwanted side effects. For all of these reasons, such attempts to demonstrate sympathetic involvement in tinnitus

were eventually dropped from further consideration. It is possible, however, that modern techniques for pharmacological manipulation of the sympathetic system and its effects on the ear might be successfully applied to a renewed examination of this hypothesis.

Nonsympathetic Mechanisms That Might Maintain Sustained Activity in the Auditory CNS. Even without sympathetic effects upon the inner ear, there are other mechanisms that might contribute to sustained low-level activation of the cochlear nerve and auditory CNS. First, there is normally a high rate of resting activity in many cochlear nerve afferents (Kiang, Watanabe, Thomas, and Clark 1965) and this activity evidently does not generate perceptions of sound in normally hearing individuals who do not experience tinnitus. If, however, there are central neurons which become sensitized due to traumatizing events at the periphery, as suggested in the previous section, then it might well be the case that resting discharge rates in cochlear nerve fibers could drive the sensitized CNS neurons to respond as though a suprathreshold acoustic stimulus were present. Because the spontaneous rates of cochlear nerve fibers in undamaged regions of the cochlea can remain high (Liberman and Kiang 1978), such neurons could continue to drive sensitized CNS neurons even after inputs from damaged portions of the cochlea had been interrupted. All that would be needed is for some portion of the CNS neurons to have sufficiently broad response areas that they receive input both from the damaged region and some relatively undamaged region. Evidence that some CNS neurons display broadly tuned responses following peripheral damage (Harrison et al. 1991; Salvi et al. 1992a) suggests that such neurons might serve as putative sites for sensitization-induced responding to resting activity of cochlear afferents.

Second, it is also possible that cochlear nerve fibers could generate abnormally elevated levels of spontaneous activity, thus providing input to CNS neurons, and such increased activity might generate conscious perceptions of sound whether or not the CNS neurons were sensitized. This is the now-classic hypothesis that tinnitus represents an elevation of spontaneous activity of the auditory nerve (Goodhill 1954; McFadden 1982; Stevens and Davis 1938). Evidence concerning this hypothesis remains equivocal, however, as extensive investigation in animals exposed to ototoxic drugs or to damaging levels of noise has generated mixed results. A few studies have found increases in spontaneous activity (Evans and Borerwe 1982; Salvi and Ahroon 1983), while a number of others have found either no change or else depression of spontaneous activity (Dallos and Harris 1978; Kiang et al. 1970; Liberman and Kiang 1978). If the tinnitus in noise-exposed or drug-treated humans results from elevated levels of spontaneous activity in auditory nerve fibers, it is surprising that the phenomenon is not easier to demonstrate in animal models.

Possibly a more likely source that might contribute to sustained excitation of the auditory CNS is the presence of ambient sound. Everyone who has sat quietly in a soundproof chamber to undergo audiometric testing is aware of the interfering noises created by autogenous sound sources including breathing, heartbeats, and other barely perceptible movements that can generate noise. It is clear that even when individuals are in a quiet environment, their ears are subjected to non-negligible levels of sound. Although the frequency content of such sounds is likely to be lower than the perceived pitch in most cases of tinnitus (particularly if autogenous sounds are conducted to the cochlea through sound-dampening body tissues), that objection can be overruled if tonotopic distortion increases the effectiveness of lower-frequency sounds for activating higher-frequency CNS regions, as previously described. Particularly if sensitization has occurred in CNS neurons that respond to ambient sound frequencies, it might be possible for high-frequency tinnitus of moderate or even high intensity (such as that typically reported by tinnitus sufferers) to be perceived, even though the affected individual is exposed to nothing more than very modest levels of lower-frequency ambient sound. In this connection, it should be recalled that a large percentage of individuals with tinnitus have relatively normal hearing levels below about 2 kHz (Meikle et al. 1992), and thus should be capable of hearing a considerable portion of the ambient sound.

It could be objected that severely hearing-impaired people, who often have tinnitus, will not hear much, if any, ambient sound, particularly if they have "flat" or low-frequency hearing losses. However, this group has been shown to be the group least likely to be affected by sleep disturbance due to tinnitus (Meikle, Griest, and Press, unpublished observations), a finding which might indicate that their tinnitus recedes or becomes less noticeable when ambient sound levels fall below the level of audibility for them. It is also possible that in the most profoundly hearing-impaired, CNS sensitization is especially widespread, long-lasting, or extreme in other regards, and that neural excitation responsible for tinnitus sensations maintains itself more independently of peripheral sensory inputs (in a manner similar to that of phantom limb pain).

Relation of Sensitized Neurons to Tonotopic Maps

Thus far, we have hypothesized (1) the existence of altered cochleotopic mapping, as the result of deafferentation and consequent reassignment of adjacent frequency regions to the deafferented zone; and (2) the maintenance of neural input to the deafferented zone by sensitization of CNS units that receive inputs from remaining cochlear neurons that are continuously generating impulses (either spontaneously, or in response to sympathetic activation or to low-level ambient sound). The next question is, what is the precise anatomical location within which sensitized CNS neurons would be found, and which cochlear neurons would be likely to provide the necessary input to them to maintain a sustained perception of tinnitus?

Sensitization would be expected to occur

within those CNS region(s) that normally receive input from the cochlear regions that are damaged. The well-known effects of excessive sound stimulation produce patterns of cochlear depression and damage that most often affect frequencies *above* the frequency of the input sound (Davis, Morgan, Hawkins, Galambos, and Smith 1950; Davis and Silverman 1970). Likewise, effects of ototoxic drugs commonly affect high frequencies most markedly, although cochlear damage can often be spotty and/or widespread (DeWeese, Saunders, Schuller, and Schleuning 1988). Thus, if CNS sensitization is produced by such agents it is probable (though not inevitable) that such effects would be most evident in the higher-frequency regions. That suggestion is consistent with the fact that at least 75 percent of the Tinnitus Clinic patients match the pitch of their tinnitus to frequencies above 3 kHz, as was shown in Figure 14-1.

As for the location of cochlear neurons capable of providing sustained input to sensitized neurons in the auditory CNS, they could not be neurons in the most heavily damaged or depressed cochlear regions, where both spontaneous and evoked responding are eliminated or greatly reduced (Kiang et al. 1970; Liberman and Kiang 1978). It is possible that neurons in the transition zones, for example where cochlear neurons show abnormal tuning curves, could contribute some type of sustained input to the sensitized CNS neurons, although this seems unlikely because the experimental evidence so far indicates that such neurons have elevated thresholds and reduced spontaneous activity. However, it is possible that such neurons could be excited by efferent sympathetic activity, and an interesting research topic would thus involve investigation of the effects of sympathetic stimulation upon traumatized cochlear nerve fibers. Nevertheless, it seems more likely that units with normal sensitivity, located in normal-hearing regions bordering the damaged zone(s), would generate spontaneous activity or low-level responses to ambient sound or to sympathetic excitation that might be capable of providing sustained input to sensitized CNS neurons.

If so, the tendency for cochlear damage to occur more readily in the higher frequencies would suggest that normal cochlear neurons capable of driving sensitized CNS regions would be most likely to be located in the lower-frequency border of the damaged cochlear zone. That suggestion fits well with the evidence cited earlier that tonotopic remodelling acts to shift the inputs to the CNS to frequencies *below* the normally effective range.

Presumably, if over time the cochlear damage process extends to progressively lower and lower frequencies, both the sensitization effects and the altered cochleotopic maps should reflect that trend by shifting to the appropriate border frequencies corresponding to the prevailing site of damage within the cochlea. A very interesting test of this hypothesis would be to conduct a prospective study of the alterations of tinnitus pitch over time, in individuals who undergo progressive hearing loss. Such work might serve to determine whether those individuals also experience corresponding, progressive changes in the pitch of their tinnitus.

Summary of the Model

In the model we propose for tinnitus, the concept of sensory remodelling at various levels of the CNS is combined with the concept of sensitization of central auditory neurons; the latter neurons are those that, prior to cochlear damage, were activated by frequencies corresponding to the damaged regions of the cochlea and/or the adjacent cochlear regions. The chain of events is hypothesized to be as follows:

1. Excessive acoustic stimulation or other peripheral insult causes damage or depression of cochlear nerve fibers, resulting in permanent or temporary deafferentation of some portion of the auditory CNS.
2. Deafferentation of CNS structures sets in motion the cellular events that result in distortion of cochleotopic maps by expansion of the CNS regions responding to sound frequencies that border the damaged region(s) of the cochlea.

3. Because of the characteristic tendency for the cochlea to show damage first in the higher frequencies, the border regions most likely to be over-represented in the reorganized CNS are those with frequencies *lower* than the region of greatest cochlear damage (but for small, fairly restricted lesions, both the lower and the higher frequency borders could expand into the deafferented regions of the CNS).

4. Concurrently with the tonotopic alterations described above, sensitization of some CNS neurons occurs as a result of the peripheral damage or of the noxious stimulation that caused t h e cochlear damage; although sensitization has been demonstrated most convincingly in the inferior colliculus, theoretically sensitization could occur at a number of different sites within the auditory CNS.

5. As a result of sensitization, the affected CNS neurons now tend to fire vigorously in response to low-level inputs that formerly were ineffective; such inputs from the remaining cochlear nerve fibers might include sympathetically induced activity, normal or abnormal spontaneous activity, and/or responses of cochlear nerve fibers to ambient sound.

6. The low-level inputs described above would be expected to originate mainly in the cochlear regions bordering the location of the end-organ damage.

7. Because of cochleotopic remodelling in the deafferented CNS regions, the constant activity of the sensitized CNS neurons would result in a larger-than-normal region of cortical activity, corresponding to the expanded cochleotopic representation for frequencies adjacent to (and usually lower than) those that would have excited the deafferented region prior to damage.

8. The frequency (or frequencies) that acquire expanded cortical representations in the deafferented CNS would determine the perceived pitch of the resulting tinnitus.

This model should be viewed as describing the chain of events leading to tinnitus in susceptible individuals. Some individuals will experience cochlear damage, indicated by hearing impairment, without developing tinnitus. In these individuals it is inferred that the sensitization process does not occur. Individual differences in regard to the induction of tinnitus may resemble the situation with chronic pain, in which the abnormal condition occurs only in certain individuals. Factors predisposing a given individual to develop either chronic pain or chronic tinnitus are not known, nor is it known whether certain types of damage are more likely than others to be associated with chronic sequelae in either the auditory or the somatosensory systems.

RELEVANCE OF THE MODEL TO THE PERCEIVED LOUDNESS OF TINNITUS

Clinical observations concerning the loudness of tinnitus indicate a paradoxical effect in that external tones matched to the perceived loudness of tinnitus are often only a few dB above threshold, even for tinnitus that is perceived as very intense (Fowler 1943, 1944; Graham and Newby 1962; Meikle and Walsh 1984; Roberts 1986; Vernon 1976). This discrepancy between the low levels of external matching sounds and the high subjective loudness ratings of tinnitus has been attributed to recruitment (Goodwin and Johnson 1980; Vernon 1976). The tinnitus model described above offers two possible mechanisms that might explain the paradoxical loudness of tinnitus, and either or both of these mechanisms could be operative within in any given individual.

First, sensitization of CNS elements, resulting in increased discharge rates of CNS neurons in response to low-level or spontaneous activity from cochlear regions bordering the zone(s) of peripheral damage, should cause acoustic stimuli in the corresponding frequency ranges to be perceived as louder than normal. Increases in the stimulus level would be expected to produce abnormal growth of loudness (Gerken et al. 1986; Salvi et al. 1990, 1992a, 1992b), in a manner analogous to the hyperpathic responses elicited by gentle stimulation of cutaneous regions affected by abnormal pain responses following peripheral nerve damage (Devor 1988). Sensitization of auditory CNS neurons might thus constitute a neural mechanism for loudness recruitment, and it is loudness recruitment that has most often been hypothesized as leading to the paradoxical loudness of tinnitus (Goodwin and Johnson 1980; Vernon 1976).

Second, distortion of tonotopic maps at higher levels of the auditory CNS could also account for the aberrant loudness of tinnitus. External matching sounds might be expected to sound louder than normal if they activate larger-than-normal regions owing to the hypothesized expansion of the tonotopic map. It is clear that this might be a fertile area for investigation, if and when imaging techniques for analyzing the extent of neural activity within the auditory cortex in man (Belliveau et al. 1991; Cheyne et al. 1991; Fox et al. 1988) can be performed with sufficient resolution that abnormalities or alterations in tonotopic maps can be discriminated. It is possible that such tests might provide objective evidence, not only of the areal extent of brain reorganization that may have occurred in any given individual, but also of CNS changes that may form the neural basis for loudness recruitment.

Finally, with regard to the suggestion that sympathetic efferent activation of the ear may help to maintain the sustained sensations of sound in tinnitus, it is clear that such a mechanism if substantiated could perhaps account for the fact that tinnitus, like pain, is often exacerbated by stress and fatigue (Meikle et al. 1987). Because of the idiosyncratic nature of sympathetic activity in different individuals (Koizumi and Brooks 1980; Kuntz 1953), sympathetic involvement might also help to explain the unpredictability with which different individuals having the same general pattern of peripheral hearing loss can exhibit idiosyncratic variations in regard to tinnitus pitch and localization (see section on Audiological Correlates of Tinnitus) as well as the temporal variability of their tinnitus (Meikle et al. 1987). It is conceivable that sympathetic antagonists might be

found to ameliorate or otherwise modify affected individuals' perceptions of tinnitus, and that if so a variety of useful clinical and experimental techniques might be derived from pharmacological interventions of this type.

RELEVANCE OF THE MODEL TO THE PERCEIVED LOCALIZATION OF TINNITUS

It seems quite reasonable to expect that damage-induced reorganization of sensory maps, as well as sensitizaton of central neurons, could affect not only the pitch but also the localization of tinnitus. Small alterations of subcortical structures should in fact be especially significant for sound localization, in view of the evidence that it is the *balance* between ipsilateral and contralateral activity (Brugge 1985) that determines the final sensations involving the perceived locations of sounds. Sound localization mechanisms might thus be especially vulnerable to small changes in the amount or location of CNS activity. That suggestion highlights the need for further physiological work on sound localization in animal models with experimentally damaged hearing.

In addition to these general comments, there is specific evidence from the somatosensory domain that may be relevant to individuals whose tinnitus began as a unilateral sensation and later became bilateral. In the experiments of Calford and Tweedale (1990), restricted peripheral denervation of one digit produced expanded cortical representations in the contralateral cortex, as described earlier. The contralateral cortex is the side to which somatosensory inputs normally project, thus it would be expected that any damage-induced alterations should affect the cortex opposite to the hand which received surgical deafferentation. What was unexpected in the Calford and Tweedale data was that homotopic regions in the cortex *ipsilateral* to the operated side also showed expanded representation, producing a "mirror image" of the altered sensory map on the other side of the brain. These changes occurred despite the fact that the ipsilateral somatosensory cortex never responded to stimulation of the affected digit either before or after surgery. In effect, responses in the ipsilateral cortex behaved as though they, too, had been subjected to peripheral deafferentation even though the digit on that side was in fact intact and its neural connections to the CNS were uninterrupted. The authors concluded that there is "a mechanism providing balanced transfer of changes in corresponding regions of the two hemispheres" (Calford and Tweedale 1990, p. 806).

If similar effects occur following partial or complete damage to the cochlear end organ on one side, it could provide a mechanism whereby tinnitus that is originally unilateral comes to be perceived bilaterally. This mechanism could then explain the otherwise problematic finding that many patients perceive tinnitus that has identical pitch and other spectral characteristics in both the left and the right ears.

Further support for the notion that such interhemispheric transfer may occur commonly in sensory systems comes from several lines of research into visual mechanisms. Electrophysiological recording in primary visual cortex (area 17) in the cat has indicated that neurons recorded simultaneously in homologous regions of both hemispheres can exhibit oscillatory responses that are synchronized with essentially 0° phase difference (Engel, Konig, Kreiter, and Singer 1991), and this interhemispheric synchronization appears to depend on an intact corpus callosum. In other work, the cortical representation of retinal projections could be markedly altered by retinal lesions in one eye, but only when the other eye was removed (Kaas et al. 1990). It is known that there are numerous corticocortical and other types of interconnections between the auditory regions in the two hemispheres (Brugge 1985), thus suggesting that homologous zones of auditory cortex might be subject to the same type of correlated activation or alteration as those already shown for the visual and somatosensory systems.

Clearly, there is need for further work on physiological mechanisms subserving sound localiza-tion and other forms of binaural interaction. That need is highlighted by the peculiar alterations of tinnitus that sometimes occur following intense sound stimulation. For example, one study documents the experience of an individual with bilateral tinnitus, perceived as having the identical pitch of 10 kHz in both ears, who exhibited very different recovery processes in the two ears following unilateral exposure to 500 Hz at 121 dB SPL for 21 minutes (Young and Lowry 1983). In the exposed ear, the tinnitus was absent for 3 hours following the exposure, and then returned as a complex of multiple frequencies which gradually changed from a low of 3260 Hz until the preexposure value of 10 kHz was regained 1 week postexposure. The tinnitus in the nonexposed ear also exhibited a pitch change, first to a narrow band between 6700-8000 Hz, and then fluctuating between several slightly higher noise bands until the original 10 kHz tinnitus was reinstated 4 weeks postexposure. These observations suggest that the perceived attributes of tinnitus can be influenced by exceedingly complex central integrative mechanisms.

CONCLUSION

Although the model we have suggested above may help to explain certain aspects of tinnitus, it does not address several important topics: First, nothing has been said here about the ability to mask or "cover up" tinnitus using external sounds, a procedure which can succeed in substantially reducing the tinnitus in the large majority of Tinnitus Clinic patients (Hazell et al. 1985; Vernon 1988; Vernon and Meikle 1981, 1988). At present there is essentially no explanation for the efficacy of tinnitus masking, nor have mechanisms been advanced to account for its widespread occurrence in tinnitus of widely differing characteristics and varying degrees of severity. Tinnitus masking does not appear to behave like conventional auditory masking of one external sound by another (Vernon and Meikle 1981).

Tinnitus-masking phenomena do, however, offer additional support for the hypothesis that tinnitus represents the interaction of both peripheral and central neural mechanisms. Based on work at the Tinnitus Clinic, the following observations are relevant: (1) Some, though not all, patients exhibit contralateral masking effects; (2) in a small number, dichotic masking with uncorrelated noise is more effective than diotic (i.e., correlated) masking; (3) although it might be expected that diotic masking using correlated noise should require lower sound levels than monaural masking, (because of the possibility of binaural loudness summation), the actual results are variable and idiosyncratic, some individuals actually requiring *louder* sound levels diotically to achieve masking results equivalent to those obtained with monaural stimulation (J. Vernon, personal communication). From all of these observations, the conclusion seems unavoidable that there are many idiosyncratic permutations of masking effects upon the perceived magnitude of tinnitus. The laws governing these masking effects will certainly prove to be complex, and may well involve neural processes that are as yet unknown.

The lack of knowledge is even more profound with regard to *residual inhibition*, that is, the temporary elimination or reduction of tinnitus after the masking sound is turned off. This puzzling phenomenon occurs in close to 90 percent of the patient population when masking is presented using synthesized noise bands under earphones. Residual inhibition is of potentially great neurological interest because of the fact that it can last for surprisingly long times in certain patients. Although the modal value for residual inhibition, following a standardized test using one minute of masking, is in the range 30-60 seconds, it is not uncommon for patients to experience many minutes of total silence following the offset of the 1-minute masking sound (Vernon and Meikle 1981, 1988). Especially in patients whose tinnitus has been constant and unremitting for years, such a result is unexpected, to say the least. At this stage, it is difficult to imagine what type of neural mechanism is responsible, other than to recognize that it probably belongs

within the general category of neural plasticity known as "long-term potentiation" (Briggs, Brown, and McAfee 1985; Brown and McAfee 1982; Gerken et al. 1986). As yet, however, the auditory system has not received much study in regard to neural plasticity of this type. Nevertheless, the fact that residual inhibition occurs so reliably indicates that it is an important aspect of tinnitus that requires explanation.

It is also interesting to speculate about salicylates and their role in inducing or exacerbating tinnitus. Salicylate-induced tinnitus could be accounted for by the model proposed here if the hearing impairment caused by salicylates constitutes an effective form of peripheral deafferentation. Although it is not certain that salicylate-induced tinnitus behaves in the same way as tinnitus observed in the clinical population, the available observations concerning salicylate-induced tinnitus in humans suggest that it may: Tinnitus due to salicylates is easily masked and experiences substantial residual inhibition (McFadden 1982; Meikle, unpublished observations); its sensory attributes, including its pitch, sound quality, and localization, appear to resemble those of tinnitus induced by noise and other agents that tend to depress high-frequency hearing (Brummett, Vernon, and Meikle, unpublished observations); and there is the well-known ability of salicylates to exacerbate preexisting tinnitus sensations, indicating that the process by which salicylates induce tinnitus may affect the same neural generators as those involved in tinnitus due to permanently damaging agents. It would be of interest, therefore, to investigate the central effects of salicylates in experimental animals in which the extent of cochleotopic reorganization can be evaluated.

The model that is proposed here places considerable emphasis on the role of central neural mechanisms in generating tinnitus, while at the same time suggesting ways in which peripheral auditory damage might induce or interact with those central mechanisms. One result of this conceptualization is to negate the type of thinking that seeks to categorize clinically significant tinnitus as being either "central" or "peripheral". From the diagnostic point of view an "either-or" usage of those terms would seem to be inappropriate, given the high likelihood that precise knowledge of the precipitating factors is not available for most if not all individuals who experience chronic tinnitus. Likewise from a theoretical standpoint, in view of the close interactions that are known to exist between the auditory CNS and the ear, it seems prudent to avoid presuming that such a dichotomy exists unless there is convincing neurological evidence in its favor. To take what seems to be the most generally defensible view, clinical data such as those that were summarized here suggest that tinnitus commonly represents the integration of *both* central and peripheral mechanisms.

A recent discussion of phantom limb phenomena concluded by emphasizing the dependence of conscious sensations on high-level sensory processing performed by the brain (Melzack 1992). That same emphasis also seems proper for tinnitus, embodying as it does a number of similarities to the experience of phantom limb—mimicry of external stimuli, referral to specific anatomical loci, and persistence in the face of demonstrable deafferentation. It seems appropriate therefore to quote the following lines from Melzack's discussion as they provide an elegant summing up not only for phantom limb but also for tinnitus:

> ... phantom limbs are a mystery only if we assume the body sends sensory messages to a passively receiving brain. Phantoms become comprehensible once we recognize that the brain generates the experience of the body. Sensory inputs merely modulate that experience; they do not directly cause it.

Drs. William J. Roberts and Ronald C. Kramis of the Neurological Sciences Institute, Portland, Oregon provided significant help through their many personal communications concerning sympathetically maintained pain. I thank Mara Charnell for creating the figures. This work was supported by U.S. Dept. of Education Special Project Grant #10860006.

REFERENCES

American Tinnitus Association. 1986. *Tinnitus Patient Survey.* Portland (OR): American Tinnitus Association.

Aran, J.-M. and Cazals, Y. 1981. "Electrical Suppression of Tinnitus." In D. Evered and G. Lawrenson (Eds.), *Tinnitus,* pp. 217–231. *Ciba Foundation Symposium 85.* London: Pitman.

Atkinson, M. 1944. "Tinnitus Aurium: Observations on Its Nature and Control." *Annals of Otology, Rhinology, and Laryngology, 53,* 742–751.

Beausaing-Linder, M. and Hultcrantz, E. 1980. "Early Effects of Cervical Sympathetic Stimulation on Cerebral, Ocular, and Cochlear Blood Flow." *Acta Physiologica Scandinavica, 109,* 433–437.

Belliveau, J.W., Kennedy, D.N., McKinstry, R.C., Buchbinder, B.R., Weisskoff, R.M., Cohen, M.S., Vevea, J.M., Brady, T.I., and Rosen, B.R. 1991. "Functional Mapping of the Human Visual Cortex by Magnetic Resonance Imaging." *Science, 254,* 716–719.

Berlin, C.I. and Lowe, S.S. 1972. "Differential Diagnostic Evaluation: Central Auditory Function." In J. Katz (Ed.), *Handbook of Clinical Audiology,* pp. 280–312. Baltimore: Williams & Wilkins.

Brechtelsbauer, P.B., Prazma, J., Garret, G., Carrasco, V.N., and Pillsbury, H.C. 1990. "Catecholaminergic Innervation of the Inner Ear." *Otolaryngology—Head and Neck Surgery, 103,* 566–574.

Briggs, C.A., Brown, T.H., and McAfee, D.A. 1985. "Neurophysiology and Pharmacology of Long-term Potentiation in the Rat Sympathetic Ganglion." *Journal of Physiology, 359,* 503–521.

Brown, T.H. and McAfee, D.A. 1982. "Long-term Synaptic Potentiation in the Superior Cervical Ganglion." *Science, 215,* 1411–1413.

Brugge, J.F. 1985. "Patterns of Organization in Auditory Cortex." *Journal of the Acoustical Society of America, 78,* 353–359.

Burns, W. 1968. *Noise and Man.* Philadelphia: Lippincott.

Calford, M.B. and Tweedale, R. 1988. "Immediate and Chronic Changes in Responses of Somatosensory Cortex in Adult Flying-fox after Digit Amputation." *Nature, 332,* 446–448.

Calford, M.B. and Tweedale, R. 1990. "Interhemispheric Transfer of Plasticity in the Cerebral Cortex." *Science, 249,* 805807.

Carrasco, V.N., Prazma, J., Faber, J.E., Triana, R.J., and Pillsbury, H.C. 1990. "Cochlear Microcirculation. Effect of Adrenergic Agonists on Arteriole Diameter." *Archives of Otolaryngology, 116,* 411–417.

Cheyne, D., Kristeva, R., and Deecke, L. 1991. "Homuncular Organization of Human Motor Cortex as Indicated by Neuromagnetic Recordings." *Neuroscience Letters, 122,* 17–20.

Cook, A.J., Woolf, C.J., Wall, P.D., and McMahon, S.B. 1987. "Dynamic Receptive Field Plasticity in Rat Spinal Cord Dorsal Horn following C-primary Afferent Input." *Nature, 325,* 151–153.

Dallos, P. and Harris, D. 1978. "Properties of Auditory Nerve Responses in Absence of Outer Hair Cells." *Journal of Neurophysiology, 41,* 365–383.

Dandy, W.E. 1941. "Surgical Treatment of Ménière's Disease." *Surgical Gynecology and Obstetrics, 72,* 421–425.

Davis, H., Morgan, C.T., Hawkins, J.E. Jr., Galambos, R., and Smith, F.W. 1950. "Temporary Deafness Following Exposure to Loud Tones and Noise." *Acta Otolaryngologica, 88,* Supplement, 1–56.

Davis, H. and Silverman, S.R. 1970. *Hearing and Deafness.* New York: Holt, Rinehart & Winston.

Dengerink, H.A. and Wright, J.W. 1988. "Circulation of the Inner Ear. III. The Physiology of Cochlear Blood Flow: Implications for Treatment." In A.F. Jahn and J. Santos-Sacchi, *Physiology of the Ear,* pp. 227–340. New York: Raven Press.

Densert, O. and Flock, A. 1974. "An Electron-microscopic Study of Adrenergic Innervation in the Cochlea." *Acta Otolaryngologica, 77,* 185–197.

Devor, M. 1988. "Central Changes Mediating Neuropathic Pain." In R. Dubner, G.F. Gebhart, and M.R. Bond (Eds.), *Proceedings V World Congress on Pain,* pp. 114–128. Amsterdam: Elsevier.

Devor, M. and Wall, P.D. 1978. "Reorganization of Spinal Cord Sensory Map after Peripheral Nerve Injury." *Nature, 276,* 75–76.

DeWeese, D.D., Saunders, W.H., Schuller, D.E., and Schleuning, A.J. 1988. *Otolaryngology—Head and Neck Surgery.* St. Louis: C.V. Mosby.

Donaldson, I. 1978. "Tinnitus: A Theoretical View and a Therapeutic Study Using Amylobarbitone." *Journal of Laryngology and Otology, 92,* 123–130.

Dostrovsky, J.O., Millar, J. and Wall, P.D. 1976. "The Immediate Shift of Afferent Drive of Dorsal Column Nucleus Cells Following Deafferentation: A Comparison of Acute and Chronic Deafferentation in Gracile Nucleus and Spinal Cord." *Experimental Neurology, 52,* 480–495.

Eggermont, J.J. 1984. "Tinnitus: Some Thoughts about Its Origin." *Journal of Laryngology and Otology,* Supplement 9, 31–37.

Eggermont, J.J. 1990. "On the Pathophysiology of Tinnitus: A Review and a Peripheral Model." *Hearing Research, 48,* 111–124.

Emmett, J.R. and Shea, J.J. 1980. "Treatment of Tinnitus with Tocainide Hydrochloride." *Otolaryngology,—Head and Neck Surgery, 88,* 442–446.

Engel, A.K., Konig, P., Kreiter, A.K., and Singer, W. 1991. "Interhemispheric Synchronization of Oscillatory Neuronal Responses in Cat Visual Cortex." *Science, 252,* 1177–1179.

Evans, E.F. and Borerwe, T.A. 1982. "Ototoxic Effects of Salicylates on the Responses of Single Cochlear Nerve Fibres and on Cochlear Potentials." *British Journal of Audiology, 16,* 101–108.

Evans, E.F., Wilson, J.P., and Borerwe, T.A. 1981. "Animal Models of Tinnitus." In D. Evered and G. Lawrenson (Eds.), *Tinnitus,* pp. 108–129. *Ciba Foundation Symposium 85.* London: Pitman.

Evered, D. and Lawrenson, G. (Eds.). 1981. *Tinnitus. Ciba Foundation Symposium 85.* London: Pitman.

Eysel, U.T. 1982. "Functional Reconnections without New Axonal Growth in a Partially Denervated Visual Relay Nucleus." *Nature, 299,* 442–444.

Feldmann, H. 1971. "Homolateral and Contralateral Masking of Tinnitus by Noise-bands and by Pure Tones." *Audiology, 10,* 138–144.

Fields, H.L. 1990. *Pain Syndromes in Neurology.* London: Butterworths.

Fields, H.L., Dubner, R., and Cervero, F. 1985. *Advances in Pain Research and Therapy,* Vol. 9, *Proceedings IV World Congress on Pain.* New York: Raven Press.

Fowler, E.P. 1943. "Control of Head Noises: Their Illusions of Loudness and Timbre." *Archives of Otolaryngology, 37,* 391–398.

Fowler, E.P. 1944. "Head Noises in Normal and in Disordered Ears: Significance, Measurement, Differentiation and Treatment." *Archives of Otolaryngology, 39,* 498–503.

Fox, P.T., Raichle, M.E., Mintun, M.A., and Dence, C. 1988. "Nonoxidative Glucose Consumption during Focal Physiologic Neural Activity." *Science, 241,* 462–464.

Gerken, G.M. 1979. "Central Denervation Hypersensitivity in the Auditory System of the Cat." *Journal of Acoustical Society of America, 66,* 721–727.

Gerken, G.M., Saunders, S.S. and Paul, R.E. 1984. "Hypersensitivity to Electrical Stimulation of Auditory Nuclei Follows Hearing Loss in Cats." *Hearing Research, 13,* 249–259.

Gerken, G.M., Simhadri-Sumithra, R., and Bhat, K.H.V. 1986. "Increase in Central Auditory Responsiveness during Continuous Tone Stimulation or Following Hearing Loss." In R.J. Salvi, D. Henderson, R.P. Hamernik, and V. Colletti, *Basic and Applied Aspects of Noise-Induced Hearing Loss,* pp. 195–211. New York/London: Plenum Press.

Gerren, R.A. and Weinberger, N.M. 1983. "Long Term Potentiation in the Magnocellular Medical Geniculate Nucleus of the Anesthetized Cat." *Brain Research, 265,* 138–142.

Goodhill, V. 1954. "Otologic Aspects." In "Symposium: Tinnitus—New Concepts in Etiology and Management." *Transactions of the American Academy of Ophthalmology and Otolaryngology, 58,* 529–532.

Goodwin, P.E. and Johnson, R.M. 1980. "The Loudness of Tinnitus." *Acta Otolaryngologica, 90,* 353–359.

Graham, J.T. and Newby, H.A. 1962. "Acoustical Characteristics of Tinnitus." *Archives of Otolaryngology, 75,* 162–167.

Harrison, R.V., Nagasawa, A., Smith, D.W., Stanton, S., and Mount, R.J. 1991. "Reorganization of Auditory Cortex after Neonatal High Frequency Cochlear Hearing Loss." *Hearing Research, 54,* 11–19.

Hazell, J.W.P. 1981. "Measurement of Tinnitus in Humans." In D. Evered and G. Lawrenson (Eds.), *Tinnitus,* pp. 35–48. *Ciba Foundation Symposium 85.* London: Pitman.

Hazell, J.W.P. 1987. "A Cochlear Model for Tinnitus." In H. Feldmann (Ed.), *Proceedings III International Tinnitus Seminar,* pp. 121–128. Karlsruhe: Harsch Verlag.

Hazell, J.W.P., Wood, S.M., Cooper, H.R., Stephens, S.D.B., Corcoran, A.L., Coles, R.R.A., Baskill, J.L., and Sheldrake, J.B. 1985. "A Clinical Study of Tinnitus Maskers." *British Journal of Audiology, 19,* 65–146.

Hoheisel, U. and Mense, S. 1989. "Long-term Changes in Discharge Behavior of Cat Dorsal Horn Neurones Following Noxious Stimulation of Deep Tissues." *Pain, 36,* 239–247.

House, J.W. and Brackmann, D.E. 1981. "Tinnitus: Surgical Treatment." In D. Evered and G. Lawrenson (Eds.), *Tinnitus,* pp. 204–216. *Ciba Foundation Symposium 85.* London: Pitman.

Hultcrantz, E., Nuttall, A.L., Brown, M.C., and Lawrence, M. 1982. "The Effect of Cervical Sympathectomy on Cochlear Electrophysiology." *Acta Otolaryngologica, 94,* 439–444.

Jacobs, K.M. and Donoghue, J.P. 1991. "Reshaping the Cortical Motor Map by Unmasking Latent Intracortical Connections." *Science, 251,* 944–946.

Jastreboff, P.J. 1990. "Phantom Auditory Perception (Tinnitus): Mechanisms of Generation and Perception." *Neuroscience Research, 8,* 221–254.

Jastreboff, P.J. and Sasaki, C.T. 1986. "Salicylate-induced Changes in Spontaneous Activity of Single Units in the Inferior Colliculus of the Guinea Pig." *Journal of the Acoustical Society of America, 80,* 1384–1391.

Jenkins, W.M. and Merzenich, M.M. 1987. "Role of Cat Primary Auditory Cortex for Sound Localization Behavior." *Journal of Neurophysiology, 52,* 819–847.

Kaas, J.H. 1991. "Plasticity of Sensory and Motor Maps in Adult Mammals." *Annual Review of Neuroscience, 14,* 137–167.

Kaas, J.H., Krubitzer, L.A., Chino, Y.M., Langston, A.L., Polley, E.H., and Blair, N. 1990. "Reorganization of Retino-topic Maps in Adult Mammals after Lesions of the Retina." *Science, 248,* 229–231.

Kaas, J.H., Merzenich, M.M., and Killackey, H.P. 1983. "The Reorganization of Somatosensory Cortex Following Peripheral Nerve Damage in Adult and Developing Mammals." *Annual Review Neuroscience, 6,* 325–356.

Kemp, D.T. 1981. "Physiologically Active Cochlear Micromechanics—One Source of Tinnitus." In D. Evered and G. Lawrenson (Eds.), *Tinnitus,* pp. 54–76. *Ciba Foundation Symposium 85.* London: Pitman.

Kemp, D.T. 1982. "Cochlear Echoes: Implications for Noise-induced Hearing Loss." In R.P. Hamernik, D. Henderson, and R. Salvi (Eds.), *New Perspectives on Noise-Induced Hearing Loss,* pp. 189–206. New York: Raven Press.

Kiang, N.Y.-S., Moxon, E.C., and Levine, R.A. 1970. "Auditory-nerve Activity in Cats with Normal and Abnormal Cochleas." pp. 241–268. In G.E.W. Wolstenholme and J. Knight (Eds.), *Sensorineural Hearing Loss. Ciba Symposium.* London: Churchill.

Kiang, N.Y.-S., Watanabe, T., Thomas, E.C., and Clark, L.F. 1965. *Discharge Patterns of Single Fibers in the Cat's Auditory Nerve.* Cambridge, MA: MIT Press.

Koizumi, K. and Brooks, C.M. 1980. "The Autonomic System and Its Role in Controlling Body Functions." In V.B. Mountcastle (Ed.), *Medical Physiology,* (14th Ed) Vol 1, pp. 893–922. St. Louis: Mosby.

Kramis, R.C., Gillette, R.G., and Roberts, W.J. 1991. "Post-sympathectomy Neuralgia: The Result of Concurrent Deafferentation and Sympathetically-maintained Pain Mechanisms?" *Society for Neuroscience Abstracts, 17,* 438.

Kuntz, A. 1946. *The Autonomic Nervous System,* p. 530. Philadelphia: Lea & Febiger.

Lempert, J. 1946. "Tympanosympathectomy. A Surgical Technique for the Relief of Tinnitus Aurium." *Archives of Otolaryngology, 43,* 199–212.

Liberman, M.C. and Kiang, N.Y.-S. 1978. "Acoustic Trauma in Cats." *Acta Otolaryngologica, Supplement 358.*

Livingston, W.K. 1943. *Pain Mechanisms.* New York: Macmillan.

Lonsbury-Martin, B.L. and Martin, G.K. 1981. "Effects of Moderately Intense Sound on Auditory Sensitivity in Rhesus Monkeys: Behavioral and Neural Observations." *Journal of Neurophysiology, 46,* 563–586.

Maixner, W., Dubner, R., Bushnell, C., Kenshalo, D.R. Jr., and Oliveras, J.-L. 1986. "Wide-dynamic-range Dorsal Horn Neurons Participate in the Encoding Process by which Monkeys Perceive the Intensity of Noxious Heat Stimuli." *Brain Research, 374,* 385–388.

McFadden, D. 1982. *Tinnitus. Facts, Theories, and Treatments.* Washington, DC: National Academy Press.

McMahon, S.B. and Wall, P.D. 1983. "Plasticity in the Nucleus Gracilis of the Rat." *Experimental Neurology, 80,* 195–207.

McMahon, S.B. and Wall, P.D. 1984. "Receptive Fields of Rat Lamina I Projection Cells Move to Incorporate a Nearby Region of Injury." *Pain, 19,* 235–247.

Meikle, M. and Griest, S. 1987. "The Perceived Localization of Tinnitus." In H. Feldmann (Ed.), *Proceeding III Internatioual Tinnitus Seminar,* pp. 183–189. Karlsruhe: Harsch Verlag.

Meikle, M.B. and Griest, S.E. 1989. "Gender-based Differences in Characteristics of Tinnitus." *Hearing Journal, 42,* 68–76.

Meikle, M.B. and Griest, S.E. 1991. "Computer Data Analysis: Tinnitus Data Registry." In A. Shulman (Ed.), *Tinnitus, Diagnosis/Treatment.* pp. 416–430. Philadelphia: Lea & Febiger.

Meikle, M.B. and Griest, S. 1992. "Asymmetry in Tinnitus Perceptions. Factors That May Account for the Higher Prevalence of Left-sided Tinnitus." In J.-M. Aran and R. Dauman (Eds.), *Proceedings IV International Tinnitus Seminar.*

Meikle, M.B., Griest, S.E., Press, L.S., and Stewart, B.J. 1992. "Relationships between Tinnitus and Audiometric Variables in a Large Sample of Tinnitus Clinic Patients." In J.-M. Aran and R. Dauman (Eds.), *Proceedings IV International Tinnitus Seminar.*

Meikle, M., Schuff, N., and Griest, S. 1987. "Intra-subject Variability of Tinnitus: Observations from the Tinnitus Clinic." In H. Feldmann (Ed.), *Proceedings III International Tinnitus Seminar,* pp. 175–180. Karlsruhe: Harsch Verlag.

Meikle, M. and Walsh, E.T. 1984. "Characteristics of Tinnitus and Related Observations in over 1800 Clinic Patients." *Journal of Laryngology and Otology, Supplement 9,* 17–21.

Meikle, M. and Whitney, S. 1984. "Computer-assisted Analysis of Reported Tinnitus Sounds." *Proceedings II International Tinnitus Seminar. Journal of Laryngology and Otology, Supplement 9,* 188–192.

Melding, P.S., Goodey, R.J., and Thorne, P.R. 1978. "The Use of Intravenous Lignocaine in the Diagnosis and Treatment of Tinnitus." *Journal of Laryngology and Otology, 92,* 115–121.

Melzack, R. 1992. "Phantom Limbs." *Scientific American, April.*

Mendell, L.M. 1984. "Modifiability of Spinal Synapses." *Physiological Review, 64,* 260–324.

Merzenich, M.M. and Jenkins, W.M. 1983. "Dynamic Maintenance and Alterability of Cortical Maps in Adults: Some Implications." In R. Klinke and R. Hartmann (Eds.), *Hearing—Physiological Bases and Psychophysics,* pp. 162–168. New York: Springer-Verlag.

Merzenich, M.M., Kaas, J.H., Wall, J.T., Sur, M., Nelson, R.J., and Felleman, D.J. 1982. "Progression of Change Following Median Nerve Section in the Cortical Representation of the Hand in Areas 3b and 1 in Adult Owl and Squirrel Monkeys." *Neuroscience, 10,* 639–665.

Merzenich, M.M., Nelson, R.J., Stryker, M.P., Cynder, M.S., Shoppmann, A., and Zook, J.M. 1984. "Somatosensory Cortical Map Changes Following Digit

Amputation in Adult Monkeys." *Journal of Comparative Neurology, 224,* 591–605.

Millar, J., Basbaum, A.I., and Wall, P.D. 1976. "Restructuring of the Somatopic Map and Appearance of Abnormal Neuronal Activity in the Gracile Nucleus after Partial Deafferentation." *Experimental Neurology, 50,* 658–672.

Miller, J.M., Ren, T.Y., Laurikainen, E., Quirk, W.S., and Nuttall, A.L. 1992. "Effects of Sympathetic Stimulation on the Bilateral Cochlear Blood Flow in the Guinea Pig." *Abstracts: Association for Research in Otolaryngology, 36.*

Møller, A.R. 1984. "Pathophysiology of Tinnitus." *Annals of Otology, Rhinology, and Laryngology, 93,* 39–44.

Nodar, R.H. 1978. "Tinnitus Aurium: An Approach to Classification." *Otorhinolaryngology—Head and Neck Surgery, 86,* 40–45.

Pantev, C., Hoke, M., Lütkenhöner, B., and Lehnertz, K. 1989. "Tonotopic Organization of the Auditory Cortex: Pitch versus Frequency Representation." *Science, 246,* 486–488.

Passe, E.R.G. 1953. "Surgery of the Sympathetic for Ménière's Disease, Tinnitus, and Nerve Deafness." *Archives of Otolaryngology, 57,* 257–266.

Penner, M.J. 1980. "Two-tone Forward Masking Patterns and Tinnitus." *Journal of Speech and Hearing Research, 23,* 779–786.

Phillips, D.S., Trune, D.R., and Mitchell, C. 1990. "Solving the 'One Ear vs. Two Ears' Data Analysis Problem." *The Hearing Journal, 43,* 27–32.

Pickles, J.O. 1979. "An Investigation of Sympathetic Effects on Hearing." *Acta Otolaryngologica, 87,* 69–71.

Pons, T.P., Garraghty, P.E., Ommaya, A.K., Kaas, J.H., Taub, E., and Mishkin, M. 1991. "Massive Cortical Reorganization after Sensory Deafferentation in Adult Macaques." *Science, 252,* 1857–1860.

Rajan, R., Irvine, D.R.F., Calford, B.M., and Wise, L.Z. 1992. "Effect of Frequency-specific Losses in Cochlear Neural Sensitivity on the Processing and Representation of Frequency in Primary Auditory Cortex." pp. 119–129. In A.L. Dancer, D. Henderson, R.J. Salvi, and R.P. Hamernik (Eds.), *Noise-Induced Hearing Loss.* St. Louis: Mosby-Year Book.

Reed, G.F. 1960. "An Audiometric Study of Two Hundred Cases of Subjective Tinnitus." *Archives of Otolaryngology, 71,* 94–104.

Roberts, W.J. 1986. "A Hypothesis on the Physiological Basis for Causalgia and Related Pains." *Pain, 24,* 297–311.

Roberts, W.J. and Kramis, R.C. 1990. "Sympathetic Nervous System Influence on Acute and Chronic Pain." In H.L. Fields (Ed.), *Pain Syndromes in Neurology,* pp. 85–106. London: Butterworths.

Robertson, D. and Irvine, R.F. 1989. "Plasticity of Frequency Organization in Auditory Cortex of Guinea Pigs with Partial Unilateral Deafness." *Journal of Comparative Neurology, 282,* 456–471.

Ross, M.D. 1973. "Autonomic Components of the VIII Nerve." *Advances Oto-Rhino-Laryngology, 20,* 316–336.

Salvi, R.J. 1976. "Central Components of the Temporary Threshold Shift." In D. Henderson, R.P. Hamernik, D.S. Dosanjh, and J.H. Mills, *Effects of Noise on Hearing,* pp. 247–260. New York: Raven Press.

Salvi, R.J. and Ahroon, W.A. 1983. "Tinnitus and Neural Activity." *Journal of Speech and Hearing Research, 26,* 629–632.

Salvi, R., Powers, N.L., and Saunders, S.S. 1992a. "Functional Changes in Single Neurons in the Inferior Colliculus of the Chinchilla Following Acoustic Overstimulation." *Abstracts: Association for Research on Otolaryngology, 132.*

Salvi, R.J., Powers, N.L., Saunders, S.S., Boettcher, F.A., and Clock, A.E. 1992b. "Enhancement of Evoked Response Amplitude and Single Unit Activity after Noise Exposure." pp. 156–171. In A.L. Dancer, D. Henderson, R.J. Salvi, and R.P. Hamernik (Eds.), *Noise-Induced Hearing Loss.* St. Louis: Mosby.

Salvi, R.J., Saunders, S.S., Gratton, M.A., Arehole, S., and Powers, N. 1990. "Enhanced Evoked Response Amplitudes in the Inferior Colliculus of the Chinchilla Following Acoustic Trauma." *Hearing Research, 50,* 245–258.

Sasaki, C.T., Kauer, J.S., and Babitz, L. 1980. "Differential [^{14}C]2-Deoxyglucose Uptake after Deafferentation of the Mammalian Auditory Pathway—A Model for Examining Tinnitus." *Brain Research, 194,* 511–516.

Spoendlin, H. 1988. "Neural Anatomy of the Inner Ear." In A.F. Jahn and J. Santos-Sacchi, *Physiology of the Ear,* pp. 201–219. New York: Raven Press.

Spoendlin, H. and Lichtensteiger, W. 1966. "The Adrenergic Innervation of the Labyrinth." *Acta Otolaryngologica, 61,* 423–434.

Stevens, S.S. and Davis, H. 1938. *Hearing. Its Psychology and Physiology.* New York: Wiley.

Tonndorf, J. 1980. "Acute Cochlear Disorders: The Combination of Hearing Loss, Recruitment, Poor Speech Discrimination, and Tinnitus." *Annals of Otology, Rhinology, and Laryngology, 89,* 353–358.

Tonndorf, J. 1987. "The Analogy between Tinnitus and Pain: A Suggestion for a Physiological Basis of Chronic Tinnitus." *Hearing Research, 28,* 271–275.

Tukey, J.W. 1977. *Exploratory Data Analysis.* Reading, MA: Addison-Wesley.

Vernon, J.A. 1987. "Assessment of the Tinnitus Patient." In J.W.P. Hazell (Ed.), *Tinnitus,* pp. 71–95. Edinburgh: Churchill Livingstone.

Vernon, J.A. 1988. "Current Use of Masking for the Relief of Tinnitus." In M. Kitahara (Ed.), *Tinnitus. Pathophysiology and Management,* pp. 96–106. Tokyo: Igaku-Shoin.

Vernon, J.A. 1976. "The Loudness (?) of Tinnitus." *Hearing and Speech Action, 44,* 17–19.

Vernon, J.A. and Meikle, M.B. 1985. "Clinical Insights into Possible Physiological Mechanisms of Tinnitus." In E. Myers (ed.), *New Dimensions in Otorhinolaryngology—Head and Neck Surgery,* Vol. 1, pp. 439–446. New York: Elsevier Science Publishers.

Vernon, J. and Meikle, M. 1988. "Measurement of Tinnitus: An Update." In M. Kitahara (Ed.), *Tinnitus: Pathophysiology, Diagnosis and Treatment,* pp. 36–52. Tokyo: Igaku-Shoin.

Vernon, J.A. and Meikle, M.B. 1981. "Tinnitus Masking: Unresolved Problems." In D. Evered and G. Lawrenson (Eds.), *Tinnitus,* pp. 239–262. *Ciba Foundation Symposium 85.* London: Pitman.

Wall, J.T. and Cusick, C.G. 1984. "Cutaneous Responsiveness in Primary Somatosensory (S-I) Hindpaw Cortex before and after Partial Hindpaw Deafferentation in Adult Rats." *Journal of Neuroscience, 4,* 1499–1515.

Wall, P.D. and Devor, M. 1982. "Consequences of Peripheral Nerve Damage in the Spinal Cord and in Neighboring Intact Peripheral Nerves." In W.J. Culp and J. Ochoa (Eds.), *Abnormal Nerves and Muscles as Impulse Generators,* pp. 588–603. New York: Oxford Univ Press.

Wall, P.D. and Egger, M.D. 1971. "Formation of New Connections in Adult Rat Brains after Partial Deafferentation." *Nature, 232,* 542–545.

Waxman, S.G. (Ed.). 1988. *Advances in Neurology, Vol 47: Functional Recovery in Neurological Disease.* New York: Raven Press.

Wilson, J.P. 1987. "Theory of Tinnitus Generation." In J.W.P. Hazell (Ed.), *Tinnitus,* pp. 20–45. Edinburgh: Churchill Livingstone.

Wilson, J.P. and Sutton, G.J. 1981. "Acoustic Correlates of Tonal Tinnitus." In D. Evered and G. Lawrenson (Eds.), *Tinnitus,* pp. 82–101. *Ciba Foundation Symposium 85.* London: Pitman.

Woolf, C.J. 1983. "Evidence for a Central Component of Post-injury Pain Hypersensitivity." *Nature, 306,* 686–688.

Young, I.M. and Lowry, L.D. 1983. "Incurrence and Alterations in Contralateral Tinnitus Following Monaural Exposure to a Pure Tone." *Journal of the Acoustical Society of America, 73,* 2219–2221.

CHAPTER 15

PATHOPHYSIOLOGY OF TINNITUS

AAGE R. MØLLER
University of Pittsburgh School of Medicine

INTRODUCTION

This chapter discusses some hypotheses about how specific changes in the function of the ear and the auditory nervous system may cause tinnitus. Only subjective tinnitus will be considered, which is tinnitus that cannot be heard by an observer and therefore most likely does not have an acoustic origin. Such tinnitus may be generated in any part of the inner ear or the auditory nervous system, but it is not likely to involve the normal transduction process in the cochlea that converts sound into a neural code in the individual fibers of the auditory nerve. One important goal of studies of subjective tinnitus is therefore to identify the anatomical location of the physiological abnormality that causes the sensation of a sound without the presence of a sound that reaches the ear in the normal fashion. Another important task of such research is to determine the nature of this anomaly, and to determine how the anomaly has evolved and what caused it to evolve.

The ultimate goal of such research is naturally to facilitate the development of an effective treatment. Our present, and almost total, lack of knowledge about the pathophysiology of tinnitus, together with our limited knowledge about the function of the normal auditory system, are major obstacles in developing effective methods of treatment for tinnitus.

It seems unlikely that all types of tinnitus should have the same pathophysiology, and it also seems unlikely that all types of tinnitus are generated at the same anatomical location. Thus the weak and moderately disturbing tinnitus that is common in elderly people (and particularly in people who have been exposed to noise) probably has a different pathophysiology than that of incapacitating tinnitus that prevents its victim from having a normal social life and from sleeping normally, and which often is associated with a hypersensitivity to sound that makes even moderate sounds become severely unpleasant, and often producing a sensation of pain. It therefore is not realistic to seek one single explanation of pathophysiology for all types of tinnitus.

Discussions are also presented in this chapter on some recent results pertaining to studies of patients with incapacitating tinnitus, based on intracranial neurophysiological recordings from the eighth nerve and on brainstem auditory evoked potentials (BAEP) made during microvascular decompression (MVD) operations. Similarities between tinnitus and disorders that are caused by vascular compression of other cranial nerves such as hemifacial spasm (HFS), trigeminal neuralgia (TN), and disabling positional vertigo (DPV) will be discussed. A hypothesis regarding the mechanism for the normal detection of sound will be discussed, because such a mechanism may be related to the generation of some forms of tinnitus.

WHERE IN THE AUDITORY SYSTEM IS TINNITUS GENERATED?

Much effort has been devoted to finding the cause of tinnitus in an abnormal function of the ear. The association between an abnormal function of the ear and tinnitus may have arisen from the fact that many patients with subjective tinnitus feel that their tinnitus comes from the ear. Recent studies, however, show indications that the abnormal neural activity that causes severe incapacitating tinnitus is most likely not generated in the ear or in the auditory nerve but rather more centrally in the auditory nervous system (Møller, Møller, and Yokota 1992b). Such abnormal neural activity may be generated by nuclei of the ascending auditory pathway that have become hyperactive as a result of peripherally located neural irritation or nerve pathologies. There is, however, little doubt that some forms of tinnitus are generated in the ear or in the auditory nerve. We will consider this first, and then later discuss how tinnitus may be generated in the auditory nervous system.

ABNORMAL NEURAL ACTIVITY IN THE AUDITORY NERVE

In order to understand what type of neural activity in individual fibers of the auditory nerve can produce tinnitus, it is important to know what criteria the central auditory nervous system uses to detect the presence of a sound. Generally, it has been assumed that tinnitus may arise from an increased discharge rate of nerve cells in some part of the ascending auditory nervous system. This is based on the assumption that a sound above threshold causes the discharge rate of single nerve fibers to increase, and it has been assumed that the discharge rate of auditory nerve fibers is related to the perception of the loudness of a sound.

Single auditory nerve fibers are active (have spontaneous discharges) even in total silence, and if the discharge rate is to be used as a criterion of the presence of a sound, it must obviously be interpreted by the central nervous system since no sound is actually present. The central nervous system must then detect when the discharge rate of single auditory nerve fibers exceeds a certain level, if the discharge rate of auditory nerve fibers is to be used as a criterion for a sound being present. However, the results of recent research

have placed doubt on this assumption. Thus, studies of animal models of tinnitus in which a presumed tinnitus is accomplished by the administration of acetylsalicylate or ototoxic aminoglycosides seem to indicate that these agents, as well as overstimulation with noise (Kiang, Moxon, and Kahn 1976), may cause the spontaneous activity in single auditory nerve fibers to decrease (Kiang, Moxon, and Levine 1970; Harrison and Evans 1982; Evans and Borerwe 1982). These results indicate that it is not the discharge rate of single auditory nerve fibers that causes the type of tinnitus resulting from noise exposure or drugs, and thus that tinnitus is not likely to be related to the discharge rate of single auditory nerve fibers.

There are several other reasons why it seems unlikely that the central auditory nervous system detects the presence of a sound on the basis of the discharge rate of single auditory nerve fibers. The results of studies in animals show that the discharge rate of most auditory nerve fibers in response to broadband sounds reaches a plateau at low sound levels (20 to 30 dB above threshold) (Møller 1977, 1983a,b,c)—thus well below the sound levels that are regarded to be within the physiological range. There are only a few nerve fibers in which the discharge rate increases monotonically over a large range of sound levels when studies using pure-tone stimuli (Liberman 1978). This seems to indicate that it is not the value of the discharge rate of single auditory nerve fibers as such that determines the subjective sensation of the intensity of a sound. Since it thus does not seem to be the (average) discharge that communicates information about a sound's intensity to the central nervous system, it seems more likely that it is the time pattern of the discharges that communicates this information. The waveform of a sound is coded in the discharge pattern of single auditory nerve fibers (Rose, Brugge, Anderson, and Hind 1967), and such temporal coding may also play an important role in mediating information about the presence of a sound, and maybe about the loudness of a sound (Eggermont 1990; Møller 1984). It is known that the time pattern of a sound is generally coded in the discharge pattern of single auditory nerve fibers over a range of sound intensities that includes the entire physiological range of sound intensities above threshold (Møller 1977, 1983a,b,c; Rose et al. 1967; Rose, Hind, Anderson, and Brugge 1971). This is despite the fact that the (average) discharge rate does not change noticeably when the intensity of a sound is increased about 20 to 30 dB above threshold.

That the neural activity in auditory nerve fibers is phase-locked to a sound means that the probability of firing of these nerve fibers is higher at a certain point (phase) of the waveform of a sound. The discharge pattern of single auditory nerve fibers becomes phase-locked to a sound at low intensities when there is little or no increase in the average discharge rate, and this phase-locking is maintained over the entire physiological range of sound intensities for pure tones, pairs of pure tones (Rose et al. 1967, 1971), as well as for broadband noise (Møller 1977, 1983a,b,c; deBoer 1967). The phase-locking of the discharges of single auditory nerve fibers to the time pattern of a sound thus seems to be a more robust feature of neural coding than is the discharge rate, at least for sounds in the frequency range below 5 kHz (Møller 1977, 1983a,b,c; Rose et al. 1967, 1971; Eggermont and Epping 1987).

When neural activity in many auditory nerve fibers becomes phase-locked to the waveform of a sound, it also results in the neural activity in the auditory nerve fibers that are responding to the sound becoming mutually correlated. Spontaneous neural activity of single auditory nerve fibers in different nerve fibers is regarded to be uncorrelated (Johnson and Kiang 1976). There is thus a fundamental difference between the time pattern of spontaneous neural activity and neural activity that is evoked by a sound when an ensemble of nerve fibers are observed.

When neural activity in many nerve fibers is correlated, excitation of neurons that integrate the activity from such auditory fibers will increase with the degree of phase-locking and the number of nerve fibers that carry such phase-locked activity, but the output of that nerve cell would be small if the neural activity that is integrated over many nerve fibers is uncorrelated. This is because correlated neural activity in many nerve fibers adds together in phase. By detecting correlated neural activity in many auditory nerve fibers, such neurons would have the potential of being detectors of the presence of sound, and maybe also the potential to signal the loudness of a sound to higher brain centers. The substrate for such integration is present in the cochlear nucleus, where many neurons have the property to integrate the activity in many primary auditory nerve fibers.

An hypothesis that assumes it is the correlation of neural activity in many nerve fibers that determines whether or not nerve activity is interpreted as a sound is attractive, because this measure is not dependent on fluctuations in the spontaneous discharge rate that may occur without the presence of a sound. Phase-locking is therefore a much more robust characteristic of sound-evoked neural activity in single auditory nerve fibers than is the rate of discharges in single auditory nerve fibers (Eggermont 1990; Møller 1984).

If phase-locking of auditory nerve activity can generate a sensation of sound, then any pathological process that causes phase-locking may evoke the sensation of a sound, even when no physical sound reaches the ear, thus tinnitus. Such artificial correlation could be caused by pathological communication (through ephaptic transmission) between auditory nerve fibers or between hair cells in the cochlea (Eggermont 1990; Møller 1984). It is possible that the tinnitus that results from, for instance, surgical injury to the intracranial portion of the auditory nerve, which may occur during MVD operations to relieve trigeminal neuralgia and hemifacial spasm, may be caused by an abnormal cross-transmission between nerve fibers that results in synchronization of the spontaneous neural activity in many nerve fibers. Also, acoustic tumors are often associated with tinnitus, which may worsen after removal of the tumor, probably as a result of surgical injury to the nerve. Such patients may have tinnitus together with severe hearing loss or even total deafness. It is possible that injury to the ear from noise exposure, and maybe from ototoxic antibiotics, has a similar effect, namely establishing an abnormal communication between hair cells or auditory nerve fibers.

That tinnitus indeed may result directly from neural activity in auditory nerve fibers is evident from studies that show that electrical current passed through the cochlea (and possibly the auditory nerve) can have an immediate effect of increasing/decreasing the tinnitus, depending upon the current direction (Portmann, Cazals, Negrevergne, and Aran 1979; Cazals, Negrevergne, and Aran 1977).

VASCULAR COMPRESSION OF THE EIGHTH NERVE AS CAUSE OF TINNITUS

If tinnitus in all cases was only a result of an abnormal function of the ear (or of the auditory nerve), so that neural activity was produced in the auditory nerve that was similar to that produced by sound, then it would be easy to understand the pathophysiology of tinnitus. However, it seems that the physiological abnormality that generates the tinnitus in many cases is located in the central auditory nervous system. There are, however, indications that it may be an injury to the ear or to the auditory nerve that may cause the changes in such centrally located neural structures. This concept implies that the generation of tinnitus is more complex than has been previously assumed.

It has become evident from studies of the auditory system, as well as other systems, that an injury to or stimulation (irritation) of the peripheral portion of such systems can over a period of time cause changes in more central systems that would indicate that there was a change in synaptic efficacy or a synaptic reorganization. Such changes may shift the relationship between inhibition and excitation and affect the temporal pattern of the neural response. Since inhibition normally limits the maximal sustained firing rate, a reduced inhibition may result in an abnormally high firing level of certain neurons (Pollak and Park 1993), which may explain the pain (or discomfort) many patients with tinnitus

often experience when exposed to loud sounds. Such an imbalance between inhibition and excitation may have many consequences.

Some forms of incapacitating tinnitus can be alleviated by moving a compressing blood vessel off the eighth nerve and placing a soft implant between the nerve and the vessel (Jannetta 1977, 1987; Kondo, Ishikawa, Yamasaki, and Konishi 1980, A.R. Møller, M.B. Møller, Jannetta, and Jho 1992a; Møller 1992; M.B. Møller, A.R. Møller, Jannetta, and Jho 1992). This has led to the assumption that these forms of tinnitus are caused by irritation of the auditory nerve from a blood vessel; such irritation may indeed give rise to neural activity in the auditory nerve that may be interpreted as a sound by the central auditory nervous system.

However, while this seems to be an attractive explanation for tinnitus, it does not explain the high degree of hypersensitivity that many patients with incapacitating tinnitus experience. Recent studies indicate that such incapacitating tinnitus may instead be caused by hyperactivity of some nuclei of the ascending auditory pathway (Møller et al. 1992, 1992a,b; Møller and Møller 1991). Such hyperactivity could be caused by reduced inhibition, as mentioned above.

Since these patients can be cured by moving the blood vessel off the auditory nerve, there seems little doubt that vascular irritation of the auditory nerve is implicated in generating the tinnitus. The previous assumption that such hyperactivity is brought about directly by abnormal neural activity in the fibers of the auditory nerve that is generated by the irritation of the auditory nerve from the close contact with a blood vessel does not seem to explain these forms of incapacitating tinnitus. Rather, it seems more likely that the vascular irritation over time causes changes in certain specific nuclei of the ascending auditory pathway. These changes may be in the form of altered synaptic efficacy that causes a shift in the balance between inhibition and excitation. This would explain the finding that incapacitating tinnitus often also involves an abnormal perception of sound intensity in the form of a hypersensitivity to sound that is associated with a distinct, unpleasant sensation when exposed to sounds of high intensity. Such incapacitating tinnitus is thus similar to pain.

Disorders such as TN, HFS, and DPV that can be cured by MVD of the respective cranial nerve have several features in common with certain forms of incapacitating tinnitus: The functions of the respective cranial nerves are close to normal, with only a small, if any, decrease in sensitivity of the face in patients with TN or in facial weakness in patients with HFS (Digre and Corbett 1988). Similarly, patients with tinnitus often have near normal hearing or only a slight (usually high-frequency) hearing loss, even in cases in which the tinnitus is incapacitating. Another characteristic of such incapacitating tinnitus is that it worsens over time, as typically do the symptoms in patients with HFS and TN. This may be a result of progressive injury to the auditory nerve, but it may also be explained by an increasing change in the central auditory nervous system, which is in accordance with the assumption that the development of changes in central nuclei occurs gradually over a period of time.

It follows from the discussion above that the site of lesion may not be the site of the physiological abnormality that generates the abnormal nerve activity perceived as tinnitus in patients with incapacitating tinnitus, such as that caused by vascular compression of the eighth cranial nerve. We have attempted to identify the site of the physiological abnormality of tinnitus that is caused by vascular compression of the intracranial portion of the eighth nerve using intraoperative electrophysiological recordings (Møller et al. 1992a; Møller and Møller 1991).

The intensity of the tinnitus that is experienced by the patients who have been operated upon for tinnitus using the MVD technique in our institution has been severe. Therefore, if the tinnitus of these patients had produced neural excitation similar to that evoked by a sound, one would expect that the click-evoked potentials recorded from the structures that generate the tinnitus

would display major abnormalities. It is well known that even a relatively weak broadband background noise will cause a noticeable decrease in the amplitude of the click-evoked potentials that can be recorded from the ear and the auditory nerve. However, we found in a study of 19 consecutive patients who were operated upon for incapacitating tinnitus that there were no noticeable abnormalities in the click-evoked potentials when recorded from the exposed eighth nerve, nor were there any abnormalities in the latency of peak III in the BAEP when compared with results from patients with matched hearing losses but no tinnitus (Møller 1992a; Møller and Møller 1991). Peak III of the BAEP is assumed to be generated by the cochlear nucleus (Møller and Jannetta 1981, 1983). However, the latency of peak V in 16 of these 19 patients with tinnitus who had high-frequency hearing loss was slightly (but statistically significantly) shorter than in patients with similar hearing loss but no tinnitus (the sharp tip of peak V is generated by the termination of the lateral lemniscus in the inferior colliculus [Møller and Jannetta 1982]).

It is thus surprising that the patients we studied, whose tinnitus was so severe, did not have large abnormalities in their auditory evoked potentials of the peripheral portion of the classical ascending auditory pathway. This is particularly surprising in view of the fact that almost half of the patients with tinnitus obtained a substantial relief from their tinnitus as a result of MVD of the auditory nerve (Møller 1992a; Møller and Møller 1991), thus strongly indicating that the vascular irritation of the eighth nerve indeed was related to the tinnitus. Because of the absence (or near absence) of specific and recordable signs of abnormal function of the nuclei of the ascending auditory pathway, at least as far as the lateral lemniscus, it seems reasonable to conclude that the physiological abnormalities that cause tinnitus in these patients were not a direct result of a physiological abnormality of the eighth nerve, nor does the cochlear nucleus seem to be affected. These results indicate that some nuclei of the ascending auditory pathway that are located between the cochlear nucleus and the inferior colliculus may be hyperactive. While this could be caused by an increased excitation by a reduced inhibition that might explain tinnitus, the reduced latency of peak V that we observed should be interpreted cautiously, because the differences in latency were small (although statistically significant), and because of the small number of patients studied. Thus, the small degree of abnormalities seen in the BAEP seems insufficient to explain the severe symptoms of these patients.

HOW CAN PERIPHERAL INJURIES AFFECT HIGHER BRAIN CENTERS?

There is considerable evidence from studies in animals that injury to the ear and auditory nerve can result in various types of alterations in the function of centrally located neural structures. Thus, exposure to a strong sound that results in temporary threshold shift (TTS) causes single neurons in the cochlear nucleus to have an elevated threshold for a period of time after cessation of the exposure. Excitatory tuning curves also become broader than normal (Salvi 1976; Henderson and Møller 1975), which is in agreement with the assumption that injury to the cochlea will affect the active processes in the cochlea that produce high sensitivity and sharp tuning. Single nerve cells in the cochlear nucleus usually display inhibitory response areas on both sides of their excitatory areas, similar to what is seen in primary auditory nerve fibers. It is interesting that the inhibitory areas of cochlear nucleus units become more depressed than the excitatory areas as a result of temporary threshold shift that is induced by overexposure to sound. These inhibitory response areas can be demonstrated by presenting a constant tone at a unit's characteristic frequency, at an intensity that is above threshold, at the same time as a second tone with variable frequency and intensity is used to probe areas of inhibition. A reduction in the inhibitory area may result from a decrease in the spontaneous discharge rate of single auditory nerve fibers that have inhibitory influence on neurons in the cochlear nucleus.

It has been shown that overstimulation by a sound may increase the excitability of neurons in the inferior colliculus (Salvi, Perry, Hamernik, and Henderson 1982; Salvi, Saunders, Gratton, Arehole, and Powers 1990), which could be explained either by a reduction of the inhibitory influence on neurons in the inferior colliculus or an increased excitation of more caudal nuclei.

If it is assumed that it is the spontaneous activity of specific auditory nerve fibers that maintains a proper level of inhibition in the auditory system (for instance, in the inferior colliculus), then a reduction in such spontaneous activity could explain the tinnitus that immediately follows an overexposure to sound. The gradual decrease of such tinnitus over a period of time could be explained by the gradual restoration of normal spontaneous activity in auditory nerve fibers. It is most likely auditory nerve fibers tuned to high frequencies that have such inhibitory influence on inferior collicular neurons. A decrease in the spontaneous activity of such auditory nerve fibers may then have the same effect on centrally located nuclei as an increased excitation. This may explain why both increased spontaneous activity and decreased spontaneous activity of auditory nerve fibers may cause tinnitus. It has thus been shown in animals experiments that deprivation of input to the ascending auditory system (by destruction of the cochlea) can cause a decrease in the integration time of the inferior colliculus (Gerken, Solecki, and Boettcher 1991), thus an indication of hyperexcitability.

The hypothesis that tinnitus is a result of slightly decreased spontaneous activity in the auditory nerve fibers that maintain a proper level of inhibition in the inferior colliculus may explain this remarkable absence of electrophysiological signs of abnormalities from the auditory nerve and from the farfield potentials of the brainstem nuclei in patients with incapacitating tinnitus.

It seems evident from the results reported above that vascular compression in itself does not generate sufficient abnormal nerve activity to account for the degree of tinnitus experienced by patients whose tinnitus can be alleviated by MVD operations. The irritation of the auditory nerve from the close contact with a blood vessel may in such patients generate neural activity which over time alters the balance between inhibition and excitation in specific nuclei of the ascending auditory pathway. This may occur by altering synaptic efficacy in nuclei of the ascending auditory pathway that occurs over time.

It is known that inhibition mediated by GABA is responsible for the decrease in the firing rate of some inferior collicular neurons when the stimulus level is increased beyond a certain value (Pollak and Park 1993) (thus giving these neurons a non-monotonic, stimulus-firing rate function). If GABA-induced inhibition is necessary to control firing of inferior collicular neurons when the stimulus level is increased above a certain level, reduction of such inhibition may explain the hypersensitivity to sound that many patients with incapacitating tinnitus experience. Thus, the application of bicuculline, which is a GABA antagonist, increases the sound-driven discharge rate by several hundred percent (Pollak and Park 1993). Although it is not known if an increased discharge rate of inferior collicular neurons will cause the sensation of tinnitus, it may indicate that pharmacological agents that enhance GABAergic receptors (such as benzodiazepines) may cause a reduction in the firing of inferior collicular neurons that is perceived as tinnitus. Similarly, substances that modulate the effect of excitatory amino acids, such as baclofen, may have a similar effect and thus be candidates for treating certain forms of tinnitus.

The hypothesis that changes in some central auditory nuclei are induced over time by the irritation of the auditory nerve from a blood vessel is supported by the observation that the results of MVD operation on 72 patients (31 female, 41 male) were dependent on the duration of the patients' symptoms (Møller et al. 1992). In this study the outcome of the MVD operation on the patients' tinnitus was classified as "excellent,"

"much improved," "slightly improved," "no change," and "worse." The overall success rate was: excellent and much improved, 40.3%; slightly improved, 11.1%; no change, 48.6%; only one person became worse (as a result of an injury to the auditory nerve that also caused a hearing loss). It is important to note that those patients who experienced an outcome that was "excellent" and "much improved" following MVD operations had had their tinnitus for an average of 2.8 years, while those who had "no change" had had their tinnitus for an average of 7.1 years. It thus seems to be more difficult to relieve tinnitus if the patient has had the condition for a long time. This is similar to what is the case for trigeminal neuralgia (TN) (Apfelbaum 1984).

Somewhat surprisingly, the success rate for women was considerably better than that for men (54.8% of 31 female versus 29.3% of 41 male subjects in this study). This difference between women and men is statistically significant. The reason for this large difference is not known, but it is known that reproductive hormones stimulate the secretion of GABA (McGinnis, Gordon, and Gorski 1980; Perez, Zucchi, and Maggi 1986). It has previously been shown that the latencies of the individual peaks in the BAEP vary during the menstrual cycle of women who are of reproductive age (Dehan and Jerger 1990; Elkind-Hirsch, Stoner, Stach, and Jerger 1992), thus indicating that female reproductive hormones influence inhibition and excitation in the brainstem auditory pathways. These results of MVD operation on patients with tinnitus may be taken as further indications of the influence of reproductive hormones on the relation between inhibition and excitation in the central nervous system.

IS THE EXTRALEMNISCAL AUDITORY NERVE SYSTEM INVOLVED IN INCAPACITATING TINNITUS?

In view of the small abnormalities in the auditory evoked potentials in patients with incapacitating tinnitus, we have suggested that the physiological abnormality that causes this type of tinnitus and the hypersensitivity to sound often associated with severe tinnitus may not be located in the classical ascending auditory pathway at all, but rather in the extralemniscal system (Møller et al. 1992b; Møller and Møller 1991). The extralemniscal auditory system, also known as the nonspecific system (Graybiel 1972), branches off the lemniscal system at the level of the inferior colliculus. It projects to the association cortices rather than to the primary auditory cortex, as is the case for the lemniscal system (Graybiel 1972; Aitkin 1986). The extralemniscal system has been studied to a lesser degree than the traditional ascending auditory system, but it is known that neurons in the extralemniscal system respond much less specifically to sound stimulation than do neurons in the lemniscal system; this is why the extralemniscal system is also known as the nonspecific system (Graybiel 1972; Aitkin 1986).

Some neurons in the extralemniscal system receive input not only from the auditory system but also from the somatosensory system. Some of the neurons in the extralemniscal system therefore respond to somatosensory stimulation in addition to auditory stimulation (Aitkin 1986; Thompson, Smith, and Bliss 1963; Hotta and Kameda 1963). We therefore assumed that it should be possible to manipulate the sensation of tinnitus in one way or another by stimulation of the somatosensory system, if the extralemniscal system is involved in incapacitating tinnitus (Møller and Møller 1991). To test this hypothesis, we stimulated the median nerve electrically in patients with severe (incapacitating), moderately severe, and weak tinnitus, and asked each patient to report any change he or she might experience in his or her tinnitus (Møller et al. 1992b). Six of 26 patients with tinnitus experienced a decrease in loudness of their tinnitus and less annoyance when their median nerves were stimulated. Of these 6, 4 had severe tinnitus, 1 had moderate tinnitus, and 1 had mild tinnitus. In 4 patients, the tinnitus increased as a result of electrical stimulation of the median nerve (2 of these 4 patients had severe tinnitus, 1 had moderate

tinnitus, and 1 had mild tinnitus). There were no statistical differences between the hearing thresholds of the patients who experienced an increase, decrease, or no effect on their tinnitus from electrical stimulation of the median nerve. Of those who did not experience any change, 8 had severe tinnitus, 2 had moderate tinnitus, and 2 had mild tinnitus. The classification of "severe," "moderate," and "mild" tinnitus was based on the patients' own subjective evaluation of their tinnitus using a similar classification as described by Reed (1960) and M.B. Møller and colleagues (1992).

People without tinnitus also experience a change in the loudness of certain sounds as a result of electrical stimulation of the median nerve. In a study in which repetitive clicks (at 40 pps) or broadband noise of different intensities were presented to one ear it was found that in most subjects the tinnitus loudness increased (Møller et al. 1992b). The change was largest for high-intensity clicks, and the change decreased when the stimulus intensity was decreased. When 40 pps clicks were presented at 105 dB Pe SPL (about 68 dB SL), the mean equivalent to change in loudness was an increase of 2.2 dB + 1.0 dB in the 12 subjects of the study. The effect of electrical stimulation of the median nerve was less when the clicks were presented at a lower intensity. The loudness of broadband noise at 90 dB SPL was only increased by an equivalent of 0.5 dB + 1.2 dB (mean value of 12 subjects). The effect was less when the contralateral median nerve was stimulated, and the change in the perceived loudness was greatest when the median nerve was stimulated at a rate of 2 pps; the effect was only slightly less at stimulus rates of 4 and 10 pps. In these studies of patients with tinnitus and subjects without tinnitus, the electrical stimulation was presented at an intensity at which the individuals experienced a strong tingling sensation but no pain (Møller et al. 1992b).

These results were interpreted to show that the extralemniscal auditory system may normally be involved in the perception of loud (unpleasant) sounds. However, that effect is different from the involvement of the extralemniscal system in patients with incapacitating tinnitus and (acoustic) sounds because the perception of acoustic sounds increases as a result of median nerve stimulation while the sensation of tinnitus decreases in some patients.

CONCLUSIONS

It seems evident that there are many different causes of tinnitus, and that the location of the physiological abnormality that causes the tinnitus may be different for different types of tinnitus. While it seems evident that some types of tinnitus are generated in the ear *or* in the auditory nerve, there is recent evidence that indicates that the pathophysiology of severe incapacitating tinnitus is more complex, and that the neural activity that gives rise to this type of tinnitus is different from that elicited by sound. This is supported by the observation that there is a disagreement between the results of loudness matching in the determination of the intensity of tinnitus and its annoyance level, thus supporting the hypothesis that the neural activity causing tinnitus is different in character from the neural activity evoked by a sound. There is evidence indicating that the location of the physiological abnormality generating this type of severe tinnitus is located much more centrally in the auditory nervous system. The hypothesis that incapacitating tinnitus that can be cured by microvascular decompression (MVD) of the auditory nerve may develop due to a change over time in synaptic efficacy causing an imbalance between excitation and inhibition is supported by these recent studies of incapacitating tinnitus.

The finding that some types of incapacitating tinnitus may be cured by vascular decompression of the auditory nerve intracranially indicates that such tinnitus has a similar etiology as other disorders that are caused by vascular compression of other cranial nerves, such as TN, HFS, and DPV. The fact that MVD of patients with incapacitating tinnitus does not have the same success rate as MVD of TN, HFS, and DPV is puzzling. There are also indications that more than one abnormality

may be required for incapacitating tinnitus to develop, as has been suggested for TN, HFS, and DPV. We do not know what such "other factors" may be. The finding that the extralemniscal system, of which we have very little knowledge, may be involved in some forms of tinnitus requires more studies to be performed before this hypothesis can be confirmed.

REFERENCES

Aitkin, L. 1986. *The Auditory Midbrain, Structure and Function in the Central Auditory Pathway.* Clifton, NJ: Humana Press.

Apfelbaum, R.I. 1984. "Surgery for Tic Doloureux." *Clinical Neurosurgery, 31,* 357–368.

Cazals, Y., Negrevergne, M., and Aran, J.-M. 1977. "Electrical Stimulation of the Cochlea in Man: Hearing Induction and Tinnitus Suppression." *Journal of the American Audiological Society, 3,* 209–213.

de Boer, E. 1967. "Correlation Studies Applied to the Frequency Resolution of the Cochlea." *Journal of Auditory Research, 7,* 209–217.

Dehan, C.P. and Jerger, J. 1990. "Analysis of Gender Differences in the Auditory Brainstem Response." *Laryngoscope, 100,* 18–24.

Digre, K. and Corbett, J.J. 1988. "Hemifacial Spasm: Differential Diagnosis, Mechanisms, and Treatment." In E. Tolosa (Ed.), *Advances in Neurology, Volume 39, Facial Dyskinesia,* pp. 151–176. New York: Raven Press.

Eggermont, J.J. 1990. "On the Pathophysiology of Tinnitus: A Review and Peripheral Model." *Hearing Research, 48,* 111–124.

Eggermont, J.J. and Epping, W.J.M. 1987. "Coincidence Detection in Auditory Neurons: A Possible Mechanism to Enhance Stimulus Specificity in the Grassfrog." *Hearing Research, 30,* 219–230.

Elkind-Hirsch, K.E., Stoner, W.R., Stach, B.A., and Jerger, J.F. 1992. "Estrogen Influences Auditory Brainstem Responses during the Normal Menstrual Cycle." *Hearing Research, 60,* 143–148.

Evans, E.F. and Borerwe, T.A. 1982. "Ototoxic Effects of Salicylate on the Responses of Single Cochlear Nerve Fibers and on Cochlear Potentials." *British Journal of Audiology, 16,* 101–108.

Gerken, G.M., Solecki, J.M., and Boettcher, F.A. 1991. "Temporal Integration of Electrical Stimulation of

Auditory Nuclei in Normal-hearing and Hearing-impaired Cat." *Hearing Research, 53,* 101–112.

Graybiel, A.M. 1972. "Some Fiber Pathways Related to the Posterior Thalamic Region in the Cat." *Brain Behavior and Evolution, 6,* 363–393.

Harrison, R.V. and Evans, E.F. 1982. "Reverse Correlation Study of Cochlear Filtering in Normal and Pathological Guinea-pig Ears." *Hearing Research, 6,* 303–314.

Henderson, D. and Møller, A.R. 1975. "Effect of Asymptotic Threshold Shift in Neural Firing Patterns of the Rat Cochlear Nucleus." *Journal of the Acoustical Society of America,* 57, 53(A), Abstract.

Hotta, T. and Kameda, K. 1963. "Interactions between Somatic and Visual or Auditory Responses in the Thalamus of the Cat." *Experimental Neurology, 8,* 1–13.

Jannetta, P.J. 1977. "Observations on the Etiology of Trigeminal Neuralgia, Hemifacial Spasm, Acoustic Nerve Dysfunction and Glossopharyngeal Neuralgia. Definitive Microsurgical Treatment and Results in 117 Patients." *Neurochirurgia* (Stuttgart), *20,* 145–154.

Jannetta, P.J. 1987. "Microvascular Decompression of the Cochlear Nerve as Treatment of Tinnitus." In H. Feldmann (Ed.), *Proceedings III International Tinnitus Seminar,* pp. 348–352. Karlsruhe: Harsch Verlag.

Johnson, D.H. and Kiang, N.Y.-S. 1976. "Analysis of Discharges Recorded Simultaneously from Pairs of Auditory Nerve Fibers." *Biophysical Journal, 16,* 719–734.

Kiang, N.Y.-S., Moxon, E.C., and Kahn, A.R. 1976. "The Relationship of Gross Potentials Recorded from Cochlea to Single Unit Activity in the Auditory Nerve." In R.J. Ruben, C. Elberling, and G. Salomon (Eds.), *Electrocochleography,* pp. 95–115. Baltimore: University Park Press.

Kiang, N.Y.-S., Moxon, E.C., and Levine, R.A. 1970. "Auditory-nerve Activity in Cats with Normal and Abnormal Cochleas." In G.E.W. Wolstenholme and J. Knight (Eds.), *Sensorineural Hearing Loss,* pp. 241–268. London: Ciba Foundation, J.A. Churchill.

Kondo, A., Ishikawa, J., Yamasaki, T., and Konishi, T. 1980. "Microvascular Decompression of Cranial Nerves, particularly the Seventh Cranial Nerve." *Neurologia Medico-Chirirgica* (Tokyo), *20,* 739–751.

Liberman, M.C. 1978. "Auditory-nerve Response from

Cats Raised in a Low-noise Environment." *Journal of the Acoustical Society of America, 63,* 442–455.

McGinnis, M.Y., Gordon, J.H., and Gorski, R.A. 1980. "Time Course and Localization of the Effects of Estrogen on Glutamic Acid Decarboxylase Activity." *Journal of Neurochemistry, 34,* 785–792.

Møller, A.R. 1977. "Frequency Selectivity of Single Auditory Nerve Fibers in Response to Broadband Noise Stimuli." *Journal of the Acoustical Society of America, 62,* 135–142.

Møller, A.R. 1983a. *Auditory Physiology.* New York: Academic Press.

Møller, A.R. 1983b. "Use of Pseudorandom Noise in Studies of the Frequency Selectivity: The Periphery of the Auditory System." *Biological Cybernetics, 47,* 95–102.

Møller, A.R. 1983c. "Frequency Selectivity of Phase-locking of Complex Sounds in the Auditory Nerve of the Rat." *Hearing Research, 11,* 267–284.

Møller, A.R. 1984. "Pathophysiology of Tinnitus." *Annals of Otology, Rhinology, and Laryngology, 93,* 39–44.

Møller, A.R. 1992. "Central Neurophysiological Processes in Tinnitus." In J.-M. Aran and R. Dauman (Eds.), *Proceedings of the Fourth International Tinnitus Seminar, Bordeaux, 1992.* Amsterdam: Kugler & Ghedini Publications.

Møller, A.R. and Jannetta, P.J. 1981. "Compound Action Potentials Recorded Intracranially from the Auditory Nerve in Man." *Experimental Neurology, 74,* 862–874.

Møller, A.R. and Jannetta, P.J. 1981. "Compound Action Potentials Recorded Intracranially from the Auditory Nerve in Man." *Experimental Neurology, 74,* 862–874.

Møller, A.R. and Jannetta, P.J. 1982. "Evoked Potentials from the Inferior Colliculus in Man." *Electroencephalography and Clinical Neurophysiology, 53,* 612–620.

Møller, A.R. and Jannetta, P.J. 1983. "Auditory Evoked Potentials Recorded from the Cochlear Nucleus and its Vicinity." *Journal of Neurosurgery, 59,* 1013–1018.

Møller, A.R. and Møller, M.B. 1991. "Auditory Nerve Compound Action Potentials (CAP) and Brainstem Auditory Evoked Potentials (BAEP) in Patients with Intractable Tinnitus." In *Proceedings of the Symposium on Tinnitus, Midwinter Meeting of the Associa-*

tion for Research in Otolaryngology (held in St. Petersburg, FL, February 3, 1991), Abstract.

Møller, A.R., Møller, M.B., Jannetta, P.J., and Jho, H.D. 1992a. "Compound Action Potentials Recorded from the Exposed Eighth Nerve in Patients with Intractable Tinnitus." *Laryngoscope, 102,* 187–197.

Møller, A.R., Møller, M.B., and Yokota, M. 1992b. "Some Forms of Tinnitus May Involve the Extralemniscal Auditory Pathway." *Laryngoscope, 102,* 1165–1171.

Møller, M.B. 1987. "Vascular Compression of the Eighth Nerve as a Cause of Tinnitus." In H. Feldmann (Ed.), *Proceedings III International Tinnitus Seminar, Muenster, 1987,* pp. 340–347. Karlsruhe: Harsch Verlag.

Møller, M.B., Møller, A.R., Jannetta, P.J., and Jho, H.D. 1992. "Vascular Decompression Surgery for Severe Tinnitus: Selection Criteria and Results." *Laryngoscope, 103,* 421–427.

Perez, J., Zucchi, I., and Maggi, A. 1986. "Sexual Dimorphism in the Response of the GABAergic System to Estrogen Administration." *Journal of Neurochemistry, 47,* 1798–1803.

Pollak, G.D. and Park, T.J. 1993. "The Effects of GABAergic Inhibition on Monaural Response Properties of Neurons in the Mustache Bat's Inferior Colliculus." *Hearing Research, 65,* 99–117.

Portmann, M., Cazals, Y., Negrevergne, M., and Aran, J.-M. 1979. "Temporary Tinnitus Suppression in Many through Electrical Stimulation of the Cochlea." *Acta Otolaryngologica, 87,* 249–299.

Reed, G.F. 1960. "An Audiometric Study of 200 Cases of

Subjective Tinnitus." *Archives of Otolaryngology, 71,* 94–104.

Rose, J.E., Brugge, J.F., Anderson, D.J., and Hind, J.E. 1967. "Phase-locked Response to Low-frequency Tones in Single Auditory Nerve Fibers of the Squirrel Monkey." *Journal of Neurophysiology, 30,* 769–792.

Rose, J.E., Hind, J.E., Anderson, D.J., and Brugge, J.F. 1971. "Some Effects of Stimulus Intensity on Response of Auditory Fibers in the Squirrel Monkey." *Journal of Neurophysiology, 34,* 685–699.

Salvi, R.J. 1976. "Central Components of the Temporary Threshold Shift." In D. Henderson, R.P. Hamernik, D.S. Dosanjh, and J.H. Mills (Eds.), *Effect of Noise on Hearing,* pp. 247–260. New York: Raven Press.

Salvi, R.J., Perry, J., Hamernik, R.P., and Henderson, D. 1982. "Relationship between Cochlear Pathologies and Auditory Nerve and Behavioral Responses following Acoustic Trauma." In R.P. Hamernik, D. Henderson, and R.J. Salvi (Eds.), *New Perspectives on Noise-Induced Hearing Loss,* pp. 165–188. New York: Raven Press.

Salvi, R.J., Saunders, S.S., Gratton, M.A., Arehole, S., and Powers, N. 1990. "Enhanced Evoked Response Amplitudes in the Inferior Colliculus of the Chinchilla following Acoustic Trauma." *Hearing Research, 50,* 245–258.

Thompson, R.F., Smith, H.E., and Bliss, D. 1963. "Auditory, Somatic Sensory, and Visual Response Interactions and Interrelations in Association and Primary Cortical Fields of the Cat." *Journal of Neurophysiology, 26,* 365–378.

CHAPTER 16

PSYCHOPHYSICAL OBSERVATIONS AND THE ORIGIN OF TINNITUS

M.J. PENNER
University of Maryland

R.C. BILGER
University of Illinois

Abstract

In this chapter, we examine prototypical psychophysical data involving the masking of tinnitus (Feldmann 1971). We argue that tinnitus isomasking contours may reflect isoloudness judgments, and that differences in ipsilateral and contralateral tinnitus masker levels are consistent with a cochlear origin of tinnitus. If tinnitus is due to cochlear malfunctions, then existing simulations of the normally functioning cochlea (Patterson and Holdsworth 1991) may be modified to produce tinnitus. In particular, by changing tuning and suppression functions to reflect that of tinnitus sufferers, it may be possible to produce a quantitative model of tinnitus.

INTRODUCTION

Many different otological afflictions are associated with the symptom of tinnitus. Tinnitus may accompany dysfunctions, including conductive loss (Graham and Newby 1962), Ménière's disease (Caparosa 1963; Day 1963), sensorineural hearing loss (Stevens and Davis 1938), retrocochlear lesions and brainstem tumors (Brackman 1981), and may also be a consequence of restorative surgical interventions, such as stapedectomy, fenestration, tympanoplasty, and radical mastoidectomy (Douek 1987).

By far the most common cause of tinnitus, though, is cochlear damage which may result from noise trauma or noise exposure. In fact, it has been estimated that 34 percent of the people with tinnitus also suffer from noise-induced hearing loss (Reed 1960). It is the source of such tinnitus that we discuss in this chapter: What do available psychophysical data concerning such tinnitus imply about its origin?

Before beginning to discuss the issues, some caveats are necessary. First, limiting our remarks to tinnitus associated with sensorineural hearing loss may not guarantee that the resulting tinnitus has one common origin. Indeed, tinnitus may have two coexisting sources (Penner 1989a). Second, the approach taken in this chapter is to base inferences on the psychoacoustical observations made by tinnitus sufferers. Ultimately, the origin of tinnitus is not solely a psychoacoustic question but will require physiological corroboration.

The physiological basis of tinnitus in animals and man is not yet, however, understood. Indeed, until Jastreboff and colleagues (Jastreboff, Brennan, and Sasaki 1988), it was not certain that animals perceived tinnitus. Therefore, in some publications, animals were presumed to have tinnitus after drugs, which generally induced tinnitus in humans, were administered. Even the appropriate neural code underlying tinnitus is not identified: Is tinnitus due to an incremental (Eggermont 1984; Tonndorf 1981) or an abrupt change in neural response rates (Kiang, Moxon, and Levine 1970)? In the absence of definitive physiological data and theory, psychoacoustic facts may form a basis for initial conjecture.

Based on psychophysical data involving the masking of tinnitus, the prevailing view at the present time is that tinnitus is a central signal, originating after cochlear injury and manifesting itself retrocochlearly. We will review here the masking data supporting this hypothesis and offer an alternative explanation. Other psychophysical data, such as the pitch of tinnitus or the description of it by the tinnitus sufferer, have occasionally been used as a basis for inference regarding the locus of tinnitus but such inference is speculative (Reed 1960; Goodhill 1950).

PSYCHOACOUSTIC DATA

Masking of Tinnitus

In an exemplary paper, Feldmann (1971) presented data that are consistent with the notion that tinnitus originates retrocochlearly. To understand that interpretation and to motivate another view, a brief review of masking in normal-hearing subjects and pitch matching in subjects with tinnitus will be informative.

In their classic paper, Wegel and Lane (1924) showed that a pure tone is most effectively masked by tones near it in frequency. In fact, for normal-hearing subjects, the frequency and level of an unknown masked tone may be deduced from the pattern revealed by its frequency-specific isomasking contour (masker level as a function of masker frequency). An example of the evident relation between a signal and its isomasking contour is presented in Figure 16-1. Note that there is a local minimum in masker level near the frequency of the external signal.

Fletcher (1940) postulated, as later physiologists would show (von Békésy 1960), that isomasking contours such as those in Figure 16-1 resulted, at least in part, from the cochlear interaction of the masker and the signal. Because each signal in Figure 16-1 is at a low level (10 dB SPL), it primarily activates one region of the basilar membrane (Rhode 1971). To mask the signal, a masker must activate the same region (Fletcher 1940).

Because the auditory system acts as a series of bandpass filters (Fletcher 1940), activity in a specific region is most readily produced by nearby tones. Therefore, the resulting isomasking contour displays a local minimum in the region activated by the signal, and the signal frequency can be inferred from the position of the local minimum in signal threshold. Behavioral frequency selectivity is accompanied by frequency selectivity at the neural level: The responses of a single nerve fiber, as reflected in isorate contours, are also frequency selective (Evans 1975).

Frequency selectivity in normal-hearing observers is exhibited when masking a narrowband signal. A pure-tone complex with widely spaced components or broadband noise, however, cannot be easily masked by a single pure tone or by a narrowband masker. Thus, the isomasking contour for such a signal might not display frequency selectivity.

Isomasking contours for tinnitus, even tinnitus described as tonal, are not often frequency specific (Feldmann 1971; Burns 1984; Penner 1986; Tyler and Conrad-Armes 1984), even if frequency selectivity is present for external signals in the tinnitus region (Burns 1984; Penner 1986). An example of the lack of frequency-specific masking of tinnitus accompanied by the frequency-

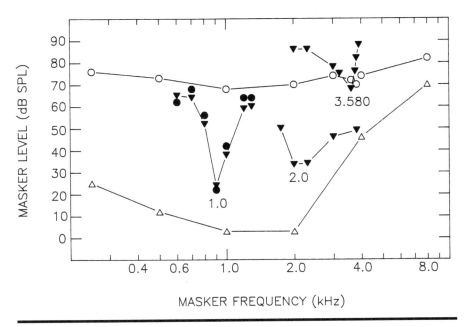

FIGURE 16-1. Isomasking contours (sinusoidal masker level as a function of masker frequency) and audiogram (sinusoidal signal level as a function of frequency). Isomasking contours for pure tones at the labeled frequencies are marked by the upside-down triangles (forced-choice procedure) and filled circles (adjustment procedure). Tinnitus isomasking contours are marked with open circles. Threshold is also graphed (triangles). The average frequency of the tone said to match the predominant pitch of the tinnitus was 3.580 kHz. (Reprinted with permission from American Speech-Language-Hearing Association.)

specific masking of external tones (at 1, 2, and 3.58 kHz) is also presented in Figure 16-1.

The lack of frequency-specific masking of tinnitus has prompted investigators to posit that tinnitus is not likely to be masked by physical interaction in the cochlea (Feldmann 1971; Burns 1984; Penner 1986; Tyler and Conrad-Armes 1984). Before accepting the conclusion that tinnitus is not masked in the cochlea, however, some additional aspects of the problem need to be considered.

Matches to Tinnitus

Tinnitus differs from external sounds in that the variability of matches of pure tones to the predominant pitch of the tinnitus obtained with the method of adjustment is rather large, often spanning several octaves (Burns 1984; Norton, Schmidt, and Stover, 1990; Penner 1983; Tyler and Conrad-Armes 1983). For example, for 10 subjects who used an adaptive psychophysical technique with the matching tone in the ipsilateral ear, Tyler and Conrad-Armes (1983) found an average within-session range of 3.2 octaves in the pure tone judged as matching the tinnitus pitch for their adaptive procedure. Data from one subject who made repeated matches to tinnitus are presented in Figure 16-2 (Penner 1983). As is usual in matches made to tinnitus, the matches were inconsistent, and for this subject, spanned nearly one octave.

Because tinnitus is seldom reliably matched to a single pure tone, it is likely to be either a fluctuant

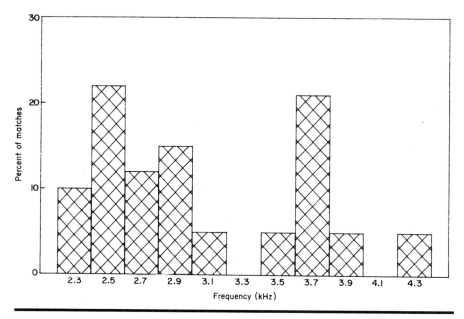

FIGURE 16-2. Distribution of matching responses for subject RP. The ordinate displays the percent of the 80 matches made to the tinnitus which lay in the 200 Hz region whose midpoint is displayed on the abscissa. (Reprinted with permission from American Speech-Language-Hearing Association.)

or a broadband signal or both. With one octave spacing between pure-tone or one-third-octave narrowband noise maskers, fluctuant and/or broadband external sounds could not reasonably be expected to be masked, raising the question of whether fluctuant, broadband tinnitus was actually masked. Could some other psychophysical judgment have been made?

LOUDNESS OF TINNITUS

In this section, we use one of the equations governing the growth of loudness for normal-hearing subjects to predict isomasking contours for tinnitus. The data fitted with the equal-loudness hypothesis are those of Feldmann (1971). Because Feldmann's data have been replicated (Burns 1984; Penner 1986; Tyler and Conrad-Armes 1984), fits to other data are redundant; therefore,

we restrict ourselves to Feldmann's seminal data in the ensuing discussion. The implication is that subjects in tinnitus masking studies may generally have been confused by the relation between masking and loudness.

For normal-hearing subjects, the relation between sensation level and loudness is known to depend in part on the absolute threshold of the sound involved. The exact relation between loudness and threshold is still disputed (Humes and Jesteadt 1991; Larkin and Penner 1989), but one popular form relates the loudness, L, in sones, of a pure tone with pressure P to the threshold pressure, p_0, by the equation

$$L = k(P-p_0)^p \qquad (16\text{-}1)$$

where k is a constant (Luce 1959; Stevens 1966) and the exponent, p, is approximately 0.6 for frequencies from 0.5 to 8.0 kHz. Equation 16-1 is, of course, the basis of the sone scale of loudness (International Standards Organization 1959). For frequencies less than 0.5 kHz, the exponent is likely to exceed 0.6 (Hellman and Zwislocki 1968). It is by no means established that Equation 16-1 describes the growth of loudness associated with sensorineural hearing loss near threshold. Nonetheless, data from subjects with sensorineural hearing loss have been fitted with Equation 16-1 (Tyler and Conrad-Armes 1983; Penner 1984).

If two sounds, X, at pressure P_x with threshold $p_{x,0}$, and Y, at pressure P_y with threshold $p_{y,0}$, are equated for loudness, then if the exponent is constant,

$$P_x - p_{x,0} = P_y - p_{y,0} \qquad (16-2)$$

Note that Equation 16-2 has no free parameters: Neither the exponent, p from Equation 16-1, nor the constant, k, are required for predicting loudness matches. It is important to note that Equation 16-2 can be obtained from Equation 16-1 only if the exponent, p, remains constant for all sounds. The models in Equations 16-1 and 16-2 have been called the linear-correction power law because the threshold intensity is subtracted from the stimulus intensity prior to compression.

We chose to fit the data with the linear-correction model rather than with the modified power-law model, in which stimulus intensities are compressed prior to subtraction (Humes and Jesteadt 1991). Two reasons prompted this choice. First, loudness judgments in the modified power-law depend on the exponent, p, which was not determined individually for Feldmann's (1971) subjects or in any other published data. Although the average value of p is about 0.6 (Stevens 1955), and that value is employed by the International Standards Organization (1959), much data attests to individual variability in the exponent (McGill 1974; Reason 1968; Stevens and Guiaro 1964). Therefore, we used a model that did not require a subject-specific value. Second, the main difference between the linear-correction power model and the modified power model with compressed internal noise is the rate of the rise of loudness

near absolute threshold. Thus, the differences in the two models will only affect the fits for matching tones which are near their absolute thresholds, a situation which is not generally the case for Feldmann's data (Feldmann 1971).

We also chose a model that depends only on the thresholds of the stimuli involved in the match. Several recent models of loudness growth are phrased in terms of both the dynamic range and the thresholds of the stimuli (Larkin and Penner 1989; Lim, Rabinowitz, Braida, and Durlach 1977; Pavel and Iverson 1981). The dynamic range models are more accurate predictors of the underlying processes than are simple threshold models, if only because there is an extra parameter, the dynamic range, used to fit the data. In general, loudness judgments are too variable to provide unequivocal support for one formulation or another and the range and threshold are not independent of each other. For these reasons, we employ the simpler linear correction model to fit the tinnitus isomasking contours of Feldmann (1971).

Predicting Isomasking Contours

Feldmann (1971) presents the thresholds of pure tones at the audiometric frequencies and the levels of one-third-octave bands of noise centered at the audiometric frequencies which "mask" the tinnitus. The fits of Equation 16-2 to the data from Feldmann are presented in Figure 16-3.

In Figure 16-3, the audiogram of the subject was used to determine $p_{x,0}$. This means that the threshold of the pure tone is taken as a proxy for the threshold of the one-third-octave band noise. If the third-octave bands fell within a critical band, then the proxy would be accurate. To the extent that the noise exceeds a critical band, the approximation is in error. Our approximation is similar in principle to that of Bilger and colleagues (Bilger, Nuetzel, Rabinowitz, and Rzeckowski 1984) who estimate the threshold of babble (broadband stimuli) from absolute audiometric thresholds. In the present case, because the threshold is much less than the level of the "masking" noise, the ex-

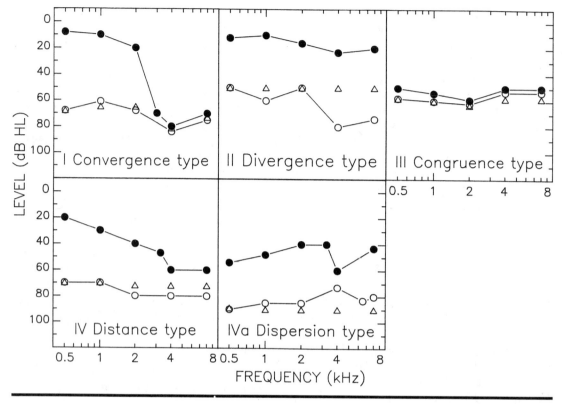

FIGURE 16-3. Different types of "masking" contours for tinnitus. The filled circles represent the thresholds of the pure tones, the open circles represent the levels of third-octave bands of noise which mask tinnitus, and the triangles represent the predictions from Equation 16-2. The data in the figure are Feldmann's (1971).

act value of threshold does not generally markedly affect the patterns of the isomasking predictions except for frequencies exceeding 4 kHz in the convergence-type isomasking contour.

Because the modified power law (Humes and Jesteadt 1991) compresses the thresholds prior to subtraction, its predictions would be dependent on threshold. Even though the fits of the modified power law might be superior to those seen in Figure 16-3, that model cannot be applied to the data because the compression factor is not known. Therefore, the level of sounds at other frequencies that are predicted to match the loudness of the 0.5

kHz "masker" was determined using Equation 16-2 and plotted in Figure 16-3.

The fits of Equation 16-2 were not applicable to 125 and 250 Hz noise bands, because the exponent is greater in these regions than elsewhere. It is the ratio of the exponents at the low and high frequencies which would be needed to make the predictions at 125 and 250 Hz. Failure of Equation 16-2 to fit equal-loudness contours at low frequencies when tinnitus is the standard has been previously noted (Penner 1984).

There is general agreement that the loudness of a band of noise grows somewhat more rapidly than the loudness of a 1 kHz pure tone. However, loudness matches between a pure tone and noise are highly variable. Not only is there variability between subjects, but different matches are obtained depending on whether the subject adjusts the tone or the noise (Zwicker 1958). Because there is scant data on the growth of loudness of noise and because the exponent governing the growth of loudness is unimportant if it remains constant, Equation 16-2 was employed as a first approximation whenever the noise was within the frequency region in which the exponent in Equation 16-2 remained constant for pure tones.

As can be seen from Figure 16-3, for all but the divergence-type contour, the predicted isoloudness contours are within 10 dB of Feldmann's (1971) data. The failure of the isoloudness model to fit the divergence-type contour is noteworthy and will be dealt with later.

Feldmann (1971) also positioned the masker in the ear contralateral to monaural tinnitus and found that tones or noise bands of only moderate

intensity masked the tinnitus in the contralateral ear. The intensity required to mask tinnitus was sometimes smaller in the ear without the tinnitus, suggesting that tinnitus may be centrally masked. If, however, the data reflected a contralateral loudness judgment, then Equation 16-2 could again be used to predict the "masker" level in the contralateral ear. Fits of the isoloudness model to the data from Feldmann's Figure 16-2 are presented in Figure 16-4. As can be seen in Figure 16-4, the linear correction model predicts that the intensity required for a tone to be judged as loud as the tinnitus is less in the contralateral than in the ipsilateral ear.

Another masking phenomenon which may be of use in inferring the origin of tinnitus is that of Penner, Brauth, and Hood (1981). They showed that tinnitus becomes audible in noise which previously masked it. They offered two explanations: Either the neural activity underlying the tinnitus does not adapt, or the tinnitus is a central signal that becomes audible in noise because the periph-

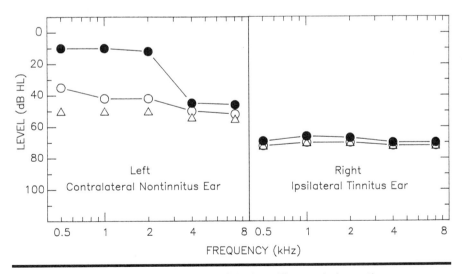

FIGURE 16-4. Contralateral "inhibition" of tinnitus. The symbols are the same as those in Figure 16-1. The data in the figure are Feldmann's (1971). The subject reported tinnitus in the right ear only.

eral auditory system adapts to the noise. Because these data are consistent with either a central or a peripheral origin of tinnitus, they do not preclude the view espoused here that tinnitus may have a peripheral origin.

DISCUSSION

There is one discrepancy between our predictions and Feldmann's (1971) masking contours. While four of Feldmann's masking contours are nicely fitted with the isomasking model embodied in Equation 16-2, the fifth, the divergence type, is not. We will first discuss this inconsistency and then examine the general issue of the masking of tinnitus.

The audiogram associated with the divergence-type masking contour is the only one which is not markedly abnormal. Indeed, the audiogram is within 20 dB HL for all frequencies except 4 kHz. Penner (1988, 1989a,b) has presented data consistent with the interpretation that some forms of tinnitus are due to spontaneous otoacoustic emissions (SOAEs), acoustic energies which can be detected when a sensitive miniature microphone is inserted into the ear canal. SOAE-caused tinnitus has been documented only in subjects with nearly normal hearing, and Penner even presented some data indicating that internal tones of cochlear origin may cause tinnitus when SOAEs cannot be measured (Penner 1992). The audiogram associated with the divergence-type contour is essentially normal, suggesting that SOAE-caused tinnitus could be a possibility.

Several other pieces of circumstantial evidence linking the divergence-type contour and SOAE-caused tinnitus are also noteworthy. First, about 4 percent of the members of a tinnitus self-help group had SOAE-caused tinnitus (Penner 1990). Feldmann (1971) estimates that 3 percent of subjects with tinnitus display a divergence-type masking contour. Thus, there is rough agreement between Feldmann's estimate of the prevalence of the divergence-type masking contour and Penner's (1990) estimate of the prevalence of SOAE-caused tinnitus. Second, SOAEs are most common in the 1

to 2 kHz region (Bilger, Matthies, Hammel, and Demorest 1990) where Feldmann's divergence-type masking contour displays a 10 dB local minimum, as would be expected if an SOAE near 1 kHz were masked. These observations do not unequivocally link SOAEs to the divergence contour, but, coupled with the reasonably close fits to the other contours, they do raise the question of whether some combination of masking SOAE-caused tinnitus and loudness matching to other forms of tinnitus might produce all the observed isomasking contours.

It is easier to reconcile the discrepancies between the data and the predictions for the divergence-type contour than to understand why subjects in the tinnitus-masking experiment might be making loudness judgments. Although we are not able to offer a definite answer, psychophysical findings for normal-hearing subjects provide a framework in which the question may be pursued.

Consider the mechanism involved in masking a single external tone. In one popular excitation model, masking is thought to be a "swamping" of the neural activity evoked by the signal on the neural channels which respond to the signal (Moore and Glassberg 1982). If the tinnitus were a broad-band and fluctuant signal, then the neural activity it evokes would encompass many neural channels, some sporadically. With the neural activity alternating abruptly over channels that respond to tones ranging over several octaves, masking of tinnitus might be hard to distinguish from fluctuations in the tinnitus itself. In these circumstances, the tinnitus "masker" might merely produce the same overall excitation as the tinnitus, but not necessarily in any specific channels. Thus, overall excitation might be equated with masking. Because excitation is likely to be related to loudness (Zwicker 1958, 1963), the masking contours could represent isoloudness contours with the tinnitus serving as the standard.

The excitatory masking analogy is a speculative hypotheses consistent with the notion that tinnitus isomasking contours may be tinnitus isoloudness contours. Undoubtedly, other hypotheses consistent with isoloudness also exist. The purpose of this chapter is not to enumerate and test all hypotheses, but merely to cast reasonable doubt on the idea that tinnitus isomasking contours necessarily represent masking in the ordinary sense.

The intuition motivating the loudness hypothesis is the observation that, although the audiograms of Feldmann's (1971) subjects differ substantially, their isomasking contours are nearly horizontal lines. The patterns are therefore reminiscent of equal-loudness contours obtained for loud pure tones (Robinson and Dadson 1956). Additionally, equal-loudness contours obtained when tinnitus serves as the standard and an external comparison tone is adjusted to match its loudness are also generally horizontal lines (Penner 1984).

If tinnitus were not masked, then arguments based on the tinnitus isomasking contours are also suspect. For example, the lack of correspondence of the Wegel and Lane (1924) masking contours and the tinnitus isomasking contours has led to the conclusion that tinnitus is not masked in the cochlea or that the pattern of activity responsible for tinnitus is not identical to the pattern evoked by an external stimulus. The difference in ipsilateral and contralateral tinnitus masker levels has led to the conclusion that tinnitus is masked centrally. There is also another interpretation: Perhaps the tinnitus was not masked.

The arguments presented thus far are controversial because they are based on correlative, circumstantial evidence. However, the locus of tinnitus must ultimately be physiologically verified, and prior to that milestone, conclusions related to the origin are likely to be speculative. The notion that the available data are consistent with a cochlear origin of tinnitus means that explicit predictions concerning its psychophysics become possible.

FUTURE DIRECTIONS

If tinnitus were a peripheral signal, as Stevens and Davis (1938) originally postulated and as the psychophysical data may permit as a possibility, then extant simulations of the peripheral auditory system provide a logical route for modeling tinnitus, if the model's parameters are modified to accommodate changes in auditory functions due to hearing loss.

There are many ways in which the psychophysics of subjects with tinnitus and sensorineural hearing loss differ from that of normal-hearing subjects. In terms of modelling tinnitus, two differences are likely to be particularly salient: Auditory filters (i.e., isomasking contours) in such subjects are broader (Florentine, Buus, and Zwicker 1980; Zwicker and Schorn 1978) and suppression regions narrower (Penner 1980). Isomasking contours have already been discussed and represent the data which result from banks of auditory filters. The topic of lateral suppression has not yet been described and it is to that topic which we now turn.

Evidence favoring lateral suppression was presented by Houtgast (1972): The response of the auditory system to a tone of a given frequency can be reduced (suppressed) by particular tones at different frequencies. These data are consistent with the physiological data of Kiang (1968), which show that the neural response rate to two tones can be less than to one. In general, suppression and tuning regions covary (Robertson 1976): the narrower the suppression region, the wider the isomasking contour. Penner (1980) has shown that tinnitus sufferers did not exhibit two-tone suppression in the tinnitus region. She argued, as Ruggero and colleagues (Ruggero, Rich, and Freyman 1983) did subsequently to explain SOAEs, that the lack of suppression in regions of hearing loss might cause an imbalance in the suppression and excitation characteristics. Such an imbalance could produce excess spontaneous activity in adjacent regions and the excess activity, if narrowband, could cause SOAEs, or if broadband, could be perceived as tinnitus.

This word picture may be made concrete by incorporating it into the model of Patterson and Holdsworth (1991). Patterson and Holdsworth have presented a model of multichannel neural activity corresponding to broadband signals. The model transforms sounds into an "auditory image" which is intended to be the internal likeness of the sound. The components of the model comprise a cochlear simulation which includes a filterbank, compression and suppression mechanisms. By altering the suppression and excitation regions, in accord with the data from subjects with tinnitus and sensorineural hearing loss, we may be able to modify the model so that it will produce tinnitus.

Testing the model is not difficult and is underway in the laboratories of both Penner and Feth. The internal auditory image for each individual subject is constructed from his threshold sensitivity, isomasking contours, and suppression regions. Regions of excess activity displayed by the simulation should correspond to the tinnitus region. The tinnitus region may be experimentally measured in a tinnitus pitch-matching paradigm (Penner and Bilger 1992). Furthermore, the isomasking contours and the isoloudness contours should also be predictable from the internal auditory representation.

The thesis of this chapter is that tinnitus may originate in the cochlea. Because of cochlear malfunction, an imbalance in the tuning and suppression regions may give rise to excess activity known subjectively as tinnitus (Penner 1980). By offering a reinterpretation of masking data, traditionally thought to indicate that tinnitus has a retrocochlear origin, we open the door to applying extant models of cochlear functioning to the phenomenon of tinnitus.

Some of this research was supported by grants from the National Institutes of Health (1 R01 DC00068 to MJP and DC00174 to RCB). Additional support was received from the University of Maryland.

REFERENCES

Békésy, G. von. 1960. *Experiments in Hearing.* E.G. Wever (Ed.) New York: McGraw-Hill.

Bilger, R.C., Matthies, M.L., Hammel, D.R., and Demorest, M. 1990. "Genetic Implications of Gender Differences in the Prevalence of Spontaneous Otoacoustic Emissions." *Journal of Speech and hearing Research, 33,* 418–432.

Bilger, R.C., Nuetzel, J.M., Rabinowitz, W.M., and Rzeckowski, C. 1984. "Standardization of a Test of Speech Perception in Noise." *Journal of Speech and Hearing Research, 32,* 32–48.

Brackman, D.E. 1981. Panel discussion. In A. Schulman (Chairman), *Proceedings of the First International Tinnitus Seminar. Journal of Laryngology and Otolaryngology, Supplement, 4,* 143–144.

Burns, E.M. 1984. "A Comparison of Variability among Measurements of Subjective Tinnitus and Objective Stimuli." *Audiology, 23,* 426–440.

Caparosa, R.T. 1963. "Medical Treatment for Ménière's Disease." *Laryngoscope, 73,* 666–672.

Day, K.M. 1963. "Twenty-five Years Experience with Ménière's Disease." *Laryngoscope, 73,* 693–697.

Douek, E.1987. "Tinnitus following Surgery." n H. Feldmann (Ed.), Proceedings III International Tinnitus Seminar, pp. 64–69. Karlsruhe: Harsch Verlag.

Eggermont, J.J. 1984. "Tinnitus: Some Thoughts about Its Origin." *Journal of Laryngology and Otology, 9,* 31–37.

Evans, E.F. 1975. "The Sharpening of Cochlear Frequency Selectivity in the Normal and Abnormal Cochlea." *Audiology, 14,* 419–442.

Feldmann, H. 1971. "Homolateral and Contralateral Masking of Tinnitus by Noise-bands and by Pure Tones." *Audiology, 10,* 138–144.

Fletcher, H. 1940. "Auditory Patterns." *Review of Modern Physics, 12,* 47–65.

Florentine, M., Buus, S., and Zwicker, E. 1980. "Frequency Selectivity in Normally-hearing and Hearing-impaired Observers." *Journal of Speech and Hearing Research, 70,* 1646–1654.

Goodhill, V. 1950. "The Management of Tinnitus." *Laryngoscope, 60,* 442–450.

Graham, J.T. and Newby, H.A. 1962. "Acoustical Characteristics of Tinnitus." *Archives of Otolaryngology, 75,* 162–167.

Hellman, R.P. and Zwislocki, J.J. 1968. "Loudness Determination at Low Sound Frequencies." *Journal of the Acoustical Society of America, 43,* 60–64.

Houtgast, T. 1972. "Psychophysical Evidence for Lateral Inhibition in Hearing." *Journal of the Acoustical Society of America, 51,* 1885–1894.

Humes, L.E. and Jesteadt, W. 1991. "Models of the Effects of Threshold on Loudness Growth and Summation." *Journal of the Acoustical Society of America, 90,* 1933–1943.

International Standards Organization. 1959. *Expression of the Physical and Subjective Magnitude of Sound*, ISO/R 131.

Jastreboff, P.J., Brennan, J.F., and Sasaki, C.T. 1988. "An Animal Model for Tinnitus." *Laryngoscope, 98*, 280–286.

Kiang, N.Y.S. 1968. "A Survey of Recent Developments in the Study of Auditory Physiology." *Annals of Otology, Rhinology and Laryngology, 77*, 656–675.

Kiang, N.Y.S., Moxon, E.C., and Levine, R.A. 1970. "Auditory-nerve Activity in Cats with Normal and Abnormal Cochleas." In G.E.W. Wolstenholm and J. Knight (Eds.), *Sensorineural Hearing Loss*, pp. 241–242. London: J. and A. Churchill.

Larkin, W.D. and Penner, M.J. 1989. "Partial Masking in Electrocutaneous Sensation: A Model for Sensation Matching with Application to Loudness Recruitment." *Perception and Psychophysics, 46*, 207–219.

Lim, J.S., Rabinowitz, W.M., Braida, L.D., and Durlach, N.I. 1977. "Intensity Perception: XIII. Loudness Comparisons between Different Types of Stimuli." *Journal of the Acoustical Society of America, 62*, 1256–1267.

Luce, R.D. 1959. "On the Possible Psychophysical Law." 1959. *Psychology Review, 66*, 81–95.

McGill, W.J. 1974. "The Slope of the Loudness Function: A Puzzle." In H.R. Moskowitz, B. Scharf, and J.C. Stevens (Eds.), *Sensation and Measurement*, pp. 293–307. Dordrecht, Holland: Reidel.

Moore, B.C.J. and Glassberg, B.R. 1982. "Interpreting the Role of Suppression in Psychoacoustical Tuning Curves." *Journal of the Acoustical Society of America, 72*, 1374–1379.

Norton, S.J., Schmidt, A.R., and Stover, L.J. 1990. "Tinnitus and Otoacoustic Emissions: Is There a Link?" *Hearing Research, 11*, 159–166.

Patterson, R.D. and Holdsworth, J. 1991. "A Functional Model of Neural Activity Patterns and Auditory Images." In W.A. Ainsworth (Ed.), *Advances in Speech, Hearing and Language Processing*. London: JAI Press.

Pavel, M. and Iverson, G.J. 1981. "Invariant Characteristics of Partial Masking: Implications for Mathematical Models." *Journal of the Acoustical Society of America, 69*, 1126–1131.

Penner, M.J. 1980. "The Coding of Intensity and the Interaction of Forward and Backward Masking." *Journal of the Acoustical Society of America, 67*, 608–616.

Penner, M.J. 1983. "Variability in Matches of Subjective Tinnitus." *Journal of Speech and Hearing Research, 26*, 73–76.

Penner, M.J. 1984. "Equal Loudness Contours Using Subjective Tinnitus as the Standard." *Journal of Speech and Hearing Research, 27*, 267–274.

Penner, M.J. 1986. "The Masking of Tinnitus and Central Masking." *Journal of Speech and Hearing Research, 29*, 400–406.

Penner, M.J. 1988. "Audible and Annoying Spontaneous Otoacoustic Emissions: A Case Study." *Archives of Otolaryngology, 114*, 582–587.

Penner, M.J. 1989a. "Two Coexisting Sources of Tinnitus: A Case Study." *Journal of Speech and Hearing Research, 32*, 339–346.

Penner, M.J. 1989b. "Aspirin Abolishes Tinnitus Caused by SOAEs: A Case Study." *Archives of Otolaryngology, 115*, 871–875.

Penner, M.J. 1990. "An Estimate of the Prevalence of Tinnitus Caused by Spontaneous Otoacoustic Emission." *Archives of Otolaryngology, 116*, 418–423.

Penner, M.J. 1992. "Linking Spontaneous Otoacoustic Emissions and Tinnitus." *British Journal of Audiology, 26*, 115–123.

Penner, M.J. and Bilger, R.C. 1992. "Consistent Within-session Measures of Tinnitus Pitch and Loudness." *Journal of Speech and Hearing Research, 35*, 694–700.

Penner, M.J., Brauth, S., and Hood, L. 1981. "The Temporal Course of the Masking of Tinnitus as a Basis for Inferring Its Origin." *Journal of Speech and Hearing Research, 24*, 257–261.

Reason, J.T. 1968. "Individual Differences in Auditory Reaction Time and Loudness Estimation." *Perception Motor Skills, 26*, 1089–1090.

Reed, G.F. 1960. "An Audiometric Study of Two Hundred Cases of Subjective Tinnitus." *Archives of Otolaryngology, 71*, 94–104.

Rhode, W.S. 1971. "Observations of the Vibrations of the Basilar Membrane in Squirrel Monkeys Using the Mossbauer Technique." *Journal of the Acoustical Society of America, 49*, 1218–1231.

Robertson, D. 1976. "Correspondence between Sharp Tuning and Two-tone Inhibition in Primary Auditory Neurones." *Nature, 256*, 477–478.

Robinson, D.W. and Dadson, R.S. 1956. "A Re-determination of the Equal-loudness Relations for Pure

Tones." *British Journal of Applied Physics, 7,* 166–181.

Ruggero, M.A., Rich, N.C., and Freyman, R. 1983. "Spontaneous and Evoked Otoacoustic Emissions: Indicators of Cochlear Pathology?" *Hearing Research, 10,* 283–300.

Stevens, J.C. and Guiaro, M. 1964. "Individual Loudness Functions." *Journal of the Acoustical Society of America, 36,* 2210–2213.

Stevens, S.S. 1955. "The Measurement of Loudness." *Journal of the Acoustical Society of America, 27,* 815–829.

Stevens, S.S. 1966. "Power Group Transformations under Glare, Masking, and Recruitment." *Journal of the Acoustical Society of America, 39,* 725–735.

Stevens, S.S. and Davis, H. 1938. *Hearing, Its Psychology and Physiology.* New York: Wiley.

Tonndorf, J. 1981. "Stereocilliary Dysfunction, a Cause of Sensory Hearing Loss, Recruitment, Poor Speech Discrimination and Tinnitus." *Acta Otolaryngologica, 91,* 469–479.

Tyler, R.S. and Conrad-Armes, D. 1983. "Tinnitus Pitch: A Comparison of Three Measurement Methods." *British Journal of Audiology, 17,* 101–107.

Tyler, R.S. and Conrad-Armes, D. 1984. "Masking of Tinnitus Compared to Masking of Pure Tones." *Journal of Speech and Hearing Research, 27,* 106–111.

Wegel, R.L. and Lane, C.E. 1924. "The Auditory Masking of One Pure Tone by Another and Its Probable Relation to the Dynamics of the Inner Ear." *Physics Review, 23,* 266–285.

Zwicker, E. 1958. "Über psychologishe und methodische Grundlagen der Lauheit." *Acoustica, 13,* 194–211.

Zwicker, E. 1963. "Über die Lauheit von ungedrosselten und gedrosselten Schallen." *Acoustica, 13,* 194–211.

Zwicker, E. and Schorn, K. 1978. "Psychoacoustical Tuning Curves in Audiology." *Audiology, 17,* 120–140.

THE ANALOGY BETWEEN TINNITUS AND PAIN

A SUGGESTION FOR A PHYSIOLOGICAL BASIS OF CHRONIC TINNITUS

JUERGEN TONNDORF
Columbia University

Abstract

A new hypothesis is developed concerning the origin of chronic tinnitus. It is based on an analogy between tinnitus and intractable pain, both of their causes being seen in the deafferentation of nerve fibers. It is suggested that in the control of tinnitus the same interplay exists between large inner-hair cell fibers and small outer-hair-cell fibers, provided they are deafferented, that was demonstrated to exist between large and small deafferented fibers of the somatosensory system in the control of pain.

Tinnitus (TI) is an auditory sensation existing in the absence of an external acoustic stimulus. It is called "objective" when it can be verified by an outside observer, but "subjective" when it is only perceived by the patient (Fowler 1939; among others). This distinction has lost some of its significance with the recent demonstration of the so called "cochlear echo," that is, the audible emission of sound from the ears of a number of subjects on suitable stimulation (Kemp 1978). Although only some of these subject were able to hear the emitted sound themselves, it was proposed to limit the term "tinnitus" to the subjective form (Evered and Lawrenson 1981), an opinion shared by this writer.

It appears that TI may originate at all levels of the auditory system. It has been suggested, for example, that TI might be of peripheral origin when it can be acoustically masked, and that the unmaskable variety should be of central origin (Shulman, Tonndorf, and Goldstein 1985).

The fact that there are no outward signs has, of course, hampered research on TI. One must depend wholly on the patient's description. The sensation is described in a variety of ways as "noisy" in character, or "tonal," or as tones superimposed on noise (Hazell 1980). It may be steady or pulsating, and change in character or in quality from day to day. In acute Ménière's attacks, however, the TI is a characteristic, low-pitched ("roaring") noise.

This chapter was reprinted from *Hearing Research, 28,* pp. 271–275 (1987), with permission from Elsevier Science Publishers B.V., Amsterdam, The Netherlands.

Tonal TI most frequently is rather high-pitched. Occasionally, Bekesy audiometry can be used to demonstrate tonal TI. As soon as the audiometric sweep tone approaches the frequency of the TI, the patient attempts to attenuate the signal maximally, an error only realized when the two frequencies again begin to pull apart.

Objective signs of TI in animal models have so far been reported twice (guinea pig: Evans, Wilson, and Borerwe 1981; cat: Schreiner and Snyder 1987). Both groups of authors used salicylates in doses that produce blood concentrations evoking TI in humans. Evans and colleagues (1981) demonstrated higher than normal, spontaneous discharge rates in auditory-nerve fibers of animals so affected. Schreiner and Snyder derived the amplitude spectrum of the spontaneous activity of the whole auditory nerve. They observed (1) the overall level of the spontaneous activity increase, and (2) its dominant frequency (approx. 200 Hz) shift to higher values, thus confirming and expanding on the findings of Evans and colleagues (1981). Lidocaine i.v. and electrical stimulation via round-window electrodes reduced the salicylate-induced changes. Yet, as pointed out by Møller (1984), salicylate-induced TI is not necessarily identical to TI of other origins. And then again, as already stated, there are most likely a variety of mechanisms responsible for TI, not all of them even cochlear.

Møller (1984) used a different approach from the notions underlying the above experiments. Focusing on the "temporal" properties of discharges of auditory nerve fibers, he pointed out that in the absence of stimulation the spontaneous activity in cochlear-nerve fibers is uncorrelated, that is, completely random. Especially in low-frequency fibers, at levels before the discharge rate is actually increased, the first sign of a response is a grouping of discharges, so-called phase-locking. Møller (1984) argued that, whereas the random discharges should not generate auditory percepts, the phase-locked discharges might do so; hence, they might be perceived as TI.

Central to Møller's (1984) hypothesis is the assumption that TI is invariably associated with some lesion(s) of the auditory system, an opinion that is borne out by clinical experience and is accepted by most authors (McFadden 1982). In the majority of cases the TI is a symptom accompanying hearing loss. In fact, profoundly deaf subjects usually suffer from strong TI (Graham 1981) and the first, accidental observation of the beneficial effect of electrical stimulation on TI was made on precisely such patients (Aran and Cazals 1981). If TI is tonal, its frequency often lies on the downgoing slope of the loss curve. Occasionally, when a hearing loss could at first not be found, it was finally demonstrated in the narrow frequency intervals between the conventional octave testing steps (Berlin and Shearer 1981). Moreover, Berlin ventured the opinion that in some other cases the hearing loss might be located at frequencies beyond the normal testing range, a notion that was confirmed (Shulman et al. 1985).

Arguing that the most frequent lesion of the auditory system concerns the hair cells, this writer developed the hypothesis that "ciliary dysfunction" might lead to TI, in conjunction with hearing loss, recruitment, and loss of speech perception, all symptoms of "acute" cochlear disorders (Tonndorf 1980). In a recent survey, however, only a few cases were seen in which the alleviation of TI under the effect of electrical stimulation was accompanied by a transient improvement of the hearing threshold as the above hypothesis would have demanded (Shulman et al. 1985). Apparently, ciliary dysfunction can only account for TI in acute cochlear disorders, as was originally postulated.

In the following pages, a different hypothetical explanation will be offered, one more for TI of "cochlear" origin. It is based on an analogy between chronic TI in the auditory system and chronic intractable pain in the somatosensory system. TI may be considered the equivalent of pain (Aran and Cazals 1981). There are a number of fundamental analogies between hearing and skin sensations as was demonstrated by Békésy (1957). The similarities between pain and TI include: both are wholly subjective sensations, and both are continuous events; with time, however, they may change in quality and/or character. Both can be masked by suitable inputs, although not in all cases. This included cross-modality masking of sound by pain (Benjamin 1958) and of dental pain by sound (Licklider, personal communication). In selected cases both sensations can be alleviated, or even totally suppressed, by electrical stimulation. In both systems, the alleviation of the pathological sensation may outlast the cessation of the alleviating stimulus, a phenomenon that, with reference to TI, has been termed "residual inhibition" (Feldmann 1971). Topically applied anesthetic agents, as well as centrally acting pain suppressors, may also temporarily relieve TI. A surgically sectioned afferent nerve more often than not is not helpful in either case.

There is neither a specific system for the transmission and processing of pain nor of TI. Pain signals are transmitted along the general somatosensory pathways, and TI signals along the somatosensory pathways. In addition to their afferent sensory fibers, both systems possess an equally well-developed counterpart of efferent fibers that appears to exercise some control on the input into the afferent fibers. In both systems, the afferent, as well as the efferent, fibers make connections with thalamic centers as do, of course, those of all other sensory systems.

Since there now exists a widely accepted theory on the mechanism underlying the generation of chronic, intractable pain that is largely based on physiological evidence, it may be of interest at this point to describe it in some detail and then to examine if it might be applicable to the problem of chronic TI.

The notion of pain due to denervation goes back to the earlier, pioneering studies of Cannon and Rosenblueth (1937). They demonstrated increased spontaneous activity in denervated—so-called "deafferented" structures and/or neurons.

The gate control theory of Melzack and Wall (1965) states that from the point of input, pain signals travel along two types of afferent fibers: large-diameter and small-diameter fibers. Both of them project into the substantia gelatinosa and

onto the first central transmission (T) cells, which together make up the "gate control system." The substantia gelatinosa exerts an inhibitory effect on the T-cells via the large fibers, tending to hold the gate closed, and a propagating effect via the small fibers, tending to hold the gate open. The output of the T-cells projects onto the "action system," which in turn serves to trigger the pain sensation, provided the gate is open.

Of importance to the generation of pain is the ongoing activity in the system: The small fibers are slowly adapting and thus have a tendency to hold the gate open for prolonged periods of time; and the stimulus-evoked activity, although initially deafferented large fibers become activated relatively strongly, tending to keep the gate closed. They adapt faster and prolong stimulation so that the gate is eventually forced open by the longer lasting activity of the likewise deafferented small fibers. The large fibers may be reactivated, however, by scratching or by vibratory stimulation so that the gate is again closed to some extent. It is the relative balance between both sets of fibers at any given time that, after spatial and temporal integration, modulates the output of the T-cells integration, modulates the output of the T-cells, and thus determines the triggering of pain sensations. The well-recognized long time delay between stimulation and the onset of pain, sometimes as long as 35 x, can hardly be accounted for on the basis of slow conduction of afferent fibers, but more easily on the basis of the interplay between the two sets of fibers (Melzack and Melinkoff 1974).

Of further importance are centrally evoked effects that are activated by signals traveling up along fast afferent fibers, and, for their return, make use of the efferent system. They permit general central activities, such as attention, emotion, and memories of prior experiences, to exert control over the sensory input.

Melzack and Melinkoff (1974) also discussed a possible mechanism for the phenomenon of residual inhibition (to use the auditory term). Prolonged pain may produce permanent, or semipermanent, central neural changes, such as the formation of memory-like, reverberating loops, which a suppressing agent, electrical currents for example, might temporarily interrupt. Their studies further indicated that optimal suppression could be achieved when the pain was of peripheral origin, and a lesser effect when it was of central origin. Finally, they gave evidence for the fact that pain suppression is not a placebo effect.

We shall now attempt to apply these principles to the problem of TI.

1. As already mentioned, chronic TI in the auditory system is considered the equivalent of chronic pain in the somatosensory system.

2. The afferent auditory fibers are also of two kinds. Those supplying the inner hair cells have considerably larger diameters than those supplying the outer hair cells. If the same balance would exist between them as between the two sets of fibers carrying information on pain, cochlear-nerve deafferentation should trigger TI; the fact that each outer hair-cell fiber supplies up to ten cells, whereas each inner hair-cell fiber supplies only one cell (although together with up to twenty other fibers) may somewhat complicate the situation.

3. The easiest to account for under the present hypothesis is the TI in profoundly deaf subjects. If all hair cells are gone, both sets of fibers are deafferented. In the long run, the activity of the small diameter fibers should prevail and chronic TI should develop.

4. In most cochlear disorders, however, the outer hair cells are preferentially lost and TI and hearing loss are the most frequent accompanying symptoms of such an occurrence. In this situation, apparently, the deafferentation of the small fibers is the determining effect and it is largely unopposed by large fiber actions.

5. The phenomenon of prolonged residual inhibition after electrical suppression (up to periods of several hours) suggests that central, memory-like loops might thus be interrupted in the sense of Melzack and Melinkoff (1974).

6. Acoustic masking with its relatively short residual inhibition (typically measuring in minutes) might mechanically reactivate the large diameter, inner hair cell fibers in largely the same manner as the large diameter pain fibers are temporarily reactivated by scratching or by vibratory stimulation. This view is further supported by the fact that masking appears to be only effective in cases of TI of peripheral origin (Shulman et al. 1985). It is thus suggested that the modes of action of masking and of electrostimulation might be basically different.

7. Drugs, on the other hand, could act peripherally or centrally. Their action might be differentiated on the duration of residual inhibition, if the present hypothesis is correct.

8. Like pain, TI is to some extent under central control, most likely via the efferent system. Anxiety and lack of sleep appear to aggravate it, whereas distraction alleviates it.

9. As with pain, TI of peripheral origin is apparently easier to suppress than that of central origin.

10. Ligation of the cochlear nerve in an effort to alleviate TI is usually unsuccessful, as is that of afferent somatosensory nerves to alleviate pain. In either case the locus of deafferentation is simply moved to higher levels.

11. There is good evidence that TI suppression is not a placebo effect (Dobie, in preparation).

It would be of interest to learn if there exists a cochlear disorder to man, in which the inner hair cells are preferentially eliminated, and if so, whether, in retrospect, such patients had suffered TI or not. In animals, Dallos and colleagues (Dallos, Cheatham, and Ferraro 1974) have seen inner hair cell loss in the apical portion of guinea pigs' ears after streptomycin intoxication. Deol and Gluecksohn-Waelsch (1979) have found inner hair cells to be congenitally absent in a certain variety of "waltzing" mice, incidentally in conjunction with severe hearing loss. It would be interesting to find out if these animals suffer TI or not according to the criteria proposed by Evans and colleagues (1981) and by Schreiner and Snyder (1987).

To conclude, I would like to emphasize once more that the present hypothesis is only capable of accounting for one kind of chronic TI that, although presumable a very frequent kind, is most likely not the only one.

REFERENCES

Aran, J.-M. and Cazals, I. 1981. "Electrical Suppression of Tinnitus." In *Tinnitus, Ciba Foundation Symposium 85,* pp. 217–225. London: Pitman Books Ltd.

Békésy, G. von. 1957. "Neural Volleys and the Similarity between Some Sensations Produced by Tones and by Skin Vibrations." *Journal of the Acoustical Society of America, 29,* 1059–1069.

Benjamin, F.B. 1958. "Effect of Pain on Simultaneous Perception of Non-painful Sensory Stimulation." *Journal of Applied Physiology,* 630–634.

Berlin, C.I. and Shearer, P.D. 1981. "Electrophysiological Simulation of Tinnitus." In *Tinnitus, Ciba Foundation Symposium 85,* pp. 139–145. London: Pitman Books Ltd.

Cannon, W.R. and Rosenblueth, A. 1937. *The Supersensitivity of Denervated Structures.* New York: Macmillan.

Dallos, P., Cheatham, M.A., and Ferraro, J. 1974. "Cochlear Mechanics Nonlinearities and Cochlear Potentials." *Journal of the Acoustical Society of America, 55,* 297–605.

Deol, M.S. and Gluecksohn-Waelsch, S. 1979. "The Role of the Inner Hair Cells in Hearing." *Nature* (London), *278,* 250–252.

Dobie, R.A. In preparation. "Electrical Tinnitus Suppression."

Evans, E.F., Wilson, J.P., and Borerwe, T.A. 1981. "Animal Models of Tinnitus." In *Tinnitus, Ciba Foundation Symposium 85,* pp. 108–129. London: Pitman Books Ltd.

Evered, D. and Lawrenson, G. (Eds.). 1981. *Tinnitus, Ciba Foundation Symposium 85.* London: Pitman Books Ltd.

Feldmann, H. 1971. "Homolateral and Contralateral Masking of Tinnitus by Noise Bands and by Pure Tones." *Audiology, 10,* 138–144.

Fowler, E.P. 1939. "Head Noises and Deafness: Peripheral and Central." *Laryngoscope, 49,* 1017–1023.

Graham, J.M. 1981. "Tinnitus in Children with Hearing Loss." In *Tinnitus, Ciba Foundation Symposium 85.* London: Pitman Books Ltd.

Hazell, J.W.P. 1980. "Medical and Audiological Findings in Subjective Tinnitus." *Clinical Otolaryngology, 5,* 75–80.

Kemp, D.T. 1978. "Stimulated Acoustic Emissions from within the Human Auditory System." *Journal of the Acoustical Society of America, 64,* 1386–1391.

McFadden, D. 1982. *Tinnitus: Facts, Theories, and Treatments.* Washington, DC: National Academy Press.

Melzack, R. and Melinkoff, D.F. 1974. "Analgesia Produced by Brain Stimulation; Evidence for a Prolonged Onset Period." *Experimental Neurology, 43,* 369–374.

Melzack, R. and Wall, P.D. 1965. "Pain Mechanisms: A New Theory." *Science, 150,* 971–979.

Møller, A.R. 1984. "Pathophysiology of Tinnitus." *Annals of Otolaryngology, 93,* 39–44.

Schreiner, C.E. and Snyder, R.L. 1987. "A Physiological Animal Model of Peripheral Tinnitus." In H. Feldmann (Ed.), *Proceedings III International Tinnitus Seminar, 1987,* pp. 100–106. Karlsruhe: Harsch Verlag.

Shulman, A., Tonndorf, J., and Goldstein, B. 1985. "Electrical Tinnitus Control." *Acta Otolaryngologica, 99,* 318–325.

Tonndorf, J. 1980. "Acute Cochlear Disorders; the Combination of Hearing Loss, Recruitment, Poor Speech Discrimination of Tinnitus." *Annals of Otolaryngology, 89,* 353–358.

CHAPTER 18

COCHLEAR MOTOR TINNITUS, TRANSDUCTION TINNITUS, AND SIGNAL TRANSFER TINNITUS: THREE MODELS OF COCHLEAR TINNITUS

HANS PETER ZENNER
ARNE ERNST
University of Tübingen

INTRODUCTION

Cochlear physiology has been significantly changed over the last decade. The identification of outer hair cells as the source of active amplification in auditory transduction led to some implications upon which the present paper is based. Four hypotheses of the generation of cochlear tinnitus are described in detail. Although an objective assessment of the tinnitus patient is not yet possible, it seems reasonable to speculate on the role of cochlear mechanisms in the pathogenesis of tinnitus and to outline therapeutic concepts based on these ideas.

PHYSIOLOGICAL BACKGROUND

Sound Preprocessing of the Cochlea

The cochlea is no longer regarded as a passive sound receiver. On the contrary, the active motility of outer hair cells (OHCs) enables the cochlea to preprocess the sound signal mechanically before it is transduced by the inner hair cells (IHCs). OHCs are capable of producing active, fast AC and slow DC movements (Figure 18-1) (Brownell, Bader, Bertrand, and Ribaupierre 1985; Zenner, Zimmerman, and Schmitt 1985; Zenner, Zimmer-man, and Gitter 1987, 1988a,b; Flock, Flock, and Ulfendahl 1986; Zenner 1986b; Kachar, Brownell, Altschuler, and Fex 1986; Ashmore 1987; Canlon, Brundin, and Flock 1988; Brundin, Flock, and Canlon 1992).

The slow DC movements (Zenner et al. 1985; Zenner 1986b, 1988) are supposedly aimed at actively displacing the site of the cochlear partition, including the basilar membrane and the organ of Corti in the direction of the tympanic or vestibular scale. This mechanism provides a controlled adjustment of the working angle of the stereocilia and an automatic gain control during changing sound pressure levels (Zenner 1986a,b; LePage, Reuter, and Zenner 1992a). Furthermore, the slow motility might contribute to a mechanical control of the fast AC motility.

There is presently a controversy about how the information generated by high-frequency sound events can be processed, since IHC (and the subsequent release of their efferent transmitters) as well as afferent nerve fibers (and their action potentials) cannot follow sound signals of a higher frequency cycle-by-cycle. In speech signals, the various tones (frequencies) of a voice carry only limited speech information. By contrast, a great part of the speech information is included in the

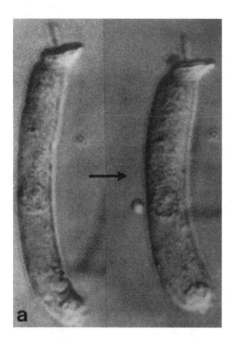

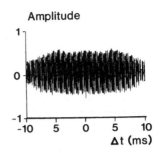

Amplitude

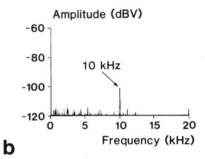

Amplitude (dBV)

10 kHz

Frequency (kHz)

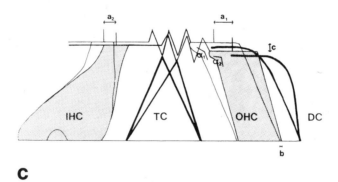

c

IHC   TC   OHC   DC

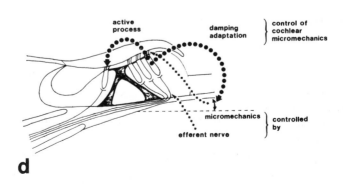

d

active process   damping adaptation   control of cochlear micromechanics

micromechanics controlled by

efferent nerve

FIGURE 18-1. Active motility of outer hair cells. *(a)* Slow motility of an isolated outer hair cell of guinea pig cochlea with a shortening of the cell body and a tilting of the cuticular plate (from Zenner, Zimmerman, and Gitter 1988a). *(b)* High-frequency motility of an isolated outer hair cell as measured with a double photodiode. The power density spectrum is displayed, characterizing a frequency of motility of 10 kHz (from Gitter, Rudert, and Zenner 1992; Zenner et al. 1988a). *(c)* Schematic figure of the transverse (a_1) and radial (a_2) active movements of OHC within the organ of Corti as seen by means of video microscopy. Due to its anatomical position, a shortening of the OHC body is transformed into two directed movements: (i) in a radial shear movement (a_1), the CP with the stereocilia slides laterally in the plane of the RL (a_1), whereas the lower part of the cell partly rotates in the same direction (b); (ii) by a transverse movement (c). Furthermore, a dynamic tilting of the CP due to a change from angle $a_1 > a_2$ is required to explain the missing displacement of the stereociliary bundle in relation to the apical surface of the CP. By contrast, the stereocilia and CP are displaced as an ensemble. The combined active transverse and radial OHC movement is mechanically coupled to the mechanically passive IHCs, which are driven by a_1 of the OHC. The decrease of the movement amplitudes from the inner row of the OHCs to the IHCs ($a_2 < a_1$) suggests the presence of a compliance in the region of TC (IHC-inner hair cell, OHC-outer hair cell, TC-tunnel of Corti, CP-cuticular plate) (from Reuter and Zenner 1990). *(d)* Signal transfer from outer to inner hair cells. The movement of outer hair cells leads to an amplification of the travelling wave. The tips of the amplified travelling wave are perceived by the inner hair cells and finally transduced (from Zenner 1986c).

precise changes of frequency—for example, modulations (van Netten and Khanna 1993)—and the amplitude of the voice's sound in time. These changes are distinctly slower than the oscillations of the carrier frequency. They are largely contained in the envelope, but not in single oscillations, of a sound frequency. Thus, it cannot be excluded that OHCs respond to the envelope of the sound signal by DC movements, and therefore to changes in the frequency and the amplitude of the sound in time. In accordance with this hypothesis, the information of a sound signal with a higher carrier frequency can be actively encoded as a low-frequency, mechanical DC component by the OHCs which subsequently can be transduced by the IHCs (Zenner and Ernst 1993). This hypothesis is supported by the recently described motile DC responses of OHC to mechanical AC stimuli (Figure 18-2) (Reuter and Zenner 1990; Brundin et al. 1989).

In addition, OHCs can respond by fast, active AC movements to an electrical stimulation up to 30 KHz (Brownell et al. 1985; Ashmore 1987; Zenner et al. 1987, 1988a). The shortening and elongation of the cellular body is characterized by a complex movement of the organ of Corti under in-situ conditions. This movement consists of an upward and downward displacement of the reticular lamina (Khanna, Ulfendahl, and Flock 1989; Reuter and Zenner 1990), and also of radial displacements of the cuticular plate including the stereocilia (Reuter and Zenner 1990). This seems to be an appropriate mechanism to enforce actively the traveling wave cycle-by-cycle by one-hundred-fold at low and moderate sound pressure levels. Thus, the active traveling wave is not a linear "inverse reflection" of the sound only, but displays profound nonlinear characteristics. The active traveling wave shows a particularly sharp tip (Sellick, Patuzzi, and Johnstone 1982; Khanna

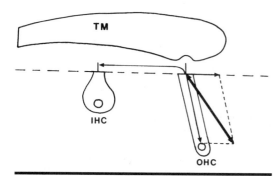

FIGURE 18-2. Transfer of the vibratory signal induced by the hypermotility of cochlear OHCs to neighboring IHC. The hypermotility of outer hair cells (OHCs) leads to unintentional motor movements in a radial and transverse direction. The resulting force is indicated by the thick arrow. An unintentional vibratory signal also results, which is to be transduced to the inner hair cells (IHCs) by fluid coupling, tectorial membrane (TM), as well as reticular lamina (RL), coupling (Reuter and Zenner 1990). This signal is perceived by the IHCs, transduced, and a tinnitus results.

and Leonard 1982; LePage and Johnstone 1980), which is thought to be recognized by the IHCs. In turn, this leads to a high-frequency selectivity as a prerequisite of speech intelligibility (Figure 18-2).

Sound Transduction and Ion Channels

OHCs and IHCs can transduce sound signals mechano-electrically. But IHCs only transfer the sound signal via an afferent transmitter to afferent nerve fibers. In OHCs, the transduced signal contributes supposedly to the control of the active movements in the organ of Corti. OHCs are characterized by a resting membrane potential of about –70 mV, IHCs by about –25 to –45 mV (Dallos 1986; Russell 1983). After sound exposure to the living animal, Russell and colleagues (1986b) recorded a phasic AC modulation of the receptor potential and an additional, sound pressure-dependent depolarizing DC component. The AC component, which is symmetrical relative to the resting poten-

tial, could also be registered in OHCs up to 70 dB SPL. There could be observed a hyperpolarizing asymmetry between 70 and 110 dB; below 110 dB a depolarizing asymmetry (DC component) of up to 5 mV can also be observed (Figure 18-3).

OHCs require essential ion channels to generate the receptor potential. They were described for the first time by Gitter and colleagues (Gitter, Zenner, and Frömter 1986) and Ashmore (1986) in OHCs of mammals. We used the patch-clamp technique to describe an apical, unspecific cation channel facing the endolymphatic space that allows potassium ions to flow along the electrochemical gradient into the interior of the OHCs. In addition, we described lateral potassium channels facing the perilymphatic side. The most important one is a voltage-sensitive, C-type channel (Gitter et al. 1986, 1992a). Ashmore (1986) probably described the same channel when reporting it to be calcium activated. In addition, he described potassium ions as the ionic basis of the receptor potential. We developed a simple model based on these investigations to describe the contribution of these ion channels to the process of auditory transduction (Zenner and Gitter 1987b). It has similarities to a hypothesis valid for submammalian hair cells (Hudspeth 1985), which are not motile, however (Figure 18-3).

According to this hypothesis, the displacement of hair cells in relation to the tectorial membrane (TM) results in a displacement of the stereocilia (directly in OHCs and indirectly in IHCs). Subsequently, potassium-conducting ion channels in the stereociliary membrane or in the apical cell membrane are opened to allow a potassium influx into the cytoplasm of the hair cell. The positive charges lead to a depolarization of the cytoplasmic potential. The depolarization causes an increase of the intracellular calcium which triggers the DC motility in OHCs, or the release of the afferent neurotransmitter in IHCs. The depolarization increases the open probability of a potassium channel of the lateral cell membrane (C-type channel in OHCs), allowing potassium ions to flow from the cytoplasm into the perilymph. Hence, the receptor cell is repolarized.

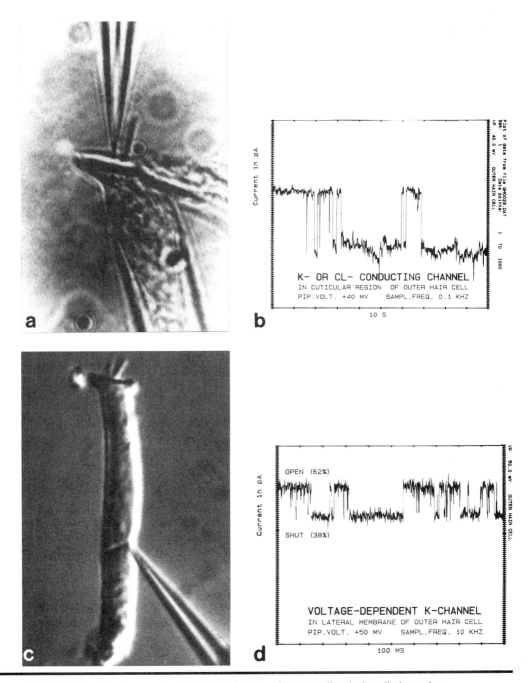

FIGURE 18-3.   Mechano-electrical transduction of mammalian hair cells based on the existence of ionic channels (a, c). Patch-clamp investigations of the apical and lateral cell membrane of guinea pig OHCs to identify ionic channels: *(b)* Trace of the unspecific apical ionic channel measured in (a); *(d)* Trace of the lateral, C-

(continued)

MAMMALIAN HAIR CELL

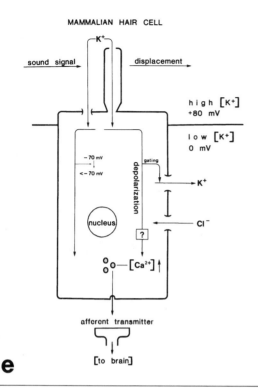

e

FIGURE 18-3. continued
type potassium channel measured in (c) (from
Gitter et al. 1986). *(e)* Schematic figure of the
mechano-electrical transduction of mammalian
hair cells: A deflection of the stereocilia leads to
an opening of apical, unspecific ionic channels
which allows endolymphatic potassium to enter
the cytoplasma of OHC. As a result, the OHC is
depolarized. The depolarization opens the lateral,
C-type potassium channel which allows
potassium from the cellular interior to flow into
the perilymph. Thus, the cell is re- or
hyperpolarized. In case of IHC, the transient
change of the receptor potential induces a
release of the afferent transmitter. The receptor
potential possibly controls the hair cell motility in
OHC (from Zenner and Gitter 1987b).

COCHLEAR TINNITUS

It is only a matter of speculation whether disturbances of receptor potential, ion channels, or active motility can lead to a subjective tinnitus, since
tinnitus cannot be verified objectively. Thus, the
following models are based on investigations of
the function and pathophysiology of OHCs without final experimental evidence for their involvement in tinnitus generation (Table 18-1).

Cochlear Motor Tinnitus

Tinnitus is usually accompanied by a sensorineural
hearing loss in a corresponding frequency range
(Hazell 1984). The frequently observed positive
recruitment phenomenon can be referred to a loss of
the nonlinearity of the cochlear micromechanics.
Thus, a positive recruitment phenomenon implies a
contribution of the OHCs in the disease, since they

TABLE 18-1. Overview of the Different
Types of Cochlear Tinnitus

I. Cochlear motor tinnitus

    – Hypermobility (activation type)

    – Hypomobility (inhibition type)

    – DC motor tinnitus (distortion of fast
      movements, static deflection of the
      stereocilia, uncoupling of the tectorial
      membrane)

    – Efferently induced motor tinnitus

II. Transduction tinnitus

    – Pathological deflection of the stereocilia

    – Ion channel disorders

III. Biochemical signal transfer tinnitus

IV. Other mechanisms of tinnitus

    – Protein biosynthesis disorder

    – Impairment of transmitter metabolism

are suggested to be the cellular basis of the cochlear nonlinearity (LePage and Johnstone 1980).

Hypermobility. Recently we suggested uncontrolled active AC movements of OHCs as an underlying mechanism in tinnitus (Zenner 1987). When OHCs were partly uncoupled in situ from the adjacent cells in a pathophysiological model of the guinea pig, they responded by overamplified vibrations to an electrical stimulus corresponding to the cochlear microphonics (CM). Due to the mechanical isolation, the pathological hypermobility of these OHCs cannot induce an otoacoustic emission in vivo. However, these oscillations of OHCs can supposedly be perceived by neighboring IHCs (LePage, Reuter, and Zenner 1992b), which leads to a tonal or narrowband tinnitus (Figure 18-4). In temporal bone sections from some patients with tinnitus and a hearing disorder, a partial OHC degeneration was found. We found a pathological increase of the AC motility in OHCs when their degeneration was induced experimentally (LePage et al. 1992a, in press). The motility was only abolished by the death of the cell. Hence, a pathological hypermotility of a degenerating OHC might be the basis of a motor tinnitus in some of the patients (Figure 18-4). Our observations correspond to an earlier speculation by Kemp (1981) suggesting that distortions and lesions around one or a few OHC result in a changed pattern of the physiological vibrations of the cochlea. Gold (1948) and Evans and colleagues (Evans, Wilson, and Borerwe 1981) presumed a disturbed active, cochlear mechanic with a positive feedback out of control in tinnitus (Figure 18-5). The presently suggested type of hypermobility in cochlear motor tinnitus is supported by these earlier hypotheses, since the active movements of OHCs correspond very well to the active cochlear mechanics.

Electromechanical Hypermobility. An uncontrolled, pathological AC movement of OHCs is not only possible at the level of a mechanical decoupling in the reticular lamina, but also in case of a disturbance of the electrical control mecha-

nism in OHCs (electromechanical motor tinnitus). Two electrical control mechanisms of the AC motility of OHCs are suggested on the basis of the present experimental evidence.

An AC movement can be elicited by

1. high-frequency changes of the cellular potential and of the transduction current (Ashmore 1987; Santos-Sacchi 1989), or
2. by an extracellular electrical field (Zenner et al. 1987a,b, 1988a).

Cellular potential and transduction current, respectively, can be attributed to the mechano-electrical transduction process. Therefore, pathological alterations of the transduction process with a subsequent activation of the AC motility may become responsible for a motor tinnitus. A candidate for a physiological, extracellular electrical field that triggers the AC movement of OHCs can be the rather vulnerable CM. Local changes in CM, or distortions, can easily be expected and may induce an uncontrolled, local activation of the AC motility of OHC.

When electrical control of AC motility of OHCs is insufficient, it seems to be unlikely that a mechanical decoupling of the OHCs from the reticular lamina occurs at the same time. Thus, an otoacoustic emission should become evident in addition to the tinnitus, because the signal should spread along the cochlear partition. However, OAE corresponding to tinnitus are an extremely rare clinical entity (Zwicker 1979). A recent paper by Plinkert and colleagues (1990) demonstrated in a rare case with a common origin of a tinnitus and spontaneous otoactoustic emission by the same frequency characteristics and their simultaneous suppression (Figure 18-5). A changed OAE activity has also been reported for a noise-induced tinnitus (Kemp 1981, 1986). The above outlined electromechanical mechanism of tinnitus combined with OAE is only infrequently observed in clinical practice. However, 73 percent of the patients of a Tinnitus Clinic show a sensorineural hearing loss, too (Hazell 1984; Hazell, Graham, and Rothera 1985). A majority of these patients

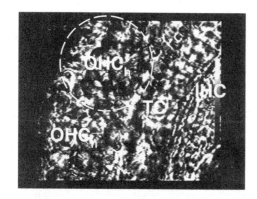

a

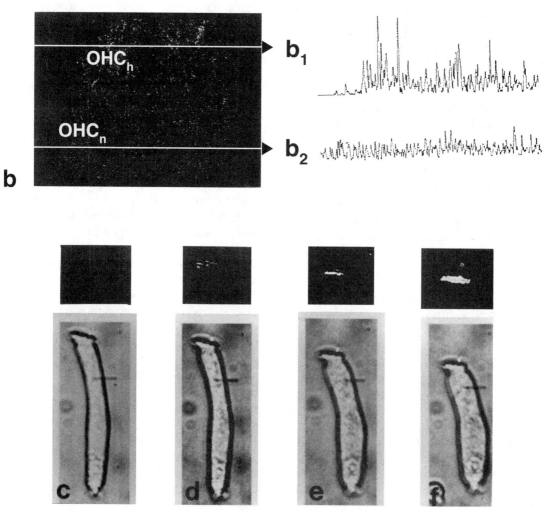

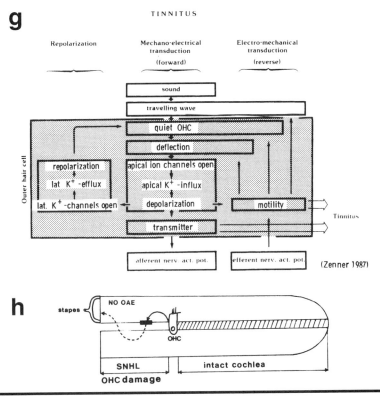

FIGURE 18-4. Hypermotility of a group of OHC as source of a motor tinnitus. *(a)* Surface view of a cochlear explant of the guinea pig during electrical stimulation: On the video screen, hypermotile (OHC_h) and normal OHCs (OHC_n) can be clearly differentiated while moving (TC - tunnel of Corti, IHC - inner hair cells), but not in the present static photograph. Thus, movement characteristics are displayed in (b). Hypermotile OHC are suggested to be sources of a motor tinnitus. Bar - 10 μm. *(b)* Digital subtraction analysis of the same cochlear explant as shown in (a): the higher intensity after digital subtraction indicates hypermotile OHCs (OHC_h) which can be easily recognized. By contrast, the remaining partition of the explant has a low-intensity profile resulting from normal OHCs (OHC_n). Line b_1 shows an intensity scan along hypermotile OHCs, line b_2 is the scan along the normal OHCs. It should be noted that the trace in b_1 has a considerably higher intensity than the trace in b_2 as evidence of hypermotility. *(c–f)* Increase in amplitude of the AC movement of an outer hair cell where it is slowly shortened during a degeneration: (c) Subthreshold stimulation of an OHC before the onset of degeneration. The digital subtraction analysis (above) does not indicate any movement. (d) Beginning of degeneration of an OHC: The digital subtraction analysis (above) shows a motility that is accompanied by a drastically enhanced amplitude with increasing degeneration in (e) and (f). The increase of amplitude corresponds to a hypermobility and is regarded as a source of tinnitus (Zimmermann and Zenner 1992, in preparation). *(g)* Schematic figure of mechano-electrical and electro-mechanical transduction in OHCs that enables the control of OHC motility. Arrows indicate possible localizations of pathological changes contributing to a motor tinnitus (open arrows) (from Zenner 1987). *(h)* Schematic drawing of a cochlea with a hypermotile OHC in a patient with tinnitus and high-frequency sensorineural hearing loss. The cochlear region of this hearing loss is characterized by a cochlear partition painted pale. It is suggested that a loss of amplification of the traveling wave, that is, induced by a lesion of OHCs, is responsible. Subsequently, the vibration induced by a hypermotile, tinnitus-producing OHC is not transported as a retrograde traveling wave to the stapes. Thus, no otoacoustic emission is generated. On the other hand, the vibration is perceived by the neighboring IHCs as well as a tinnitus.

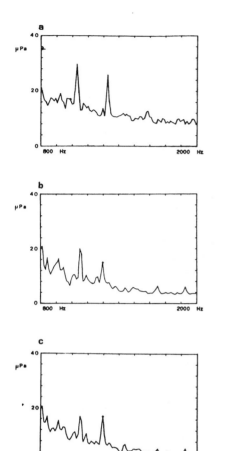

FIGURE 18-5. Power density spectra of continuous SOAEs in a patient with isofrequent tinnitus. The abscissa shows the frequency range where emissions occurred. The ordinate is scaled as sound pressure in the ear canal. Two tonal emissions were recorded in (a) left and (b) right ear, and (c) spectrum of the right ear after several days (from Plinkert, Gitter, and Zenner 1990).

suffer from a tonal or low-band tinnitus of the middle or high frequencies which corresponds to the sensorineural hearing loss. One prerequisite to measure otoacoustic emissions within the outer ear canal is their reverse transport along the cochlea. Thus, the middle and outer ear can only be reached

when the high-frequency range of the cochlea is physiologically intact (Wit 1993; Avan, Bonfils, Loth, Teyssou, and Menguy 1993; Lonsbury-Martin, Whitehead, and Martin 1993; Probst and Harris 1993). But this, unfortunately, is not the case in most of the tinnitus patients, so uncontrolled AC movements of the OHCs are not expected to lead to an otoacoustic emission, even in case of a physiological mechanical coupling to the reticular lamina.

Hypomobility. It seems credible that a partial inhibition of AC motility leads to a tinnitus. If the partial inhibition of the AC motility results in a distortion of the active vibrations at the same time, the altered OHCs should emit distortion products as active mechanical signals. They could be received by IHCs, suggesting the occurrence of a tinnitus (Figure 18-6). It should be considered that acetylsalicylic acid can interfere with the AC movements of isolated OHC (Dieler, Shehata-Dieler, and Brownell 1991).

DC Motor Tinnitus. A further tinnitus-inducing motor disorder of OHC might be an incorrect (e.g., inhibited) or an unwanted, slow movement of OHCs (Zenner 1987). These situations can be simulated with isolated OHCs as well as by in-situ or in-vivo experiments (Zenner 1986b,c; Zenner and Gitter 1989; LePage et al. 1992b, in press). The result may be a lack of control of the physiological AC oscillations, allowing a hypermobility or distortions of the fast AC motility. These products can in turn contribute to a motor tinnitus as described above (Figure 18-4). It can be concluded, furthermore, that uncontrolled DC movements of OHCs lead to a shift in the normal position of the reticular lamina, which changes the operation angle of the OHC stereocilia. This experimental evidence supports a speculation of Evans and colleagues (1981), who postulated a static shearing of the stereocilia, as observed in our experiments, leading to an elevated current flow across the OHCs. This is correlated to an increased release of afferent transmitters in IHCs.

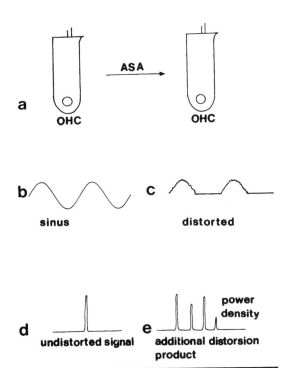

a OHC — ASA → OHC

b sinus   **c** distorted

d undistorted signal   **e** additional distorsion product   power density

FIGURE 18-6. Cochlear model of tinnitus induction by acetylsalicylic acid (ASA) by interference with the electromotility of OHC. *(a)* Schematic drawings of OHCs in the absence or presence of ASA (10). Sinusoidal movement of the unaltered OHCs. *(b)* Sinusoidal movement of the unaltered OHCs. *(c)* Postulated distorted movement of the ASA-treated OHCs. The distortions of the initial sinus signal can be recognized as extremely higher in frequency. *(d)* Postulated power density spectrum of the distortion products from (b) confirms the additional high-frequency part compared to the spectrum (d). The high-frequency parts of the distorted wave in *(e)* are perceived by the frequency specific IHCs and a tinnitus results (model based upon data from Dieler et al. 1992).

Moreover, the in-situ as well as the in-vivo experiments demonstrated in a number of cases a decoupling of the OHC stereocilia from the TM as a result of the DC motor response of OHCs at large amplitudes (Zenner and Gitter 1989). Tonndorf (1980) speculated that this decoupling might be responsible for a uncontrolled shearing of the stereocilia.

Efferently Induced Motor Tinnitus. Ninety percent of the efferent cochlear nerve fibers terminate at the level of the OHCs (Spoendlin 1969). There is increasing evidence of their role in influencing the frequency selectivity and sensitivity of the cochlear (Siegel and Kim 1982; Liberman and Brown 1986): A control of the DC motility of OHCs seems to be most likely (Zenner 1986a). The efferent nerve fibers are largely a part of the crossed olivocochlear bundle. They have an impact on the physiology of the OHCs, at least via nicotinergic acetylcholine (AchR) and $GABA_A$ receptors (Plinkert, Heilbronn, and Zenner 1991a; Plinkert, Gitter, and Zenner 1991b). OHCs with nicotinergic AchR are characterized by a shortening after efferent stimulation (Brownell et al. 1985; Plinkert et al. 1991a). When they have GABA receptors, a stimulation results in a hyperpolarization and a subsequent elongation of the cells (Plinkert et al. 1991b; Gitter et al. 1992 in press). These responses are supposedly the micromechanical basis of a contralateral tinnitus suppression.

DC Motor Tinnitus. Specific disorders of efferent nerve fibers seem to be possible in the olivary complex, along the cochlear nerve, and at the synapse between the efferent ending and the OHCs. The synapses display a complex molecular arrangement, which makes it credible that in some instances either a single step or a complex functional pattern can be severely impaired. This loss of functional integrity might cause an uncontrolled or even completely abolished DC motility, thus allowing the above described DC motor tinnitus. Eggermont (1983) has already speculated on the efferent contribution to the lack of physiological control of OHC oscillations without knowing definitely the cochlear motor mechanism at that time. His ideas correspond to our proposed model.

"Edge Effect" Hypothesis. An attractive variation of a tinnitus model has been proposed by Hazell (1987). He suggests an overshooting in the

efferent stimulation of intact OHCs adjacent (at the edge) to lost OHCs. When this so-called "edge effect" hypothesis is linked to our present knowledge, it should be pointed out that it essentially implies a subtype of a cochlear motor tinnitus.

TRANSDUCTION TINNITUS

A pathological change of the receptor potential of IHCs leads to a release of transmitters, and thus to a change of the spontaneous activity of the cochlear nerve (Figure 18-7). This might be the correlate of an experienced tinnitus. The disorders can be attributed to both an extracellular and an intracellular mechanism. In OHCs, pathological changes of the receptor potential are expected to contribute to a motor tinnitus.

Pathological Deflection of the Stereocilia

If a pathological, passive change in the angle of the stereocilia is possible, the resulting change of the receptor current subsequently leads to a pathological receptor potential.

Ion Channel Disorders

They may include the apical transduction channel as well as lateral potassium channels (Zenner and Gitter 1987a). A leakage of the apical channel or a blockage of lateral potassium channel—both resulting in a pathological receptor potential—seem to be the most likely mechanisms for this type of tinnitus. Interestingly, the tinnitus-inhibiting effect of lidocaine may possibly be related to an influence on the OHC ion channels, in addition to the other pharmacological effects. At least in extracochlear cells, channel activity can be modulated by lidocaine (Haxhiu, Strohl, Norcia, van Lunteren, Deal, and Cherniek 1987).

A perilymphatic potassium intoxication forces the OHCs to store potassium and not release it via their lateral ion channels, resulting in a continuous depolarization of the OHCs (Figure 18-8). Potassium intoxication is to be expected in cases of an acute endolymphatic potassium leakage, such as

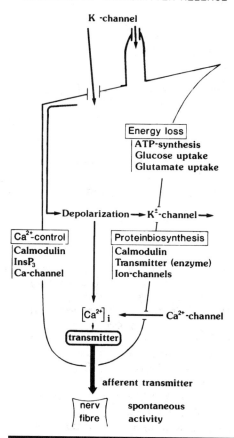

FIGURE 18-7. Biochemically induced decrease of transmitter release in cochlear hair cells (predominantly inner hair cells) can induce a biochemical signal transfer tinnitus. (from Zenner 1987)

in a sudden attack of Ménière's disease or following a trauma of the labyrinth. They are both possible candidates for the occurrence of a tinnitus (Zenner 1986a).

Electromechanical Motor Tinnitus

The active motility of OHCs is possibly controlled by the receptor potential as described above. Active extracellular and intracellular disorders leading to a changed receptor potential can induce one of the above described motor disorders in OHCs. The re-

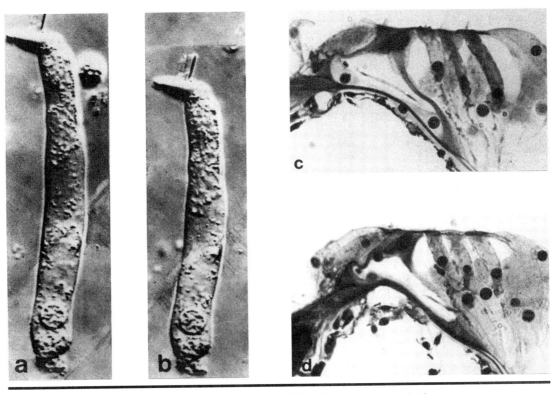

FIGURE 18-8.   Pathological contraction of OHCs after an increase in the perilymphatic K^+ concentration occurred. *(a)* OHC before and *(b)* after a K^+ intoxication. *(c)* OHC within the organ of Corti before and *(d)* during a K^+ intoxication. The shortening of the OHC can be clearly visualized in vitro (b) and in situ (d) (OHC - outer hair cells, IHC - inner hair cells) (from Zenner and Gitter 1989).

ceptor potential can be influenced at a single site of the OHCs, or by a disorder of the integrated network, resulting in a tinnitus—for example, the potassium-induced depolarization was accompanied by a contraction of the cell and a tilting of the cuticular plate (Zenner 1986a; Zenner et al. 1987b). A shift of the reticular membrane and, in rare cases, a decoupling of the stereocilia from the tectorial membrane could be observed in vivo (Zenner and Gitter 1989).

SIGNAL TRANSFER TINNITUS

The electromechanical transduction, the active motility of OHCs, the efferent control of OHCs, as well as the afferent release of neurotransmitters in

IHCs, are closely linked to the biochemical signalling cascade in auditory sensory cells.

Calcium

It seems reasonable to speculate that an important metabolic disorder of OHCs is an imbalanced level of calcium (Zenner 1987). The intracellular calcium is sensitively controlled by the second messenger inositol trisphosphate ($InsP_3$) (Schacht and Zenner 1987), the cellular potential (Ashmore and Ohmori 1990), calmodulin (Zenner 1986, 1988; Flock et al. 1986), calcium channels and, in OHCs, by AchR. There are a number of physiological roles attributable to calcium:

1. Calcium triggers the lateral C-type potassium channel that is responsible for the repolarization within the sensory transduction (Ashmore 1986).
2. Calcium is an amplifying activator of the actomyosin-driven, active DC movements of OHCs (Zenner 1986a, 1988).
3. Calcium contributes to the release of the afferent neurotransmitter in IHCs.

It is worthwhile to consider a number of single mechanisms that cause a functional loss within this complex, integrated, cellular network, and subsequently, within the calcium-dependent physiological processes. According to the proposed model, each of the three calcium-dependent processes can contribute to a tinnitus.

1. A calcium-induced disorder of the C-type potassium channel decisively influences the receptor potential and can lead to a transduction tinnitus.
2. A calcium-induced disorder of the activation of actomyosin changes the DC movement of OHCs and can cause a motor tinnitus.
3. A calcium-induced alteration of the afferent neurotransmitter release is followed by an alteration of the spontaneous activity of afferent nerve fibers, which can correlate to a tinnitus.

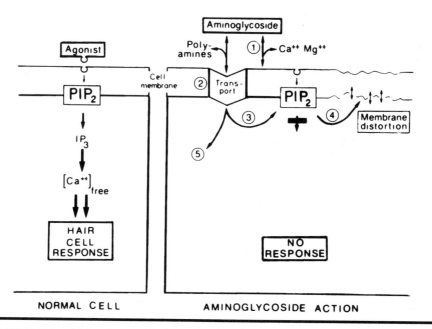

FIGURE 18-9. Molecular mechanism of aminoglycoside toxicity (right) compared to the normal cell signaling (left). *(1)* The aminoglycoside binding to the plasma membrane and displacement of cations (e.g., calcium) reversibly interferes with the calcium-dependent membrane function. *(2)* The uptake of the drug into the cell is suggested to be energy-dependent and competitive with polyamine transport. *(3)* At the cytoplasmic side, the drug is bound to PIP_2, thus inhibiting its normal function, and the cellular integrity of the plasma membrane is disrupted. Further intracellular steps of the signalling cascade—including the release of $InsP_3$ and calcium—to initiate the motile response of the OHCs are blocked (PIP_2—phosphoinositol-bis-phosphate, $InsP_3$—inositol-tris-phosphate) (according to Zenner and Schacht 1986; Schacht and Zenner 1987).

Experimental evidence confirms the hypothesized calcium changes, such as the release of $InsP_3$, and the active motility of OHCs are inhibited (Figure 18-9) by an irreversible binding of aminoglycosides to the membrane constituent phosphoinositol-bis-phosphate (PIP_2) (Zenner and Schacht 1986, Schacht and Zenner 1987). Furthermore, a blockage of AchR of OHC by receptor antagonists also results in a disordered calcium release and an inhibition of active motility (Plinkert et al. 1991a).

In some hair cells, an elevated intracellular calcium level should be decreased by the application of a calcium channel blocker. In fact, some calcium channel blockers can efficiently inhibit an artificial motility of OHCs induced by a blockage of C-type potassium channels with a subsequent repolarization blockage (Nilles and Zenner 1992, in press). These findings may explain the therapeutic effect of calcium channel blockers in some of the tinnitus patients (Figure 18-10).

The $GABA_A$ receptors of OHCs possess binding sites of benzodiazepane that amplify experimentally the hyperpolarization and the amplitude of OHC movement (Plinkert et al. 1991b). It seems reasonable that the suppression of tinnitus in some patients by drugs such as benzodiazepane or atropine is based upon the interaction with the $GABA_A$ or acetylcholine receptor, respectively (Figure 18-10).

OTHER MOLECULAR PATHOMECHANISMS LEADING TO TINNITUS

Common biochemical disorders, such as the biosynthesis of proteins, could be responsible for a reduced production of the above-mentioned cellular components (e.g., ion channel proteins, calmodulin, neurotransmitter, etc.) with the subsequent deleterious results. It can also be suggested that an impairment of production, release, or uptake of glutamate contributes to the generation of tinnitus. OHCs require glutamate to a large extent in their extracellular space. In addition, it is the most potent candidate to be the afferent neurotransmitter of the

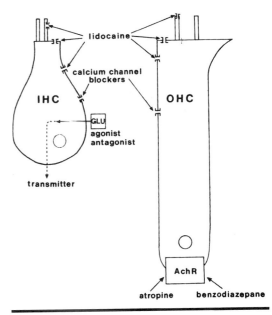

FIGURE 18-10. Schematic drawing of putative sites of action of drugs that are able to suppress subjective tinnitus in some patients (Glu - glutamate, AchR - acetylcholine receptor) (for details see text).

IHCs. The therapeutic effects of glutamate in some of the tinnitus patients might be based upon this finding (Ehrenberger and Felix 1991). In essence, the variety of these disorders can be causative for the generation of a motor, transduction, or biochemical signal transfer tinnitus.

CONCLUSION

This chapter has summarized possible molecular and cellular mechanisms which might contribute to a tinnitus (Table 18-1). They constitute a part of a highly integrated network in sensory transduction and are divided for easier understanding into three different models: active motor tinnitus, transduction tinnitus, and signal transfer tinnitus. Some steps of the pathophysiological models can even be pharmacologically influenced (lidocaine, calcium channel blocker, benzodiazepane, glutamate, atropine). This provides a rationale for the efficient suppression of tinnitus by these drugs in some of the patients.

The most evident problem of all models in tinnitus, including the ones proposed in this paper, is the lack of objective verification by measurement. Thus, the well-defined clinical situation of each patient is hardly attributable to one of the suggested models. In addition, adequate therapy—perhaps by one of the drugs considered—cannot be based upon reliable clinical findings.

We thank Drs. Reuter, Zimmermann, Plinkert, and LePage for their help in preparing the manuscript by generously providing some of the figures.

REFERENCES

Ashmore, J.F. and Meech, R.W. 1986. "Ionic Basis of Membrane Potential in Outer Hair Cells of Guinea Pig Cochlea." *Nature, 322,* 368–371.

Ashmore, J.F. 1987. "A Fast Motile Response in Guinea Pig Outer Hair Cells; The Cellular Basis of the Cochlear Amplifier." *Journal of Physiology, 388,* 323–347.

Ashmore, J.F. and Ohmori, H. 1990. "Control of Intracellular Calcium by ATP in Isolated Outer Hair Cells of the Guinea-pig Cochlea." *Journal of Physiology, 428,* 109–131.

Avan, P.A., Bonfils, P., Loth, D., Teyssou, M., and Menguy, C. 1993. "Exploration of Cochlear Function by Otoacoustic Emissions—Relations with Pure-tone Audiometry." *Progress in Brain Research, 97,* 67–75.

Brownell, W.E., Bader, C.R., Bertrand, D., and Ribaupierre, Y. 1985. "Evoked Mechanical Responses of Isolated Cochlear Outer Hair Cells." *Science, 227,* 194–196.

Brundin, L., Flock, Å., and Canlon, B. 1989. "Sound-induced Motility of Isolated Cochlear Outer Hair Cells is Frequency-specific." *Nature, 342,* 814–816.

Brundin, L., Flock, Å., Khanna, S.M., and Ulfendahl, M. 1992. "The Tuned Displacement Response of the Hearing Organ is Generated by the Outer Hair Cells." *Neuroscience, 49*(3), 607–616.

Canlon, B., Brundin, L., and Flock, A. 1988. "Acoustic Stimulation Causes Tonotopic Alterations in the Length of Isolated Outer Hair Cells from the Guinea Pig Hearing Organ." *Proceedings of the National Academy of Science USA,* 7033–7035.

Dallos, P. 1986. "Neurobiology of Inner and Outer Hair Cells—Intracochlear Recordings." *Hearing Research, 22,* 185–198.

Dieler, R., Shehata-Dieler, W.W., and Brownell, W.E. 1991. "Concomitant Salicylate-induced Alterations of Outer Hair Cell subsurface Cisternae and Electromotility." *Journal of Neurocytology, 20,* 637–653.

Eggermont, J.J. 1983. "Tinnitus: Some Thoughts about Its Origin." *Journal of Laryngology and Otology, Suppl. 9,* 31–37.

Ehrenberger, K. and Felix, D. 1991. "Glutamate Receptors in Afferent Cochlear Neurotransmission in Guinea Pigs." *Hearing Research, 52,* 73–76.

Evans, E.F., Wilson, J.P., and Borerwe, T.A. 1981. "Animal Models of Tinnitus." *Tinnitus, Ciba Foundation Symposium 85,* 108–138. London: Pitman Books, Ltd.

Flock, Å., Flock, F., and Ulfendahl, M. 1986. "Mechanisms of Movement in OHC and a Possible Structural Basis." *Archives of Otorhinolaryngology, 243,* 83–90.

Gitter, A.H., Frömter, E., and Zenner, H.P. 1992a. "C-Type Potassium Channels in the Lateral Cell Membrane of Guinea Pig Outer Hair Cells." *Hearing Research, 60*(1), 13–19.

Gitter, A.H., Rudert, M., and Zenner, H.P. 1992b, in preparation. "Modulation of Cell Length and Force Generation of Cochlear Outer Hair Cells by Extracellular Electrical Potentials."

Gitter, A.H., Zenner, H.P., and Frömter, E. 1986. "Membrane Potential and Ion Channels in Isolated Outer Hair Cells of Guinea Pig Cochlea." *Journal of Otology, Rhinology, and Laryngology, 48,* 68–75.

Gold, T. 1948. "Hearing II: The Physical Basis of Action of the Cochlea." *Proceedings of the Royal Society of London,* Vol. 35, 492–498.

Haxhiu, M.A., Strohl, K.P., Norcia, M.P., van Lunteren, E., Deal, E.C. Jr., and Cherniek, N.S. 1987. "A Role for the Ventral Surface of the Medulla in Regulation of Nasal Resistance." *American Journal of Physiology,* R494–R500.

Hazell, J.W.P. 1984. "Spontaneous Cochlear Acoustic Emissions and Tinnitus." *Journal of Laryngology and Otology, Supplement 9,* 106–110.

Hazell, J.W.P. 1987. "A Cochlear Model for Tinnitus." In H. Feldmann (Ed.), *Proceedings III International*

Tinnitus Seminar, pp. 121–130. Karlsruhe: Harsch Verlag.

Hazell, J., Graham, J., and Rothera, M. 1985. "Electrical Stimulation of the Cochlea and Tinnitus." In R. Schindler and M. Merzenich (Eds.), *Cochlear Implants.* New York: Raven Press.

Hudspeth, A.J. 1985. "The Cellular Basis of Hearing—The Biophysics of Hair Cells." *Science, 230,* 745–752.

Kachar, B., Brownell, W.E., Altschuler, R., and Fex, J. 1986. "Electrokinetic Shape Change of Cochlear Outer Hair Cells." *Nature, 322,* 365–367.

Kemp, D.T. 1981. "Physiologically Active Cochlear Micromechanics—One Source of Tinnitus." In *Tinnitus, Ciba Foundation Symposium 85,* pp. 54–81. London: Pitman Books, Ltd.

Kemp, D.T. 1986. "Otoacoustic Emissions, Travelling Waves and Cochlear Mechanisms." *Hearing Research, 22,* 95–104.

Khanna, S.M. and Leonard, D.G.B. 1982. "Laser Interferometric Measurements of Basilar Membrane Vibrations in Cats." *Science, 215,* 305–306.

Khanna, S.M., Ulfendahl, M., and Flock, Å. 1989. "Modes of Cellular Vibration in the Organ of Corti." *Acta Otolaryngologica (Stockholm), Supplement 467,* 183–188.

LePage, E.L. 1989. "Functional Role of the Olivocochlear Bundle: A Motor Unit Control System in the Mammalian Cochlea." *Hearing Research, 38,* 177–198.

LePage, E.L. and Johnstone, M.B. 1980. "Non-linear Mechanical Behavior of the Basilar Membrane in the Basal Turn of the Guinea Pig Cochlea." *Hearing Research, 2,* 183–189.

LePage, E., Reuter, G., and Zenner, H.P. 1992a, in press. "Tip Threshold: Outset of Motor Response." *Hearing Research.*

LePage, E., Reuter, G., and Zenner, H.P. 1992b, in press. "Fiber Optic Mechanical Measurements of Summating Displacements in Guinea Pig Cochlear Explant Suggest an Adaptive Role for the Outer Hair Cells." *Hearing Research.*

Liberman, M.C. and Brown, M.C. 1986. "Physiology and Anatomy of Single Olivocochlear Neurons in the Cat." *Hearing Research, 24,* 17–36.

Lonsbury-Martin, B.L., Whitehead, M.C., and Martin, G.M. 1992. "Distortion Produces Otoacoustic Emissions in Normal and Impaired Ears: Insights into Generation Processes." *Progress in Brain Research, 97,* 77–90.

Nilles, R. and Zenner, H.P. In preparation.

Plinkert, P.K., Gitter, A.H., and Zenner, H.P. 1990. "Tinnitus-associated Spontaneous Otoacoustic Emissions—Active Outer Hair Cell Movements as a Common Origin?" *Acta Otolaryngologica (Stockholm), 110,* 342–347.

Plinkert, P.K., Gitter, A.H., and Zenner, H.P. 1991b. "GABA$_A$-Receptors in Cochlear Outer Hair Cells." *Hearing Research, 53,* 131–140.

Plinkert, P.K., Heilbronn, E., and Zenner, H.P. 1991a. "A Nicotinic Acetylcholine Receptor-like Á-Bungarotoxin Binding Site on Outer Hair Cells." *Hearing Research, 53,* 123–130.

Probst, R. and Harris, F. 1993. "A Comparison in Transiently evoked and Distortion-product Otoacoustic Emissions in Humans." *Progress in Brain Research, 97,* 91-99.

Reuter, G. and Zenner, H.P. 1990. "Active Radial and Transverse Motile Responses of Outer Hair Cells in the Organ of Corti." *Hearing Research, 43,* 219–230.

Russell, I.J. 1983. "Origin of the Receptor Potential in Inner Hair Cells of the Mammalian Cochlea—Evidence for Davis' Theory." *Nature, 301,* 334–336.

Russell, I.J., Cody, A.R., and Richardson, G.P. 1986a. "The Responses of Inner and Outer Hair Cells in the Basal Turn of the Guinea-pig Cochlea Grown in Vitro." *Hearing Research, 22,* 199–216.

Russell, I.J., Richardson, G.P., and Cody, A.R. 1986b. "Mechanosensitivity of Mammalian Auditory Hair Cells in Vitro." *Nature, 321,* 517–519.

Santos-Sacchi, J. 1989. "Asymmetry in Voltage-dependent Movements of Isolated OHC from the Organ of Corti." *Journal of Neuroscience, 9,* 2954–2962.

Schacht, J. and Zenner, H.P. 1987. "Evidence that Phosphoinositides Mediate Motility in Cochlear Hair Cells." *Hearing Research, 31,* 155–160.

Sellick, P.M., Patuzzi, R., and Johnstone, B.M. 1982. "Measurements of Basilar Membrane Motion in the Guinea Pig Using the Mößbauer Technique." *Journal of the Acoustical Society of America, 72,* 131–141.

Siegel, I. and Kim, B. 1982. "Efferent Neural Control of Cochlear Mechanics? Olivocochlear Bundle Stimulation Affects Cochlear Biomechanical Nonlinearity." *Hearing Research, 6,* 171–182.

Spoendlin, H. 1969. "Innervation Patterns in the Organ of Corti of the Cat." *Acta Otolaryngologica, 67,* 239–254.

Tonndorf, J. 1980. "Acute Cochlear Disorders: The

Combination of Hearing Loss, Recruitment, Poor Speech Discrimination and Tinnitus." *Annals of Otology, 89,* 353–358.

van Netten, S.M. and Khanna, S.M. 1993. "Mechanical Demodulation of Hydrodynamic Stimuli Performed by the Lateral Line Organ." *Progress in Brain Research, 97,* 45–51.

Wit, H.P. 1993. "Amplitude Fluctuations of Spontaneous Otoacoustic Emissions caused by Internal and Externally Applied Noise Sources." *Progress in Brain Research, 97,* 59–65.

Zenner, H.P. 1986a. "K$^+$-induced Motility and Depolarization of Cochlear Hair Cells. Direct Evidence for a New Pathophysiological Mechanism in Ménière's Disease." *Archives of Oto-Rhino-Laryngology, 243,* 108–111.

Zenner, H.P. 1986b. "Motile Responses in Outer Hair Cells." *Hearing Research, 22,* 83–90.

Zenner, H.P. 1986c. "Aktive Bewegungen von Haarzellen: Ein neuer Mechanismus beim Hörvorgang." *HNO, 34,* 133–138.

Zenner, H.P. 1986d. "Molecular Structure of Hair Cells." In R.A. Altschuler, D.W. Hoffmann, and R.P. Bobbin, *Neurobiology of Hearing: The Cochlea,* pp. 1–21. New York: Raven Press.

Zenner, H.P. 1987. "Modern Aspects of Hair Cell Biochemistry, Motility and Tinnitus." In H. Feldmann (Ed.), *Proceedings III International Tinnitus Seminar,* pp. 52–57. Karlsruhe: Harsch Verlag.

Zenner, H.P. 1988. "Motility of Outer Hair Cells as an Active, Actin-mediated Process." *Acta Otolaryngologica, 105,* 39–44.

Zenner, H.P. and Ernst, A. 1993. "Sound Processing by AC and DC Movements of Cochlear Outer Hair Cells." *Progress in Brain Research, 97,* 21–30.

Zenner, H.P. and Gitter, A.H. 1989. "Transduktions- und Motorstörungen cochleärer Haarzellen bei M. Menière und Aminogykosidschwerhörigkeit." *Laryngology, Rhinology, and Otology, 68,* 533–584.

Zenner, H.P. and Gitter, A.H. 1987a. "Die Schallverarbeitung des Ohres." *Physik in unserer Zeit, 18,* 97–105.

Zenner, H.P. and Gitter, A.H. 1987b. "Possible Roles of Hair Cell Potential and Ionic Channels in Cochlear Tinnitus." In H. Feldmann, (Ed.), *Proceedings III International Tinnitus Seminar,* pp. 306–310. Karlsruhe: Harsch Verlag.

Zenner, H.P. and Schacht, J. 1986. "Hörverlust durch Aminoglykosid Antibiotika: Angriff am membranbaustein PIP$_2$ in äußeren Haarzellen als Wirkungsmechanismus." *HNO, 34,* 417–423.

Zenner, H.P., Arnold, W., and Gitter, A.H. 1988b. "Outer Hair Cells as Fast and Slow Cochlear Amplifiers with a Bidirectional Transduction Cycle." *Acta Otolaryngologica, 105,* 457–462.

Zenner, H.P., Zimmermann, U., and Gitter, A.H. 1987. "Fast Motility of Isolated Mammalian Auditory Sensory Cells." *Biochemical and Biophysical Research Communications, 149,* 304–308.

Zenner, H.P., Zimmermann, R., and Gitter, A.H. 1988a. "Active Movements of the Cuticular Plate Induce Sensory Hair Motion in Mammalian Outer Hair Cells." *Hearing Research, 34,* 233–240.

Zenner, H.P., Zimmermann, U., and Schmitt, U. 1985. "Reversible Contraction of Isolated Mammalian Cochlear Hair Cells." *Hearing Research, 18,* 127–133.

Zwicker, E. 1979. "A Model Describing Non-linearities in Hearing by Active Processes with Saturation at 40 dB." *Biological Cybernetics, 35,* 243–250.

INDEX